What People Are Saying About the Holford Diet

My entire family started the Holford Diet six weeks ago. When we began I thought it would be difficult. The thought of cooking three meals a day with all these new foods was daunting. But it's been so easy. We used to be total chocaholics—eating sweets and chocolate every day. None of us have eaten any chocolate or sweets since starting the diet. It's a miracle—and we've had no cravings. I would never have believed it possible. My daughter—who loses weight very slowly—has lost 13 pounds. I've lost 17 pounds, my husband has lost 18 pounds, and my son—who is not so overweight—has lost 11 pounds. All this has happened in the last six weeks.

The other thing is the energy. I am diabetic and was always exhausted. I could have spent every day in bed. Now my energy level is incredible. We are all feeling great.

My blood sugar level used to be high—between 11 and 18. It now stays between 4 and 8 (the optimum is 7). My blood sugar is well under control and I've been able to reduce my medication. I would recommend this diet to everybody. It is so much easier than I thought. This is literally the answer to my prayers. As a family, we are more relaxed and feel so much better. It's made a big, big difference to us all.—*Linda B.*

I have been a vegetarian for fifteen years and have always battled to keep the pounds off. I read the Holford Diet book and it is really the first diet that makes sense. I now understand so much more about a balanced vegetarian diet. I have managed to lose 17 pounds in three months and I feel wonderful. I weigh myself once a week and I always feel apprehensive—because the one thing that never happens on this diet is feeling hungry. I always imagine that I have eaten too much to have lost any weight. But the pounds are still going. Patrick Holford is my hero!—*Barbara C.*

My husband and I started the diet last week. I have already lost 9 pounds and my husband has lost 6 pounds. We're both thrilled with the quick results. My husband is insulin resistant—according to his doctor—and we are both severely overweight. The menus in the Holford Diet book are excellent and my husband doesn't even feel as if he's on a "diet"—because he has enough snacks and his blood sugar is stable. Thank you for making the transition to a healthy eating plan so easy!—*Tina H.*

I have been on the Holford Diet for just over eight weeks. My objectives when going on the diet were to lose a couple of pounds. More importantly, I just wanted to feel better. During my time on the diet I have lost a staggering 15 pounds and feel like a brand-new person. I don't even think of the Holford

Diet as a diet—for me it is just the absolute best way to eat. I will continue to eat like this for the rest of my life.—*Irene S.*

I have had a problem with my weight for twenty years—ever since the birth of my first baby. Over that time I have been on every diet imaginable. An unbearably slow loss of weight would be followed by putting it all back on when I could go hungry no longer. There was always this insinuation that I was cheating or being a glutton. Anger would follow despair as I looked at these super dieters who had given up all of this junk and lost pounds. I have never eaten junk food and thought my diet was pretty well balanced, but still the weight crept on. I discovered I had a wheat intolerance and gave up chocolate, coffee, and beef over the last few years. Still the weight crept on. And then I found the Holford Diet and lost 22 pounds in two months. The revelation was sugar balance. Once I regulated my blood sugar levels the weight just fell off. Why did no one ever tell me before? This is not a difficult way to eat and I don't starve or feel hungry at all. My body feels in balance for the first time—obviously sugar was my nemesis. I would recommend this way of eating to anyone. Even if you aren't that overweight it gets your body working properly. Thanks very much Patrick!—*Sheila W.*

In the past I tried just about every diet I heard of—even when I knew it wasn't particularly good for me. I have done food replacement diets, calorie counting, Atkins, Low-Fat, WeightWatchers—the lot! Within four days of starting the Holford Diet I felt much clearer and more alert—without the fuzziness I'd lived with for years. Then I started feeling more flexible. By the second week I was sleeping much better. I'm more optimistic, my mood is better, and my energy is much higher. I've lost 12 pounds in the first four weeks. As a result of this success I have the motivation to change my eating for good. My husband has also started—but not so strictly—and has lost 8 pounds in three weeks. On the Holford Diet I am rarely hungry and have no desire to give up—which is what happened in the past. I would recommend the Holford Diet to anyone who is serious about losing weight and gaining health.—*Diana A.*

I am married with five children. I'm fifty years old and have been diagnosed with multiple sclerosis. I exercise regularly and have done so all my life. In the last few years—despite increased training—I have struggled to lose any weight or have an impact on my body fat. On the Holford Diet I noticed weight loss almost immediately. There has been an increase in my energy levels and I feel no hunger pains. I also feel more alert. My husband has decided to go on the diet after seeing my weight loss and increased energy.

—*Tania B.*

THE Holford

LOW GL

DIET

....

THE *Holford* LOW GL DIET

Lose Fat Fast
Using the Revolutionary
Fatburner System

PATRICK HOLFORD

ATRIA BOOKS
New York London Toronto Sydney

While all the nutrients and dietary changes referred to in this book have been proven safe, those seeking help for specific medical conditions are advised to consult a qualified nutrition therapist, clinical nutritionist, doctor, or equivalent health professional. The recommendations given in this book are intended solely as education and information, and should not be taken as medical advice. Neither the authors nor the publisher accept liability for readers who choose to self-prescribe.

All supplements should be kept out of reach of infants and young children.

ATRIA BOOKS

1230 Avenue of the Americas
New York, NY 10020

Copyright © 2005 by Patrick Holford

Published by arrangement with Piatkus Books, Ltd.

Originally published in Great Britain in 2005 by Piatkus Books Limited

All rights reserved, including the right to reproduce
this book or portions thereof in any form whatsoever.
For information address Piatkus Books Limited,
5 Windmill Street, London WIT 2JA

Library of Congress Cataloging-in-Publication Data
Holford, Patrick.
    The Holford low GL diet : lose fat fast using the revolutionary fatburner
system / Patrick Holford.
        p.   cm.
    Includes bibliographical references and index.
    ISBN-13: 978-0-7432-8722-7
    ISBN-10:   0-7432-8722-3
    1. Low-carbohydrate diet—Recipes.   2. Reducing diets.   3. Glycemic
index.   4. Diet.   I. Title.
RM237.73.H65   2006
641.5'6383—dc22   2005057224

First Atria Books trade paperback edition February 2006

10 9 8 7 6 5 4 3 2 1

ATRIA BOOKS is a trademark of Simon & Schuster, Inc.

Manufactured in the United States of America

For information regarding special discounts for bulk purchases,
please contact Simon & Schuster Special Sales at
1-800-456-6798 or business@simonandschuster.com

Ⓖ is the registered trademark of Patrick Holford, 2004

CONTENTS

Part Three
....

THE ACTION PLAN

Part Four
....

FOOD: MENU PLANS AND RECIPES

Part Five
....

HIDDEN BENEFITS

Appendices

ACKNOWLEDGMENTS

This book has been a continual evolution over the past ten years and I would like to thank both the people who have been involved at every stage, and the many scientists around the world who have contributed to our understanding of weight loss and blood sugar. Most of all, I'd like to thank the thousands of people who have tried my Fatburner approach and volunteered for the trials you'll read about. No doubt this approach will continue to evolve, thanks to your invaluable feedback.

Specifically, I'd like to thank nutritionists Natalie Savona, Deborah Colson, and Fiona Macdonald-Joyce (thank you for your excellent recipes!), all trained at the Institute for Optimum Nutrition, and Paul Bedford from the YMCA for his help with the exercise chapters. I would also like to thank Gill, Anna, and Barbara at Piatkus and Kelly and the team at Atria for their skillful and patient editing.

Finally, I'd like to thank Gaby, my wife, for being a guinea pig and putting up with my crack-of-dawn lifestyle that gives birth to books!

GUIDE TO ABBREVIATIONS AND MEASURES

VITAMINS

1 gram (g) = 1,000 milligrams (mg) = 1,000,000 micrograms (mcg, also written μg).

All vitamins are measured in milligrams or micrograms. Vitamins A, D, and E used to be measured in International Units (IUs), a measurement designed to standardize the various forms of these vitamins that have different potencies.

100 IUs of vitamin A   = 30.3mcg
100 IUs of vitamin D   = 2.5mcg
100 IUs of vitamin E   = 67mg
1 pound (lb.)   = 16 ounces (oz.)
2.2 lb.   = 1 kilogram (kg)
1 pint   = 0.6 liters
1.76 pints   = 1 liter
In this book calories means kilocalories (kcals).

BRITISH (IMPERIAL)	METRIC	BRITISH (IMPERIAL)	METRIC
1 oz.	28g	5 oz.	142g
2 oz.	57g	6 oz.	170g
3 oz.	85g	7 oz.	198g
4 oz.	113g	8 oz.	227g

BRITISH (IMPERIAL)	METRIC	METRIC	USA
1 teaspoon (0.17 oz.)	5ml	5g	1 teaspoon
1 dessertspoon	10ml	10g	2 teaspoons
1 tablespoon (0.5 oz.)	15ml	14.3g	1 tablespoon
2 tablespoons (1 oz.)	30ml	28.35g	2 tablespoons
4 fl. oz.	112.5ml		½ cup
1 cup (8 oz.)	1 cup (225 ml)	225ml	
4/5 imperial pint (16 oz.)		450ml	2 cups (1 pint)
4/5 imperial quart	900ml		1 quart
4/5 imperial gallon	3.6 liters		1 gallon
1 pound (lb.)	454g		1 pound

CONVERSION SUMS

Ounces to grams:
Multiply ounce figure by 28.3 to get number of grams.

GRAMS TO OUNCES:

Divide gram figure by 28.3 to get number of ounces.

OUNCES TO MILLILITERS:

Multiply ounce figure by 30 to get number of milliliters.

CALORIES

Carbohydrate has 3.75 calories per gram.
Protein has 4 calories per gram.
Fat has 9 calories per gram.

In each part of the book, you'll find numbered references. These refer to research papers listed in the References section at the end of each part, and are there for readers who want to study this subject in depth.

PREFACE

Are you fed up with fat and the fad diets that claim to vanquish it?
You may have spent years embarking on every weight-loss diet going—cut out entire food groups, followed the culinary habits of far-flung tribes, spent a fortune on "miracle" foods. But, however wonderful these regimes seemed when you began them, the fact that you picked up this book probably means that none of them gave you what you need: a diet for life.

Chances are, you're still carrying unshed pounds, but that's just for starters. You may also feel gnawingly hungry much of the time, exhausted, and beset by cravings. And, above all, fed up with hollow promises and "sure-fire" methods that are soon unmasked as just another gimmick.

Ten years ago I proposed a way out of this wilderness. *The New Fatburner Diet* pinpointed the secret to successful weight loss and weight control: balancing blood sugar.

Put simply, when your blood sugar is too high you turn the excess into fat, and when your blood sugar is too low, you feel lethargic. So you may grab a sugary, refined snack to boost your energy, only to find that you sink back into exhaustion soon afterward—while piling on more weight. This pattern of eating can be seriously bad for your health: once a person is obese, his or her risk for the severe blood-sugar-imbalance diabetes actually increases 77 times. That's the bad news.

But there's good news. You can break out of this vicious circle forever. And, when you do, the pounds fall off easily, and your energy springs back to optimum levels.

Evolution of an idea

This discovery grew out of a growing conviction that I developed gradually at the Institute for Optimum Nutrition. I founded ION in the mid-1980s with the support and encouragement of the two-time Nobel Prize–winner Dr. Linus Pauling, who famously declared that "optimum nutrition is the medicine of the future."

A friend of Einstein's, Pauling was to chemistry what Einstein was to physics. I established ION in the spirit of this remarkable nutritional pioneer. With the ION team, I worked with hundreds of overweight people to find the key to losing weight.

Back then, of course, calorie counting was the sacred cow of weight loss. The dominant belief was that the number of calories you ate, minus what you burned off through exercise, ended up as a blob of fat around your middle. Diets aimed to cut calories—usually by cutting fat, since fat has the most calories per gram.

But I was seeing something very different—that eating different *kinds* of foods, such as what we call low-glycemic-load foods, can lead to more weight loss per calorie than high-glycemic-load foods. At the time, it was sheer heresy.

However, we were right. There are specific foods and food combinations that cause rapid weight loss, and I used this knowledge to devise the Fat-burner System. I soon realized that people who balanced their blood sugar not only lost weight—they also kept it off, felt superb, and had all the signs of improved health and vigor.

They happily slipped into a new way of eating, but, more important, they found that it works for life—the food is so delicious and varied that boredom and hunger are just not an issue. Hundreds of thousands of people followed the system with great success, and numerous scientific trials have validated the initial research.

Today's Holford Diet takes this tried-and-tested method into another dimension. With ongoing advances in nutrition, and feedback from users, it is now a cutting-edge guide to optimal health that's also a breeze to follow. And there are gourmet recipes for everything from snacks to banquets. All this, and weight loss too!

Beyond Atkins

Overall, we owe a lot to the late Dr. Atkins, who boldly stated that you could lose more weight by eating a high-protein, high-fat, low-carbohydrate diet. He claimed, as I do, that obesity results from losing blood sugar control. And he knew that the body's "cleanest" fuel is carbohydrate, which is simply digested down into glucose—the substance your cells run on.

Fat and protein, however, are much harder to metabolize and turn into usable fuel, so Atkins proposed that you'd lose some of the energy or calories they contain as ketones—breakdown chemicals—in the urine. In this way, he said, you could eat more calories and still lose weight.

Atkins was on the right track, but for the wrong reasons, and so was his diet. Despite all the hype, we now know why high-protein diets work. It isn't because fat and protein are so hard to break down for energy that you lose calories by eating them. This theory has been proved wrong.

High-protein diets work for a very simple reason. People actually eat less. You tend to feel much fuller when you eat meat and cheese than when you eat carbohydrates, because a high-protein diet does control blood sugar. However, there are some serious problems with this approach, as we'll see. Meanwhile, there is an easier, safer, healthier, and tastier way to lose weight— and you'll see results in just 30 days.

On your marks, get reset . . .

I say 30 days because, if your blood sugar is out of balance (and there's a 95 percent chance of that if you are overweight), it takes up to 30 days to "reset" your system to work properly. Then the pounds really melt away—although you'll be losing weight and gaining energy from day one.

How can you tell whether you've lost control of your blood sugar? Check out this page from the food diary of someone who has.

Woke up tired. Staggered out of bed on remote control to the coffeepot. Made a strong cup of coffee. Had a piece of toast and jam. Avoided eating anything substantial till lunch to cut down on calories. Got really hungry. Craved some bread, pasta, cookies. Had a big bowl of tuna pasta for lunch. Wanted something sweet to end the meal. Felt depressed in the afternoon and really lethargic. Had another coffee and some chocolate. Felt better.

Got home and had some toast. Meant to go to the gym but felt too tired. . . .

If this sounds like you, let me ask you a few simple questions.

- Do you find it hard to get going in the morning without a cup of tea or coffee, a cigarette, or something sweet—cereal or toast with jam?
- Do you crave something sweet after meals?
- Does your energy dip during the day, and do you find yourself craving a stimulant (such as tea, coffee, a cigarette, or chocolate) or something sweet?
- Do you feel too tired to exercise?
- Does your mood go up and down?
- Are you gradually gaining weight and finding it hard to lose, even though you're not noticeably eating more or exercising less?

If you answer yes to any of these questions, the Holford Diet is perfect for you.

It is also radical enough to change the way you eat and live—which might prompt you to ask who I am, and why you should trust what I have to say. The fact is, the kernel of the Holford Diet began as a personal experience that transformed my life long before I even set up ION.

Life study

When I was 19 and studying psychology at York University, I met two extraordinary nutritionists, Brian and Celia Wright. Like Linus Pauling, they had realized that most disease was the result of suboptimum nutrition. At the time I found this hard to swallow, but, being an adventurous spirit, I asked them to devise a diet for me.

So there I was, a university student, eating a virtually wheat-free diet, masses of fruit and vegetables, and taking a daily handful of supplements shipped from the United States (they weren't yet available in Britain). A far cry from the usual fish and chips, cigarettes, and pints of beer! My colleagues, friends, and family thought I was crazy. But I persisted.

Within two months I had lost nearly fifteen pounds, which have never returned; my skin, which had resembled a lunar landscape, cleared up; and my regular migraines virtually vanished. But most noticeable of all was the extra energy. I no longer needed so much sleep, my mind was much sharper and my body full of vitality. I started to investigate this "optimum nutrition," and I haven't stopped since.

I set up ION, which is an independent, nonprofit charity with no funding from food, supplement, or drug companies, and it has grown into Europe's largest and most respected training school for nutritional therapists. Here are some of the breakthroughs:

- In 1986 I researched zinc and proved that it was Britain's most deficient mineral. Deficiencies can cause bad skin, poor appetite control, depression, and even schizophrenia. In those days virtually no one had even heard of zinc, there was no RDA for it, and few supplements contained it.
- In 1988 we ran an experiment, filmed by the BBC's *Horizon* program and published in *The Lancet,* that proved vitamin supplements could boost children's IQ by a massive 9 percent. This was a world first.
- In the 1990s we showed that antioxidants reduce cancer, heart disease, and Alzheimer's and slow down the aging process. No one had heard of antioxidants then, but now they're the big buzzword.
- In 1998 I wrote *The Optimum Nutrition Bible,* now translated into 15 languages and sold in 30 countries, with sales at over a million copies.
- In 1993 I went public as saying that HRT (Hormone Replacement Therapy) causes breast cancer and advised women to use safer and equally effective natural alternatives. (An estimated 20,000 women in Britain developed breast cancer because of HRT between 1994 and 2004 alone.)
- In 2003 I put the spotlight on homocysteine—an amino acid more important than cholesterol, your blood pressure, and even your weight as a gauge of health. It is your single most important health statistic, measuring exactly where you are on the scale from superhealth to heading for an early grave.

In short, I've been walking my talk for 25 years—during which time my weight, size, blood pressure, pulse, and cholesterol level haven't gone up a single point.

So, after a quarter of a century at the cutting edge of diet and health—having studied thousands of research trials, tested my theories on myself and on more than 200,000 people, and gained more than a million readers world-wide—I can say with confidence that there is a simple way to lose weight, feel and look great, and stay young. And that is the Holford Diet.

How to use this book

Part One gives you the background, and tells you why this diet is scientifically proven, safer, and better for you. It also reveals why it will give you the quickest, safest, easiest, and most sustainable weight loss, as well as increased energy and better skin, mood, and concentration.

Part Two explains the five key principles of the Holford Diet—which are just as applicable to kids as to adults—and how to discover your good foods and bad foods. Once you've read this you'll understand why the Fatburner System is the state-of-the-art weight-loss and maintenance strategy.

Part Three tells you exactly what you need to do on the Holford Diet, and answers all your practical questions.

Part Four gives you scores of easy, delicious fatburning recipes and menus to enjoy.

Part Five covers the hidden benefits of the Holford Diet.

Wishing you the best of health, and looking forward to seeing less of you!

Patrick Holford
October 2004

Part One

·····················

Dieting—
The Bottom Line

Why the Holford Diet Works

Imagine this.

You've just woken up. You feel full of energy. Your mind is clear. You get up, have a healthy breakfast and, throughout the day, your energy is good, your mood is stable, you're mentally sharp, and your concentration is good. You haven't experienced a single craving. You haven't had energy dips or gotten cranky and irritable.

But that's just the *inside* story. You also look great. Your weight is more or less where you want it to be. You're well toned. Your skin has a healthy glow. People often comment on how slim and well you look and how young you look for your age. You feel young, both physically and mentally. And this is how you feel every day!

Welcome to the new you. This is not only how you could be, this is how you should be. More important, it's how you will be when you follow the Holford Diet. And all it takes to see a dramatic difference is 30 days.

I realize that you may have spent the last decade trudging through a succession of diets with nothing to show for it but a slimmed-down bank balance and more fat than you started with. Every bookstore bristles with "miracle" weight-loss techniques and "guaranteed" recipes for everything from longevity to cellulite control. So I know you may be feeling cheated by claims and promises that have never panned out. Why, then, should you believe what I'm saying?

You can be thin *and* healthy

This is why. The Holford Diet works because it is much more than just a way to lose weight. It is a holistic system for attaining optimum health—and a healthy, self-regulating body is naturally slim.

The fact is that many of the people who discover my diet, follow it, and write to me reporting substantial weight loss didn't set off to lose weight in the first place. They wanted to be healthy and thought the optimum nutrition approach made sense. And, as their health improved, the pounds dropped off. Optimum health, they found, also means optimum weight.

The body will naturally reach its ideal weight given the chance. You'll eat less if your blood sugar is stable, and your metabolism will be better able to burn off excess weight.

I have yet to see any diet work better in the long run than this approach. I teach doctors, healthcare practitioners, and nutritionists all over the world, but none is as slim, energetic, and healthy as the thousand nutritionists we have trained at ION—the Institute for Optimum Nutrition.

At ION, decades of work with more than 100,000 volunteers first revealed how overall health determines weight, by showing that overweight is a symptom of a much wider condition. We sometimes call it "21st-century-itis."

Exhaustion, moodiness, depression, bloating—21st-century-itis is a response to our polluted, urbanized, speeded-up world, and overweight is a common symptom. Could you be suffering from it? Check yourself out by answering the questions below, scoring 1 point for each yes answer.

ARE YOU:

- ☐ Tired most of the time?   (80%)
- ☐ More than 7 pounds over your ideal weight, and rising?   (74%)
- ☐ Prone to PMS?   (64%)
- ☐ Suffering from poor memory and concentration?   (43%)
- ☐ Quite often sad or depressed?   (46%)
- ☐ Plagued by dry skin, in need of daily moisturizers?   (56%)
- ☐ Having difficulty sleeping?   (53%)
- ☐ Often feeling anxious or stressed?   (64%)
- ☐ Prone to indigestion or bloating after food?   (62%)

☐ Often constipated—that is, you rarely go twice a day?   (90%)

☐ Suffering from dark circles or bags under your eyes?   (54%)

In Britain, the average person checks seven boxes. The percentages on the right are of people who answered yes in our MyNutrition health and diet survey of more than 30,000 people—Britain's largest ever—which we carried out in 2004.

You may have checked a few boxes yourself. And the reality of being, say, tired all day, uncomfortably overweight, and feeling ill is no joke. Remember, though, that all this could change in just 30 days. Your load could be significantly lightened. And three months on the Holford Diet will leave you completely free of these symptoms, as well as up to 28 pounds lighter.

A diet for life

The point is that we already know how to cure 21st-century-itis, and that is my goal for you. I want you to lose weight fast, keep losing weight until you reach your goal, and maintain your weight once you get there—but always within the context of optimum energy and well-being. This is what you can look forward to:

- Within 7 days you will start to lose pounds as quickly as you'll gain energy.
- Within 20 days you'll notice your skin has dramatically improved.
- Within 30 days you'll be starting to feel like a new you.
- And within three months? You will have seriously undamaged your health.

Of course, if you just want to lose weight there are plenty of ways to do it. I've studied them all. I was there with the rise and fall of the F Plan Diet, the Hip & Thigh Diet, the Atkins Diet, and many others. I advised Rosemary Conley as I believed her diets were dangerously low in essential fats. I challenged Dr. Atkins when the science just didn't seem to add up.

I know the pros and cons of all of them. I know why high-protein diets work better for some but not for others, and don't work in the long run. I've tested Atkins dieters and I believe that his regime can actually seriously damage health. I know why you can lose weight on low-fat diets, only to end up with dry and wrinkly skin. I know why most diets leave you exhausted. Most of all, I know why the pounds you lose keep coming back!

For me to get excited about a diet that claims to be successful, it must fulfill the following criteria:

It works in both the short and the long term

Instant results may be thrilling, but they're usually not sustained. The body can't burn more than 2 pounds of actual fat in a week, unless you go into starvation mode. I look for a steady loss of 6 to 10 pounds a month, or 28 pounds in three months, or 112 pounds in a year—if you've got that much to lose—with no rebound weight gain. That said, you can lose up to 6 pounds of excess water if you're eating foods to which you've developed an intolerance. That's why some people lose 7 pounds in the first week of the Holford Diet.

You never feel hungry

If a diet leaves you feeling famished, you won't stick to it. So from day one it has to satisfy your appetite. The Holford Diet specifically recommends the foods scientifically proven to best satisfy your appetite, and I'm going to tell you exactly which those foods are.

It's enjoyable

If you can't eat a wide variety of foods or have to actively avoid eating certain food groups, a diet will start to feel boring very fast, and it will be neither enjoyable nor sustainable. The framework of my diet, the Fatburner System, allows a cornucopia of delectable foods containing good fats, protein, and carbohydrates. You'll be able to eat bread and pasta, mayonnaise, meat—the works. You'll just pay more attention to quality and quantity.

It's safe

I'm not interested in helping people lose weight by cheating the body. Sure, you can lose weight with diet pills, or by cutting out all carbohydrates, but it just isn't good for you and, in the end, crime doesn't pay. The only side effect I want you to experience is improved health.

It makes you feel great

If a diet is working with the body's design, not against it, you should start to feel better, with more energy, improved mood and concentration, and better skin within days.

There's no rebound weight gain

You can lose weight by massively restricting food intake—but the body thinks it's gone into starvation mode and slows down your metabolism. So, as soon as you start eating enough for your needs, the pounds boomerang back. The same is true of stimulants such as caffeine. They can suppress your appetite so you can lose weight in the short term, but in the end they slow down your metabolism. As you'll see, these can give short-term weight loss, but rebound weight gain.

It's easy to follow

At the end of the day, if a diet becomes as easy and natural as breathing, you'll stick to it for life. So, if the food is delicious, is easy to find and prepare, and leaves you satisfied and feeling wonderful, you're far more likely to make it part of your life.

The word from the weight-loss trenches

The Holford Diet scores 10 out of 10 for each of these criteria. But you don't have to take just my word for it. Here are the stories of a handful of the many thousands who have followed the Fatburner System.

Linda H. was just 5 feet, 2 inches tall, but had gradually expanded sideways in her twenties. She had tried every diet under the sun and finally settled on WeightWatchers, with some success. She had been a member of WeightWatchers for five years and had managed, with much sacrifice, to get down to and maintain a weight of 122 pounds. But she found she couldn't get below this. She wasn't quite at the right weight for her and it was a frustrating impasse. Then she discovered the Fatburner System:

> *On your diet I began to lose weight at once. Within 30 days I came down to 8 stone 4 [116 pounds]—a thing I thought impossible! However, I was totally unprepared for the new energy levels. I cannot believe how marvelous I feel—I am no longer tired no matter what I do or how active I am. I have stopped falling asleep at odd moments when I relax. I no longer feel bloated and tired after eating. Your diet has changed my life!*

Carol P. had been gradually gaining weight, year after year. When she turned 60 she realized her weight was out of control:

I felt too fat and it was hard to bend over and tie the laces on my walking boots. I was getting out of breath going up hills and I started to worry about that. I decided to do your diet and the exercises. I cut out nearly all wheat, ate mainly oat porridge for breakfast, and cut out biscuits [cookies] and cakes. I also cut out caffeine, had less alcohol—just the odd glass of wine. I lost 30 pounds steadily over six months. Also, my stomach used to really stick out! It doesn't do that anymore. I think wheat was making me bloat. Now I have wheat occasionally, but not every day.

What I liked about your approach is the understanding of the human psyche and the reality of living. You don't have to be a total puritan and you don't get hungry. If I were hungry, I'd have a piece of fruit. What I needed was a diet for life. I'm not so strict now on the exercise, but still generally follow the dietary principles. I definitely feel a lot better. I like the way my body looks. I have more energy. I feel happy and my mood is more even. I will have no problem staying on this general routine for life.

Wayne P. had been gaining almost 14 pounds a year, and was now seriously obese. He realized he had to do something about it:

As a teenager I was very fit. By the age of 17 I was playing ice hockey for England. When I hit my twenties and went to work I stopped exercising, but kept eating and drinking—curries, lager, and takeaways. I reckon I put on close to a stone for every year I was alive. By the age of 33 I was 27 stone 9 pounds [287 pounds] and basically addicted to junk food. I met Patrick when I became a volunteer for ITV's Tonight with Trevor McDonald, testing whether junk food was addictive. I started following Patrick's Fatburner System.

In the first four months I lost 32 pounds, a little more than 2 pounds a week, and I'm still losing weight, week by week. I'm still following the Fatburner principles, and I'm not even that strict. I eat more fresh food and less packaged food and snack more on fruit. My downfall is drinking—I still knock back a few lagers and a bottle of wine on the weekends. But I feel better. I have more energy. I feel happier and more comfortable and have gone down two sizes. I'm also becoming more active and my weight is still reducing.

What many people following my diet love most, apart from the inevitable weight loss, are the unexpected dividends. I receive letters like the following on a regular basis:

Since following your diet I have totally cured my migraines.

For eight years I suffered incredibly badly from rheumatoid arthritis. I could barely walk without suffering from pain and exhaustion. Following your advice has enabled me to control arthritis and to lead a full and active life: I am eternally grateful for that.

I was both surprised and pleased to see a rapid reduction in the wrinkly skin under my eyes.

Following your diet and supplements my cholesterol has dropped from 255 to 190. My GP couldn't believe it!

I used to have constant pain in my knees and joints, could not play golf or walk more than 10 minutes without resting my legs. Since I've been following your advice my discomfort has decreased 95 to 100 percent. I never would have believed my pain could be reduced by such a large degree, with no return, no matter how much activity in a day or week.

Within two weeks, I had much more energy. My mood is very positive— no panic or depression. I feel buoyant, energetic, and enthusiastic. I haven't had any colds or infections. I'm sleeping much better, my PMS is much better. I experienced no breast tenderness in my last period, and no mood swings or tearfulness.

And this is how you should feel all the time. I call it 100 percent health, and there's no reason why you can't claim it for yourself. You can lose weight and feel great.

You know the definition of insanity? To keep doing the same things and expect different results. And that's what millions are doing—eating the same foods and expecting to feel better and magically shed the excess pounds. But the real magic lies in a very different means to this end.

The science of slimming

Your body has evolved over millions of years to work perfectly with a certain kind of diet. Our ancestors weren't fat, because they ate this optimum diet, as do the lucky ones such as the Hunzas in the Himalayas, whose average life span is over 100 and who never get fat or suffer from diabetes, heart disease, cancer, Alzheimer's, or any other of the diseases plaguing the 21st century. This is, in all its essentials, my diet.

If you follow the Fatburner System, you will lose weight, gain energy, improve your skin, sharpen your mind, balance your mood—and add years to your life, and life to your years. Now let's look at why.

The science behind the Holford Diet is very simple. Your body is designed to burn glucose for energy; the glucose is carried by blood to the cells. Carbohydrates such as grains and fruits are broken down into glucose in the body. But carbohydrates figure hugely in today's typical Western diet, and if you eat too much of them—particularly the refined type—you'll end up with more blood glucose than you need. You'll then store the excess as fat.

If your blood glucose levels are even, you'll have a steady supply of energy and a healthy but balanced appetite. This is the reason you'll have no problem maintaining the right weight. But, if your blood glucose levels are sometimes high, sometimes low, you'll see the beginnings of 21st-century-itis. When levels are too high, you'll lay down fat; when they're too low, you'll feel lethargic, and it will be harder to burn fat. A quarter of all people, and nine out of ten people with weight problems, have difficulty keeping their blood sugar level even. The result is exhaustion and overweight.

And this is just the beginning. Obese people are 77 times more at risk of developing diabetes than nonobese people—a statistic that alone tells you how strongly linked weight gain is to blood sugar control.

So the best way of losing weight is to regain blood glucose control, which heralds the return of your body's ability to burn fat. You'll lose weight effortlessly without having to starve, and gain health and vitality at the same time.

The five key principles

The Holford Diet is based on five key principles, which, taken together, form the fastest, safest, and most effective way to lose weight and gain health. Each is explained in detail in Part Two, but let's take a look at them now.

1: BALANCE YOUR BLOOD SUGAR

This is the crux: once you achieve it, weight loss is inevitable. Keeping your blood sugar balanced depends not only on what you eat, but also on how and when you eat it. In Chapter 7, I'll explain exactly which foods and food combinations stabilize your blood sugar best and help to burn fat. I'll be introducing you to something called the *glycemic load,* or ⒼⓁ, of a food. This is a much superior method of measuring a food's suitability than "carbohydrate points" or the "glycemic index" (GI).

To put it simply, GI is a *qualitative* measure that tells you whether the carbohydrate a food contains is "fast-" or "slow-" releasing. It doesn't tell you, however, how much of the food is carbohydrate. Carbohydrate points, or grams of carbohydrate, are *quantitative* measures that tell you how much of the food is carbohydrate, but they don't tell you what that carbohydrate does to your blood sugar. The ⒼⓁ of a food is the quantity times the quality of its carbohydrate, and that is the best way of telling you how much weight you'll gain if you choose that food.

You may be amazed by some of the foods that have a high ⒼⓁ score. But it's important to know the truth: if you understand why you gain weight, you'll hold the key to losing it. Cornflakes and corn chips, for instance, have a very high ⒼⓁ, while ice cream and peanuts do not. One single date has the same effect on your blood sugar and weight as a whole pint of strawberries. So be ready for some surprises.

Your goal will be to limit your ⒼⓁ to 40 a day—that's 10 per meal and 5 each for two snacks. So knowing your ⒼⓁ is essential. Just look at this comparison of two typical breakfasts.

BREAKFAST	ⒼⓁ		ⒼⓁ
A bowl of steel-cut oats (1 oz.)	2	A bowl of cornflakes	21
Half a grated apple	3	A banana	12
A small container of yogurt	2	Milk	2
Milk	2		35
	9		

The two may seem broadly similar, but in ⒼⓁ terms they are worlds apart. The Fatburner breakfast on the left will cut your blood glucose load, and your propensity to store fat, by no less than a third. It will push your body's metabolism one giant step toward fatburning and away from fat storing—and you will feel fuller and more energetic for longer.

And there will be immense variety to choose from. Part Four is packed with zesty, delicious recipes and menus, including Crunchy Thai Salad, Cod Roasted with Lemon and Garlic, Chicken Tandoori, and even Beef Burgers. In case you're wondering, I've done all the adding up of ⒼⓁs for you. You'll find that "ⒼⓁ awareness" swiftly becomes second nature; before you know it you'll be doing your own mixing and matching of low- foods at every meal.

You'll note that the fatburning breakfast combines oatmeal and yogurt. Mixing carbohydrates with proteins is another important way of regulating blood sugar, and again, very easy to master. There's a full discussion in Part Two, but, basically, it means you'll eat low-Ⓖ carbohydrates with good-quality protein—for example, brown basmati rice with organic chicken, whole wheat pasta with wild salmon, or rye toast with scrambled eggs.

Fiber plays a starring role, too, because a food's fiber content lowers its Ⓖ. So you'll find plenty of high-fiber choices, from beans to brown rice. Last, *when* you eat is very important. Unlike most diets, which are snackless deserts, mine will encourage you to eat two snacks a day along with your three meals.

2: EAT GOOD FATS AND AVOID BAD FATS

Essential fatty acids (or EFAs) may be a bit of a buzzword these days, but they thoroughly deserve their celebrity status. These are the "good fats" I've talked about for years, and, although it may seem counterintuitive, there's evidence that eating them can actually help you to lose weight.

The reason is very simple. Your body and brain depend on omega-3 and omega-6 EFAs. In fact, excluding water, one quarter of your brain is made up of omega-3s. So almost nothing works well without them. Your brain can't function, so omega-3 deficiency leads to lower IQ, poor memory, and a tendency to depression. Your hormones go up the creek, possibly leading to mood swings, PMS, sugar cravings, and weight gain. Your skin shrivels, and your heart and arteries suffer.

This is why these fats are called essential. And, since we can't manufacture them ourselves, it's as if our body and brain are designed to seek them out. We literally have an instinct to eat fat. We are instinctively drawn toward the creamy texture of fats, sauces, cheese, and cream, and not only this: the body's "fat sensors" are in your mouth, there to tell you when you've hit nutritional gold. Think about it. If the body needs anything (water, air, essential fats, vitamins) there's always an instinct that makes you crave it. That's why fat-free diets are such a titanic struggle for most of us.

But our need for fats has also spawned a legion of "bad" fats—fried fat, processed fat in junk food, saturated fats, even "fake" fats. When you eat EFAs, your body's fat sensors tell the brain that your essential fat needs are satisfied. But when you eat bad fats, your fat sensors are not satisfied, even though your eyes and taste buds may have been fooled into believing you've eaten the fats that you need. The sensors respond much more strongly to essential fats than to processed or saturated fats. So, if you've packed away a burger and chips or several doughnuts, you'll find yourself craving fats the next day because your body hasn't received what it needed. And you'll keep on craving them until it has.

The Holford Diet gives you exactly the right kind and amount of essential fats, not only to help you stay healthy and glowing (and cellulite free!), but also to reduce your desire to eat unhealthy fatty foods. But that's not all. The essential fats also tune up your metabolism and help you burn unwanted fat. So it's not true to say that a calorie of *any* fat has the same effect on weight gain. You'll hear the whole story and the latest research in Chapter 8.

3: ELIMINATE YOUR HIDDEN ALLERGIES

We are all unique. Think about your friends. Their appearances may be wildly different. Some will be night owls, others skylarks. They'll have different blood types. A number may be natural carnivores, others natural vegetarians. And most of us have different intolerances or allergies to certain foods, but very few even know it. Weight gain, however, is a common reaction to foods to which we're intolerant.

It follows, then, that eliminating the food to which you are unknowingly allergic can lead to highly dramatic weight loss. Lisa M., for instance, lost 5 inches off her waist in three days and 42 pounds in three months by discovering and avoiding allergens.

Rebecca S. also lost 42 pounds simply by avoiding her food allergies. In her twenties Rebecca had a stable weight, and used to exercise three or four times a week. But in her thirties she started to pile on the pounds. Over three years her weight drifted from 140 pounds up to 182 pounds and her dress size went up to 16. "I started feeling tired and lethargic and generally unwell," she said. "I didn't have the energy to go to the gym anymore. But it seemed the foods I ate were blowing me up, which was why I thought I could have a food allergy." She decided to test herself for a food allergy, which you can do with a home test kit, involving a pinprick of blood. The results showed that she was reacting to milk, egg white, and gluten—the protein found in wheat. Within a week of excluding these foods her skin and mood improved and the weight started to fall away.

Don't think that all allergies are for life. After three months strictly avoiding the foods she'd become allergic to, Lisa reintroduced egg whites and then milk to see if there was a reaction. Now she's fine on both foods, but still reacts to wheat. "I can't tell you how much better I feel. I'm 100 percent," she said. "Eliminating my food allergies has transformed my health. I just wish I'd done it sooner." Why did she lose so much weight? Because water retention, bloating, and puffiness are all common allergic reactions, and they make you feel and look fatter.

This is great news because, once you've singled out and eliminated the "bad" foods, you can see really dramatic changes very fast. It's not unusual to lose up to 7 pounds within three or four days.

Aside from weight gain and bloating, food allergies also cause many other niggling problems—aches and pains, headaches, fatigue, mood swings, annoying skin and digestive conditions. These also go when you identify and avoid what you are allergic to. You'll find out how to pinpoint the "baddies" lurking in your larder in Chapter 9.

It's reassuring to know that, as in Rebecca's case, most food allergies aren't for life. You can often "unlearn" your intolerances in as little as three months, which means you can reintroduce previously "bad" foods into your diet.

4: TAKE THE RIGHT SUPPLEMENTS

By now you're probably realizing that calorie intake and weight loss are not all that firmly linked. In fact, one of the biggest lies in nutrition today is "You can lose weight only by eating fewer calories."

The other is "You can get all the vitamins and minerals you need from a well-balanced diet." This is untrue. You simply can't guarantee that the nutrients you need are in your food.

Take vitamin C, which not only protects against degenerative diseases such as cancer, but also helps stabilize your blood sugar and speeds your fat-burning. At ION, we've examined more than 500 studies—including the "gold standard" type, which are randomized, double-blind, and placebo-controlled—that have led us to conclude that the optimal intake of vitamin C is 1,000 milligrams a day. This is what our jungle-dwelling, fruit-eating ancestors could have gotten from leaves, berries, and fruits.

But how much vitamin C is there in a supermarket orange? As much as 116 milligrams and as little as zero. Yes, the "average" orange contains 60 milligrams of the precious vitamin, but some contain virtually none of it! And even if your supermarket orange contains 60 milligrams, you'd need to eat 22 of them to achieve 1,000 milligrams.

So I recommend that you supplement 1,000 milligrams of C a day, along with eating vitamin C-rich foods such as strawberries. You can eat strawberries till the cows come home and never gain weight. (Not all fruits are this useful for fatburning or general health, however, as we'll see.)

There are some 30 vitamins and minerals that are essential for health, and along with vitamin C a number will help you burn fat, too. Essentially, they boost your metabolism, reprogramming your body to turn food into energy rather than fat. For example, the mineral chromium helps to even out appetite and energy dips by stabilizing your blood sugar. It's so effective that it's given to diabetics, with amazing results. There are also amino acids and herbs that really can give you an edge when it comes to losing weight. Hydroxy-citric acid, or HCA, is a herbal extract from the tamarind plant, which makes it harder for your body to turn glucose into fat. There's another herbal extract from a bean called *Griffonia,* which is naturally high in an amino acid called 5-hydroxytryptophan. Known as 5-HTP, this amino acid has an extraordinary capability to ease excessive appetite and sugar cravings.

These aren't drugs. They're nutrients, and they will help fine-tune your metabolism.

5: DO 15 MINUTES OF EXERCISE A DAY

If you exercise just to burn calories, quite frankly you might as well just not eat that piece of toast. The real value of exercise is that it helps stabilize your blood sugar levels and reduce your appetite. And the great news is that you don't have to do much to achieve this result—just 15 minutes a day, in fact.

It has been found that people who don't exercise eat more than people who do a little exercise or just have active jobs. The human body, it seems, needs physical activity to work properly in the way that it needs water or vitamins. Certain kinds of exercise boost the rate at which you burn fat for up to 15 hours afterward.

That's the immediate effect, but there's a long-term effect, too. With the right kind of exercise, you'll put on more muscle and lose fat, and a pound of muscle burns many more calories a day than a pound of fat. So every pound of fat you lose and every pound of muscle you gain increases your body's long-term ability to burn fat.

To kick-start this process, you'll do 15 minutes a day, or 21 minutes five times a week, or 35 minutes three times a week, of the right kind of muscle-building and fatburning exercise. And, fortunately, the fatter and less fit you are right now, the easier it will be to get the same benefits! For example, if you are overweight and underfit, jogging half a mile slowly can burn 300 calories, while if you are fitter and lighter you'd need to jog a mile.

• • • • • •

Following these five principles is easy and enjoyable—yet they'll revolutionize the way you live, simply because of the way you'll feel and look, day by day. And, if you feel and look great, that's the best motivation for making it a diet for life.

Meanwhile, the dieting industry continues to make money from you by selling quick fixes that are destined to fail. That's what keeps you coming back for more. How many diets have you been on, and how many have worked? I want to make sure that the Holford Diet is the last diet you'll ever go on.

Why So Many Diets Fail

Dieting can be like negotiating a minefield of misconceptions. Many methods for losing weight have no basis in science whatsoever—so, if your dieting life has been one long string of depressing failed attempts, it's hardly surprising.

Here I'd like to debunk some of these methods and expose them as myths. That way, you'll have the knowledge to prevent a life of yo-yo dieting and long-term health problems.

Myth number 1: You can lose weight only by eating fewer calories or exercising more.

Yes, it is true that you'll lose weight if you eat fewer calories and exercise more. But the real picture is a lot more complex than this.

Take fat. Since fat has 9 calories per gram, compared with approximately 4 per gram for protein and carbohydrate, the most successful original low-calorie diets were low-fat diets. Then the world woke up to the fact that some fats, such as the omega-3 essential fatty acids, are necessary for health. So we realized it wasn't so smart to cut out all the fats from our diets.

Meanwhile, the facts reveal something very puzzling about our calorie consumption.

People are eating less. Calorie consumption has gone down, and fat intake has gone down even more. Yet there's an obesity epidemic. That's a real paradox. At the same time, our consumption of sugar, refined carbohy-

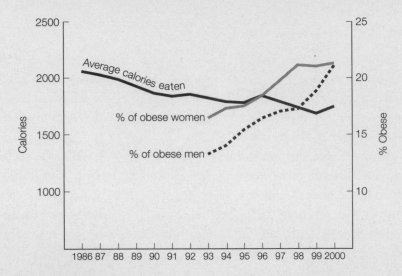

Government statistics show that the amount of calories we eat has steadily decreased over the last 15 years, while the percentage of obese people has steadily increased.

drates, and stimulants such as caffeine has risen. Could that be only coincidence?

Let's start with the big picture, using data derived from two government surveys.[1] In the figure above you will see the estimated average calorie intake (from food) of the average person in Britain over the past 15 years.

This clearly shows that we're eating fewer calories, not more, while obesity rates have tripled! And this trend runs like a thread throughout the Western world, from America to Australia. Something doesn't quite add up.

In fact, if you look globally, you won't find that calorie intake predicts obesity. For example, in the United States—where obesity is epidemic—the average daily intake is 2,360 calories. Yet in China, where obesity is exceedingly rare, the average intake is also 2,630 calories!

One possible explanation is exercise. The Chinese lead less sedentary lives than we do. But exercise alone, or lack of it, simply cannot explain why 1,000 people a day are becoming obese in the United Kingdom alone. What's more, surveys estimate that women increased their level of physical activity between 1994 and 1998, from 22 to 25 percent. For men it seems there has been little change.[2]

What's going on? We're not eating more calories. So the crucial element must be not quantity, but quality—and that's the focus of the next big diet myth.

Myth number 2: A calorie is a calorie is a calorie.

High-protein diets tried to prove this wrong, and failed. Recent studies, however, *have* proved that not all calories are the same in relation to weight loss.

Let's start with the graph below, which gives us some essential clues. You can see how our diets have changed in relation to the three main food groups—protein, fat, and carbohydrate.

As you can see, our consumption of calories from fat is decreasing, while our calories from protein and especially carbohydrates have gone up. So the culprit in the obesity epidemic we're seeing seems to be not the much maligned fat, but carbohydrates (that's sugar, grains, vegetables, and fruit) and possibly protein. Only calories from carbohydrates, however, have gone up consistently in line with increasing rates of obesity.

If carbohydrates were to blame, you'd expect countries that eat large amounts of carbohydrates to be the fattest. But that's not a hard-and-fast rule. Some of the healthiest communities in the world get 55 percent or more of their calories from carbohydrate. China, where the figure is 70 percent of calories, is a classic example. So let's go in closer and look at the *kind* of carbohydrates we are eating more of.

In the chart on the following page we are looking at the percentage of calories consumed from three kinds of carbohydrates—(added) sugar,

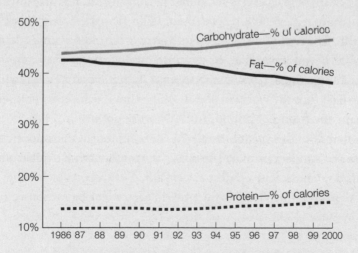

Government statistics show that over the past 15 years we have been eating less and less fat, while carbohydrate intake is on the increase.

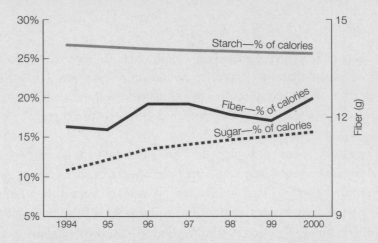

Over the past 15 years our intake of sugar has gone steadily up, while our intake of more complex carbohydrates (starch) has gone down. Fiber intake has also increased.

starch, and fiber, which is indigestible carbohydrate and has no caloric value. Fiber has gone up, which is nothing but good news and, if anything, would reduce weight because it fills you up and you eat less. But what really stands out now is our intake of sugar, which is steadily rising.

But it's highly likely that these figures relating to sugar consumption are a gross underestimation. Let's make this real. According to these figures, the average person in Britain eats 48 pounds of sugar a year. Yet according to government sources, 2.3 billion tons of sugar go into the British food supply every year.[3] That amount translates into an average of 84 pounds per person per year, almost double what the government diet survey above shows. This makes a lot more sense, because more comprehensive surveys in the United States, which tops the world in obesity, show that the annual intake of sugar there has gone from 124 pounds in 1975 to 157 pounds in 1999.

So where is all this sugar lurking? You'd be amazed at the amount not just in cakes and candy, but in soft drinks, convenience foods, chips and other salty snacks, condiments, and many breakfast cereals. Whichever way you slice it, there's obviously an awful lot of hidden sugar being consumed, and your body simply can't cope with it.

There are other problems in the calories we're getting from carbohydrates. While our intake of starch has decreased very slightly, a lot of this is refined, "fast-releasing"—what I call high- ⒼⓁ —carbohydrate, which sends your blood sugar level rocketing. White bread, cornflakes, and the like are the

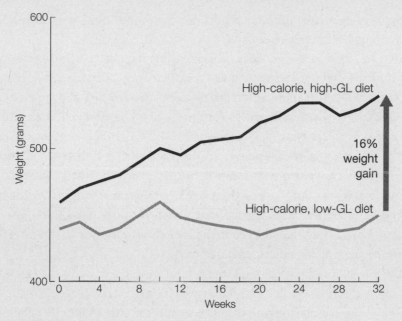

What diet works best? This chart shows weight change on high-🅖🅛 and low-🅖🅛 diets of equal calories and fat/protein/carbohydrate percentage.

nasties here. If we had the right data on starch, I believe we'd also find that we are eating more and more refined carbohydrates. And quite a few other foods, such as French fries, bananas, and dates, also carry a heavy 🅖🅛.

Now let's look at what happens to animals given identical diets in terms of calories and all other nutrients—with only one difference: 🅖🅛. In the figure above you'll see what happened to one group of rats. Half were given a high-🅖🅛 diet, the other a low-🅖🅛 diet. They couldn't cheat. They had exactly the same number of calories, and there weren't any candy stores around the corner.

In this strictly controlled study by one of the world's leading experts on weight loss, Professor Jennie Brand-Miller from the University of Sydney, the low-🅖🅛 "Fatburner" rats gained no weight.[4] But the high-🅖🅛 rats gained weight week after week, and pound after pound. By the end of 32 weeks, the high-🅖🅛 group were not only 16 percent heavier—they had gained 40 percent more body fat! A recent study, published in the medical journal *The Lancet*, found that mice on a low-🅖🅛 diet lost almost twice as much body fat in nine weeks as mice given identical nutrients with high-🅖🅛 carbohydrates instead. The low-🅖🅛 dieters were substantially leaner and slimmer.[5]

Same calories, very different results. Yet this is nothing short of heresy for conventional calorie theorists.

But, you may be asking, does the same thing happen to us? After all, rats and humans don't always respond in a similar way. The answer is yes. Researchers in the human nutrition department at South Africa's University of the Orange Free State assigned 15 volunteers to a low-Ⓖ diet and 15 others to a normal calorie-controlled diet for 12 weeks.[6] The diets contained identical numbers of calories. The two groups then switched diets for 12 more weeks. As you can see from the figure opposite, during the first 12 weeks both groups lost weight, but those on the low-Ⓖ diet lost more weight. During the second 12-week period, the group that switched to the low-Ⓖ diet lost 40 percent more weight than the group that switched to the normal diet. Yet the caloric content of both diets remained the same.

Despite all this evidence (and there's a lot more), some so-called experts still say "a calorie is a calorie" as far as weight loss is concerned. Whichever way you look at it, this is simply not true. You can lose weight by changing the quality of what you eat, even if you don't change the quantity. Of course, if you eat fewer calories of lower-Ⓖ foods, that will trigger the most rapid weight loss.

Not only that, we now know that people who eat low-Ⓖ food eat significantly less anyway, as they feel much more satisfied.[7] So, if you eat a low-Ⓖ diet, you not only lose weight, but you tend to want to eat less. It's a double whammy in your favor.

But calories can't just vanish. If two people eat the same number of calories and one, eating the high-Ⓖ diet, stores some of the calories as fat, what happens to the calories in the Fatburner? Here's the real magic. If you are not storing calories as fat, you are turning calories into energy. That is why people on the Holford Diet, such as Linda H., say, "I can't believe how marvelous I feel." I hear this kind of feedback from Fatburners all the time. You really can and you will lose weight and feel great. This is precisely why the Holford Diet works so amazingly well.

Myth number 3: If you eat a high-protein diet you lose calories in urine, so you shed more weight.

When you're on a high-protein, low-carbohydrate diet, your body switches from using carbohydrates as its primary fuel to using fat and protein instead—including the body's fat reserves. As the body burns fat, ketones—

Two groups of overweight women were given a low-calorie diet, with equivalent amounts of protein, fat, and carbohydrate. One group ate low-**ⒼⓁ** carbohydrates and the other group ate high-**ⒼⓁ** carbohydrates. Both groups lost weight, but those on the low-**ⒼⓁ** diet lost considerably more weight over 12 weeks. Those on the low-**ⒼⓁ** diet were then switched onto the high-**ⒼⓁ** diet, and vice versa. During the second period of 12 weeks, again, those on the low-**ⒼⓁ** diet lost considerably more weight.

a by-product of the process—are excreted in the urine. This process is called *ketosis.*

Supposedly, since fat and protein constitute a less efficient fuel than carbohydrate, you can eat more. The thinking is that the body will excrete some of the calories of this inefficient fuel as ketones.

Nice theory, but wrong. It is true that people do lose more weight on high-protein diets. But the reason is that they eat less on those diets. And the reason they eat less is that high-protein diets help stabilize blood sugar.

The high-protein-diet proponents, led by the late Dr. Atkins, were among the first to say that sugar makes you fat. But their solution was to say that carbohydrates are bad and protein is good, so you should eat a high-protein diet that's very low in carbohydrates. Now, a high-protein meal has a low ⓖⓛ, which as we've seen, is the key to stabilizing blood sugar, which in turn balances our appetite and helps us lose weight. But a meal with some protein and some low-ⓖⓛ carbohydrate works in the same way. There is absolutely no need to avoid or massively restrict carbohydrates to lose weight, provided you are eating the right low-ⓖⓛ kind, plus protein.

Take a look at the science. There have been two sound weight-loss trials to date published on the Atkins-type high-fat/high-protein diet versus a conventional low-fat diet. The first showed that, after six months, those on the high-fat/high-protein diet had lost 12.7 pounds, compared with 4 pounds on the low-fat diet. That's a rather unexciting half-pound a week. However, after 12 months, there was no significant difference.[8]

The other trial showed no real difference in weight loss between the high-protein approach and conventional dieting, with an average weight loss of 10 pounds after six months.[9] That's less than half a pound a week. Similarly, a review of all the high-protein/low-carbohydrate diet studies done to date concludes, "Weight loss was principally associated with decreased calorie intake." [10]

In other words, an Atkins-type diet works, but the results aren't spectacular and are due principally to eating less in general, rather than eating fewer carbohydrates. Moreover, there are problems, and even serious dangers, associated with eating high-protein/low-carbohydrate diets. I go into these in detail in Appendix 3 (see page 342), but here's an overview.

The first problem is ketosis itself. In excess, ketones can be very toxic and in extreme cases ketosis can be fatal. Reports suggest that 58 deaths have been associated with very-low-calorie, very-high-protein diets. Moreover, recent research has proved that the number of calories lost through ketosis is negligible. This makes the risk pretty high for diets based on this principle.

The diet promises more than it delivers in other ways. As I've said, I think the switch to ketosis triggers weight loss by stabilizing blood sugar, and it's known that ketosis also suppresses appetite. A low-carbohydrate diet also kick-starts weight loss because you use up your short-term stores of glucose, which are stored as glycogen, bound with water. In fact, for every pound of glycogen, you store 3 to 4 pounds of water. The net result is an immediate weight loss of up to 5 pounds—just one reason why people claim spectacular short-term weight loss. But it's not sustainable. The glycogen and water will come back, as will your appetite. Many people on high-protein diets lose weight, get bored, then gain it all back.

A diet lacking in carbohydrates such as fruit and green leafy vegetables will leave you deficient in antioxidants and vitamins, unless you are very careful about what you eat and take supplements. You won't get enough fiber, and could get constipated as a result, which can lead to digestive problems. Additionally, many people feel ill as they go through sugar withdrawal and switch to ketosis. Nausea and tiredness continue for some, making it hard to stick to the diet.

Finally, high-protein diets, especially those based on meat and milk, can be dangerous. They potentially increase the risk of bone and kidney problems and of breast and prostate cancer. And as we've seen, the weight-loss results are little different from those of conventional dieting in the long run. In my opinion the high-protein approach to stabilizing your blood sugar, and hence your weight, is certainly not worth the risk.

Myth number 4: Don't eat protein with carbohydrates. These foods fight.

"Food-combining" diets separate protein foods from carbohydrate foods. Nature doesn't. Beans, lentils, nuts, and seeds all contain both. And the healthiest nations of the world are the nut, bean, and seed eaters.

Despite this, a number of food-combining diets abound, based on the principles of Dr. Hay, a physician who wrote in the 1930s. He emphasized eating whole foods and lots of fruit and vegetables; he also advocated eating fruit separately from other foods, since, if trapped in the stomach after a steak for example, fruit can ferment. So far, so good.

He also recommended never eating carbohydrate-rich foods with protein-rich foods. So, for example, fish with rice or chicken with potatoes is out. The only study I've seen recommending that overweight or obese people follow this kind of diet showed a 3.5 percent average body-weight change over 12 weeks. Although subjects in this trial were not advised to eat less or change the kind of food they ate, there was no measure to indicate whether their weight loss was due solely to food combining or to changes in the quantity or quality of food.[11]

It is now known, however, that combining protein with carbohydrate slows down the release of sugars from a meal to the bloodstream, helps stabilize blood sugar levels, and hence helps control weight (see Chapter 7). Since the majority of overweight people have blood sugar problems, it would seem that combining protein with carbohydrate would be better, not worse for you. So, in my book, fish with rice is in, not out. This is the staple diet, along with fruits and vegetables, of numerous island and coastal peoples around the world, many of whom are exceedingly healthy and slim.

Dr. Hay's approach, if followed strictly, is probably best for those with digestive problems and worst for those with blood sugar problems. I have yet to be convinced that the benefits reported by those on food-combining diets aren't largely due to changes in the kind of foods eaten, rather than their non-combination.

Myth number 5: You can't change your metabolism.

Your metabolism is the way in which you turn your food into energy or into storage as fat. We are each programmed to respond differently to the food we eat. This programming is partly inherited: some people's metabolism rapidly turns food into fat, for instance. But your metabolism is primarily dependent on what you eat and how active you are.

Because of this, you can change both the efficiency of your metabolism and your metabolic rate—the speed at which you burn calories. Crash diets can lower your metabolic rate to half speed, for instance, while aerobic exercise can increase it tenfold and leave it raised for up to 15 hours. Where's the proof that a low-**GL** diet doesn't cause the rebound drop in your metabolic rate? In a study published in the *Journal of the American Medical Association*, two groups of overweight or obese adults were followed for two years. One group was on a low-**GL** diet, the other group followed a conventional low-fat/low-calorie diet. Each person had their metabolic rate measured once they had lost ten percent of their body weight. **The group on the conven-**

tional low-fat/low-calorie diet had almost twice the reduction in metabolic rate compared with the low-ⓖ group.[12] By changing the kinds and combinations of food you eat, you can reprogram yourself to burn fat more rapidly.

And the less fat and the more lean tissue you have, the more calories you burn off just keeping your body alive. In other words, your metabolic rate has increased, and you've changed from fatmaker to Fatburner. This is what a low-ⓖ diet will do for you.

Myth number 6: It's eating fat that makes you fat.

It isn't just fat that makes you fat. All sugar or carbohydrates and all alcohol, as well as all fats, are turned by the body into glucose. (Protein, too, can be turned into glucose, but not so easily.) Glucose, remember, is the fuel our bodies run on, and any excess is turned into fat. So too much fat, protein, carbohydrate, or alcohol can lead to fat gain and weight gain.

And, looking at fat alone, it isn't just any old fat that makes you fat. As far as your body is concerned there's a world of difference between, say, 100 calories of saturated fat from meat and 100 calories of essential fat from seeds. Saturated fat can only be burned for energy or stored as body fat. But essential fats—properly known as essential fatty acids, or EFAs—are used by the brain, the nerves, the arteries, and the skin, and balance your hormones and boost immunity into the bargain. Only if there's any left over does the body burn it or store it. So you are more likely to gain weight eating saturated fat or damaged fat in fried or processed foods than you are eating EFAs.

One big reason for this is that the body craves EFAs, precisely because it needs them to function. This craving means we are drawn to fats in general, and, as we're surrounded by saturated and processed fats the minute we enter the average supermarket, we may well end up eating them. Yet afterward the body still keeps craving fat—so we eat more fatty foods. But, if you eat EFA-rich food such as fish and seeds, you'll fully satisfy the craving and will end up eating less.

Does eating fat make you fat? Of course it does, in excess, but fat isn't the main culprit. As we saw earlier, the number of calories we eat from fat has dropped, while our intake of sugar has increased dramatically, paralleling the rise in obesity.

Low-fat diets arose out of the belief that fat is the prime culprit in weight gain. But, as with high-protein diets, there are two potential problems with this approach. First, most low-fat diets are high in carbohydrates, so sugar and refined foods replace fatty foods. This encourages a blood sugar problem that, in turn, makes it harder to maintain weight control. For this reason, very-low-fat, high-carbohydrate diets can often cause fatigue, mood swings, and sugar cravings.

The worst aspect of a low-fat diet, however, is that it cuts out EFAs. Ann Louise Gittleman is the former director of nutrition at the Pritikin Longevity Center in Florida, which emphasized low-fat eating. In her book *Beyond Pritikin,* she notes conditions in people placed on low-fat diets, such as a lack of energy, allergies, yeast problems, mood swings, and dry skin, hair, and nails, that she believed were due to the lack of EFAs.[13]

While most of us could do with cutting back on fat, the real emphasis should be on reducing foods rich in saturated fats and devoid of essential fats (meat and dairy products), and instead eating foods rich in essential fats (seeds, their oils, and fish).

Myth number 7: The best way to lose weight fast is to eat far fewer calories.

I'm dead against very-low-calorie diets and calorie counting. Not only do they encourage obsessive eating—but the math is patently wrong.

Consider this simple example. A banana has approximately 100 calories, so, if you eat a banana fewer every day for a year, you'd lose 36,500 calories. A pound of body fat is equivalent to around 4,000 calories. That means you'd lose nearly 10 pounds in the first year, 50 pounds by the fifth year, and 100 pounds after 10 years—and you'd vanish completely after 15 years!

The calorie equation for exercise is equally ridiculous. Cycle vigorously for 15 minutes each day and you will lose 10 pounds in the first year. Quite possibly. But 100 pounds after 10 years? No chance. However, according to calorie theory, merely a banana every day undoes all that hard work anyway.

According to Dr. Michael Colgan, nutritionist to many Olympic athletes, some athletes burn off more than 7,000 calories a day, but eat only 3,500 calories. Going by calorie theory alone, these athletes should have completely disappeared by now.

An investigation by Dr. Marian Appelbaum of the Bichat Hospital in Paris, of people living in famine in the Warsaw Ghetto during World War II, came up with the same contradiction.[14] With an average calorie intake of 800 calories a day, and a requirement of around 2,500 calories, a deficiency of

1,241,000 calories would have built up over two years. The average body has 30 pounds of fat, representing 120,000 calories, to dispose of. Even if all the fat were lost, what happened to the other million calories?

If you still believe it all depends on calories, listen to this. *The Sunday Times Magazine* (of London) put two similarly overweight people on diets, one on my original Fatburner Diet (approximately 1,500 calories a day), and one on the Cambridge Diet (then 330 calories). The Fatburner volunteer lost more weight after six weeks.

The missing link in the low-calorie approach is metabolism—the process of turning the fuel in food into energy that the body can use, and burning off unwanted fat. As we've seen, people's metabolisms can vary considerably. Having a slow metabolism means you'll turn more food into fat. Most obese people have slower rates of metabolism than slim people.

If you start out this way, a low-calorie diet can simply exacerbate the problem. With crash diets below 1,000 calories a day, the body sees the reduction in food as a threat, and slows down the metabolic rate by as much as 45 percent.[15] According to Dr. John Marks from Cambridge University, "As weight falls, the metabolic rate always falls too." In the short term you can lose around 7 pounds of body fluid and, if you're lucky, an absolute maximum of 2 pounds of body fat a week, which together could account for as much as 10 pounds in two or three weeks. But the minute you go back to what you were eating before, the fluid returns. And so will the fat, because your metabolic rate has slowed down, meaning that you now need to eat less food to maintain a stable weight.

This "rebound effect" is good business for mortuaries. An American report by the National Institutes of Health, using the findings of a 22-center study called the Multiple Risk Factor Intervention Trial, showed that among people whose weight varied widely over six to seven years there was a higher death rate.[16] It's also good for food-replacement programs, whose customers try crash dieting on average three times a year.

To see how dramatically unpleasant the rebound effect can be, hark back to the *Sunday Times Magazine* trial I mentioned above. Michelle, who was on the Cambridge Diet, said,

> *The first three days were torturous but from then on it got worse. Walking down the road required serious will: I was constantly exhausted and couldn't concentrate so that my work suffered badly. Weight loss came slowly—I'd expected miracles after reading the publicity boasts—but in*

the final week it finally plummeted. . . . I blew up like a balloon when I resumed eating, and seemed to retain gallons of water; conversely, "loose" skin has appeared, creating an underarm bat-wing effect. When I first stopped the diet, irresistible bingeing took over but after six weeks, with the exercise of limbs and discipline, I've managed to limit the damage to a gain of 5 pounds.

Michelle lost 10 pounds over the month and gained 5 pounds in the weeks that followed—making her net weight loss 5 pounds.

Caroline, on my Fatburner Diet, also lost 10 pounds in a month. She then put 2 pounds back on while on vacation. She commented,

One of the hardest—but best—things about it was the insistence on giving up coffee and stimulants. I had caffeine-withdrawal headaches for the first few days, but began to feel wonderful after that—alert and fit and thoroughly detoxified, with no more puffy eyes staring back from the bathroom mirror. I regained 2 pounds while on vacation but will whittle it off by eating sensibly.

The bottom line is that the body is intelligent. If you try to starve it, it will turn down your metabolic fire. If you work with its natural design, you'll burn unwanted fat easily. (By the way, you don't have to give up all stimulants and caffeine-containing drinks on the Holford Diet, but there's no question that it helps speed up weight loss. More on this in Chapter 7.)

However, very-low-calorie diets do more than make you feel bad and gain weight afterward. They can be dangerous, and the FDA now recommends that diets provide a minimum of at least 400 calories and 40 grams of protein per day for women and 500 calories and 50 grams of protein per day for men to ensure the dieter's body will not be breaking down muscle tissue or vital organs to meet calorie requirements. They do not encourage the reeducation of eating habits. And they leave you very hungry.

The solution, in the eyes of the people designing these diets, is wheat bran, which fills you up while at the same time supposedly triggers weight loss. But does that make dieters want to stick to the regime? To find out, I put ten people on a 1,000-calorie-a-day diet plus high fiber for three months. Only four lasted the course, with an average weight loss of a measly 3.25 pounds. The high dropout rate is a reflection of how difficult it is to stick to a low-calorie diet for a long period of time. In another study we put ten diet-ers on high-fiber tablets claimed to induce weight loss for a period of three months. Five completed the three months with an average weight loss of 1.5 pounds. Not very impressive.

However, some special kinds of fiber do assist weight loss, and having a high-fiber diet by eating whole foods—not by adding wheat bran—is defi-nitely good for you. This is explained in Chapter 7.

Myth number 8: Stimulants help you lose weight by reducing your appetite.

It's true that caffeine, nicotine, and the body's own adrenaline all help reduce your appetite. They do this by releasing stores of sugar held in your body. So, sure, you can lose weight by just drinking coffee—in the short term.

However, long-term use of stimulants messes up your blood sugar con-trol. Blood sugar dips lead to fatigue, mood swings, anxiety, sugar cravings, weight gain, and, of course, dependence on stimulants. The best way to con-trol your appetite, and your cravings, is to eat a low-Ⓖ diet.

Myth number 9: Diet pills work.

Every year there are new pills or potions that claim to do it all for you—starch blockers, fat blockers, appetite suppressants, diet pills. Avoid them at all costs. You can't cheat the body without paying a price.

Starch blockers inhibit the digestion of carbohydrate. The theory is that if you can't digest it, you can't gain weight. But having a whole lot of undi-gested carbohydrate in the digestive tract is bad news. It feeds the wrong kind of bugs, causing bacterial and yeast infections as well as terrible gas.

Much touted as an answer to weight loss is a supplement called *chitosan,* sometimes called the fat attractor or fat magnet, which inhibits the digestion of fat. It supposedly works because it has a positive charge and attracts fats, which have a negative charge. Once bound together with chitosan, the fat is less likely to be absorbed and passes through the body—so proponents claim—and cholesterol levels decrease.

However, three studies have found no significant differences in either weight or cholesterol levels between people taking chitosan and those taking a placebo. One study involved 30 overweight people who took chitosan or a placebo for 28 days while eating their normal diet. There was no difference in weight or cholesterol.[17] The second study, involving 51 obese women, found that the chitosan group had slightly greater cholesterol reduction than the placebo group, but there was no difference in weight loss after eight weeks.[18] Another study, with 68 obese men and women, found no improvement in weight or cholesterol.[19]

Drug companies are also cashing in on the weight-loss market with drugs that stop you from digesting fat. An example is Xenical, the drug name for a chemical called orlistat. This drug does actually work, in the sense that it reduces fat absorption. The immediate potential side effects are oily spotting, gas with discharge, oily or fatty stools, oily discharge, and an inability to control bowel movements. If that doesn't put you off, more worrisome are the effects on essential fats, so vital for heart, brain, and skin. Since EFAs are probably the most commonly deficient nutrient in the West, the last thing you want is to swallow something that stops you from using the little there is in your diet. Also, it probably isn't a good idea to have undigested fat in your digestive tract.

Some diet drugs are basically stimulants that suppress appetite and wire you up, inducing anxiety and hyperactivity. Similarly, if you drank 15 cups of coffee a day, it would also work in the short term. In the not-so-long term, stimulants mess up your body's metabolism as well as your physical, mental, and emotional health (see also myth number 8). Even if it sounds "natural," avoid any herb or supplement whose active ingredient is caffeine—and that includes guarana.

Myth number 10: There's nothing wrong with being overweight.

The health risks associated with weighing more than you should accumulate as soon as you are as little as 7 pounds overweight. With over half of people in Britain overweight and 20 percent obese, that's a lot of extra health risks.

And these are serious risks: heart disease, diabetes, kidney problems, osteoporosis, cancer, and arthritis. One study showed that about 40 percent of heart disease in women is linked to overweight, while others connect overweight to higher risks of breast cancer, arthritis, osteoporosis, and other conditions.[20] Diabetes is strongly linked to obesity.

In fact, every year obesity causes the premature deaths of 30,000 people, costs Britain's National Health Service £1 billion, and is responsible for the loss of more than 20 million working days. According to Dr. Susan Jebb of the Dunn Clinical Nutrition Centre in Cambridge in the UK, "Obesity is a serious medical condition that reduces life expectancy by increasing the risk of many chronic and potentially fatal diseases."

And with a thousand people becoming obese every day, we need to wake up to the fact that there's a disaster in the making here—but only potentially. The slope only *looks* slippery; there is a way out.

Why the Holford Diet works where others fail

You can lose weight on a low-calorie diet, a high-protein diet, a low-carb diet, or a no-fat diet. But you are stacking the odds against you. Why? Because . . .

- You get short-term weight loss as your body burns its essential store of glycogen—that's 5 pounds gone, but it all comes back!
- None of these diets satisfies your appetite better than the Holford Diet, so you have to fight hard to stay on them.
- All of these diets are highly restrictive in some way—who wants to live without carbohydrates or fats?
- None of these diets has been shown to trigger as much weight loss in the short term or the long term as the Fatburner System.

In a trial comparing the Fatburner System with Unislim—a low-calorie, high-exercise regimen with weekly support meetings—the Fatburner volunteers lost, on average, four times more weight (14 pounds in three months) than the other dieters. Every single trial by third parties proved highly successful, with many reports of additional benefits besides consistent weight loss, such as "increased alertness," "concentration improved," "no wobbly feeling," "never felt hungry," "easy to stick to," "extra energy," "thoroughly detoxified." In these trials, not one person failed to lose weight.

The original Fatburner Diet worked wonderfully well, but there's now an even faster, easier, and healthier way to chisel away at those unwanted pounds and promote your health and energy every step of the way. The Holford Diet takes about 30 days to tune up your metabolism and stabilize your blood sugar. Once this is achieved, not only will fatburning become much easier, but your weight will become much more stable and less likely to fluctuate with the odd indulgence. Although the diet may provide slightly fewer calories than you are eating now, slightly less fat, and slightly more protein, the major emphasis is on quality, and there will be plenty of it—all delicious.

Now let's summarize what *doesn't* work, and find out what does.

- The major cause of the obesity epidemic is an increase in sugar and re-fined carbohydrate consumption, not an increase in fat consumption.
- Different sources of calories have different effects on weight loss.
- Eating a low-🅖🅛 diet triggers the most rapid weight loss.
- If you eat too few calories, your metabolic rate slows down to conserve your fat, so you have to suffer to lose weight and will inevitably develop rebound weight gain.
- High-protein diets stabilize your blood sugar levels and reduce your ap-petite, but they don't work better than conventional diets and they're not good for you in the long run.
- Low-fat diets are bad for you because the body needs essential fats and keeps craving fats until it gets them.
- The best diet for long-term weight loss is a low-🅖🅛 diet, in which low-🅖🅛 carbohydrates are combined with protein and essential fats—in short, the Holford Diet.

The Inside Story on Fat

Losing extra inches is very simple. It's all about keeping your blood sugar even, a balancing act your body is designed to do. All you have to do is create the right environment for this to happen. Most people, probably including you, have unwittingly created a set of circumstances that have led your body to lose this balancing act. The result is roller-coastering blood sugar, energy, and weight.

For instance, do you need to kick-start the day with coffee, cigarettes, or something sweet? Do you gravitate toward bread, cookies, pasta, and sweet foods? Do you drink caffeinated drinks or alcohol every day? If so, the chances are you have significant dips in blood sugar. Then, when you've satisfied the craving with a big plate of pasta, a cola, a large glass of wine, or a couple of pastries, your blood sugar levels shoot up—and you dump the excess as fat.

If you lose blood sugar control, you gain weight, yet feel hungry—and exhausted—a lot of the time. If you can keep your blood sugar levels on an even keel, you'll gravitate toward your natural weight, stay there, and have a consistently high energy level.

If you have poor blood sugar control, you are three times more likely to have difficulty losing weight. That's what we found in our health and diet survey in 2004, when we surveyed 37,000 people using the Web-based MyNutrition questionnaire (see page 363 for details on how you can assess your own health using MyNutrition).[21] We also found that when you gain blood sugar control, you lose weight.

The question is, how do you regain blood sugar control? To tell you, I need to introduce you to the key players in this drama. First we'll meet the villain—insulin.

Why sugar makes you fat

The body turns carbohydrates into glucose—sugar—and conveys that glucose through the bloodstream for delivery to cells, where it's used as fuel. The trouble is that glucose is the equivalent of high-octane fuel, and dangerous stuff.

If glucose levels in the blood are too high, it can be very harmful—that's why diabetics can suffer nerve, eye, kidney, and artery damage. So as soon as

The sugar cycle. Eating sugar increases blood glucose levels. The body releases insulin into the blood to help escort glucose out and into body cells, to make energy or convert into fat. The result is low blood glucose. Either stress, which elicits the production of more adrenaline, or induced stress, caused by consuming a stimulant such as caffeine, which raises adrenal hormones, causes breakdown of stores of sugar in the liver and muscles, called glycogen, which raises blood sugar levels. Low blood glucose causes stress or cravings for either something sweet or a stimulant.

your blood sugar level shoots beyond a certain level, the body moves quickly to get the glucose out of your blood and, if you don't need it for energy, stores it as fat.

Insulin, a hormone produced by the pancreas, moves the glucose out of your blood. So why is it the villain of this story? The more frequently your blood sugar is raised, the more insulin you produce. The more insulin you produce, the more sugar you dump as fat. As a result, insulin can be thought of as the fat-storing hormone.

But there's more bad news. Having a high insulin level doesn't only encourage your body to turn food into fat, it also inhibits the body's breakdown of stored fat. So, once you're fat, you stay fat. If you're overweight, you've probably got elevated insulin levels.

Insulin is implicated in another factor that messes up your blood sugar level—insulin resistance.

In the grip of resistance

Let's say that, during the day, you're snacking or bingeing on sugary foods, drinking several cups of coffee, or smoking a few cigarettes. Every time you get a hit of sugar or a jolt from caffeine or nicotine, your blood sugar peaks. And, if this is happening a lot, more and more insulin will be rushing out to escort the glucose out of your blood as quickly as possible and into your cells. In effect, insulin will be subjecting your cells to a constant cry of "Open the door!"

Eventually the cells become so bored by hearing the same old message that it's as if they become deaf to it. So your body has to produce more and more insulin, just as if it were shouting louder and louder to be heard. The end result is that you become insensitive to your own insulin, a condition called *insulin resistance*.

According to Professor Gerald Reaven from Stanford University in California, one of the world's leading experts in blood sugar problems, the majority of obese people and 25 percent of nonobese people are insulin resistant.[22]

This means they, and quite likely you, need to produce more insulin to lower blood sugar peaks. So you will eat more carbohydrate before your body says "Stop!" and then, by the time the insulin does kick in, your blood sugar levels will have plummeted too low, leaving you once again craving something to give you a lift.

When you're in the grip of this vicious cycle, that lift is likely to be something high-⬤, such as refined pasta, and, for up to four hours afterward, insulin resistance will mess up your body's response to it. So you could either suffer from brain fog, sleepiness, and low mood after a meal, or cave in to the cravings for something to raise your blood sugar levels once more. Most people choose the latter, either eating more carbohydrate such as dessert, or homing in on a stimulant such as a cup of tea or coffee (more on this later). Meanwhile, with all these inefficient peaks and troughs in blood sugar levels, you're turning the excess glucose to fat and feeling exhausted.

But there's a more insidious downside. Remember, glucose is very damaging, so, as your insulin becomes less effective at getting it out of your bloodstream, you spend more time with too much glucose in your blood. This damages your arteries and paves the way for heart disease.

Diabetes is another direct result. This condition arises when you've become so insulin-resistant that the cells in the pancreas that make insulin become exhausted, and you can't produce enough. So you can't lower your blood sugar level very well, and some actually spills over into the urine. (Normally, the kidneys filter all glucose out, leaving it in the bloodstream, but even your kidneys have limits.) Thus, too little insulin is also bad news. As always in the body, it's a balancing act.

The plain truth is that most of us are digging our own graves with a knife and fork. But it doesn't have to be this way. The Holford Diet can literally save your life.

Your doctor can measure your own insulin resistance. Another way to get a measure on where you stand is the questionnaire below.

ARE YOU INSULIN RESISTANT?

- ☐ Are you rarely wide awake within 20 minutes of getting up?
- ☐ Do you need tea, coffee, a cigarette, or something to get you going in the morning?
- ☐ Do you really like sweet foods?
- ☐ Do you crave bread, cereal, popcorn, or pasta most days?
- ☐ Do you feel as if you need an alcoholic drink on most days?
- ☐ Are you overweight and unable to shed the extra pounds?
- ☐ Do you often have energy slumps during the day or after meals?

☐ Do you often have mood swings or difficulty concentrating?

☐ Do you often fall asleep in the early evening or need naps during the day?

☐ Do you avoid exercise because you haven't got the energy?

☐ Do you get dizzy or irritable if you go six hours without food?

☐ Do you often find you overreact to stress?

☐ Do you often get irritable, angry, or aggressive unexpectedly?

☐ Is your energy now less than it used to be?

☐ Do you get night sweats or frequent headaches?

☐ Do you ever lie about how much sweet food you have eaten?

☐ Do you ever keep a supply of sweet food close to hand?

☐ Do you ever go out of your way to make sure you have something sweet?

☐ Do you feel you could never give up bread?

☐ Do you think of yourself as addicted to sugar, chocolate, or cookies?

If you answered yes to 10 or more questions, there's a very good chance that you are insulin resistant, and struggling to keep your blood sugar level even. You are also three times more likely to have trouble losing weight. If you'd like to find out more about insulin resistance, read *The Insulin Factor*, by Antony Haynes.

You'll note that I've asked whether you need tea, coffee, or cigarettes to kick-start your day. Obviously, these have nothing to do with carbohydrates, so let's take a closer look at the role stimulants play in blood sugar chaos.

How caffeine ties you to the vicious cycle

Let's say you find yourself in an energy trough triggered by low blood sugar. You may not have eaten for a while, or you're experiencing the rebound low blood sugar that happens after a high-Ⓖ meal. One of the effects is that your body releases hormones from your adrenal glands, which sit on top of your kidneys in the small of your back. These hormones are adrenaline and cortisol, and, if your blood sugar levels are out of control, they're bad news.

You may have learned about the fight-or-flight mechanism at school. Adrenaline is the driving force behind this response, as it immediately raises your blood sugar level to give you fuel to fight back or run away. While adrenaline doesn't last long in the body, cortisol, another adrenal hormone, sticks around for much longer.

When this kind of thing happened in our prehistoric past, of course, we'd have burned off the extra glucose by either bashing that saber-toothed tiger on the head or hightailing it to the nearest cave. Our hormone levels would then return to normal, and all would be well. But the 21st-century reality is that we may simply be sitting at our office desk hungry for lunch when adrenaline and cortisol start circulating. And, if we do nothing, they'll keep doing just that, leaving us anxious and stressed.

So what's caffeine got to do with all this? This stimulant also prompts the release of adrenaline and raises blood sugar levels. So, if your levels are low, you may as easily reach for a coffee as for a doughnut.

Even more seductive are the treats that combine sugar with stimulants, such as tea or coffee with sugar, mocha drinks, chocolate, and colas. This pairing adds up to a powerful fix. Some people become more addicted to carbohydrates, others more addicted to caffeine, but most are addicted to both. Either way, they further disrupt your blood sugar control, make you more insulin resistant and keep you in the prison of seesawing weight and energy levels.

The bottom line is that the body's and brain's sensitive mechanisms for keeping your blood sugar in balance simply can't cope with a daily onslaught of sugar and other high-🅖🅛 foods and snacks, topped off with stimulants such as caffeine and nicotine. Your metabolism will respond by turning you into a fatmaker.

But there's good news. It doesn't take long to turn insulin resistance around and recover your fatburning ability. And *glucagon* is central to the process.

Enter glucagon—a Fatburner's best friend

Although it's another hormone produced by the pancreas, glucagon is the hero to insulin's villain. It is, in fact, the Fatburner's best friend, and it will get you out of the vicious cycle of seesawing blood glucose levels.

Glucagon enters the picture when your blood glucose levels are very low. It evens your blood glucose level up by telling the body to break down fat and burn it for energy. In the process, glucagon reduces any cravings for something sweet.

If insulin makes you store fat, glucagon makes you burn it. So glucagon

AVERAGE DIET

Raised **glucose** is bad for health and energy

Raised **insulin** promotes fat storage

Normal range

— blood glucose
— insulin
• • • • glucagon

Low **glucagon** minimizes fat burning

HOLFORD DIET

Normal **glucagon** promotes fat burning

Normal **glucose** promotes fat burning

Normal range

Normal **insulin** minimizes fat storage

— blood glucose
— insulin
• • • • glucagon

Blood sugar balance. When you eat a high-sugar food, your blood glucose level shoots up, which is followed by a release of insulin. Insulin helps turn glucose into fat. When you eat a low- **GL** food, your blood glucose level stays more stable, with less insulin release and relatively more glucagon.

is a fat-burning hormone. The more glucagon you produce in relation to insulin, the more you are programming yourself to burn fat.

As we've seen, if you consume the kinds of foods or stimulants that send your blood sugar rocketing, out pours the insulin and on creeps the fat. But, if you eat the kinds of food that keep your blood glucose level in check, you'll produce only small amounts of insulin and, whenever your energy is low, you'll release glucagon to burn some fat.

The Holford Diet is calculated to maximize glucagon release and minimize insulin release, thus reprogramming your metabolism to burn fat.

We've seen the inside story on hormones, sugar, and fat. Now let's frame it differently: we'll look at the dynamics of what keeps people from losing weight, and how this diet overcomes the obstacles.

- Sugar and refined carbohydrates can turn easily into fat and cause the release of an insulin overload.
- Eventually the body can become more and more resistant to insulin, leading to blood sugar peaks, followed by troughs, which lead to carbohydrate and sugar cravings.
- Insulin resistance is the hallmark of obesity and is present in most overweight people.
- Glucagon counters the effect of insulin and helps stabilize blood sugar levels and reduce appetite, sugar, and carbohydrate cravings.
- When your blood sugar level crashes, you release adrenal hormones. These further raise your blood sugar. Caffeine has a similar effect and, in the long term, encourages insulin resistance and weight gain.
- The Holford Diet promotes glucagon and reduces insulin resistance, reprogramming the body to burn fat.

4

How to Lose Weight Forever

Losing weight isn't difficult as long as you work *with* your body's design, not *against* it. As you learned in Chapter 2, you can lose weight with extreme diets, very low in fat, very low in carbohydrate, or very low in calories. But your body and your mind fight back. Your body will crave all three—fat, protein, and carbohydrate—and will signal its lack if you cut them down too far. This kind of diet fails because, in the end, your cravings win.

In fact, long-term studies have shown that dieters gain more weight than nondieters.[23] As we've seen, this is because just about any short-term extreme diet slows down your metabolism. It's because of this that many diets gradually move you from the unsustainable weight-loss phase to a more sustainable weight-maintenance phase.

The Holford Diet is sustainable from the start because it is scientifically calculated to satisfy your cravings and your appetite from Day One. It's the Rolls-Royce of diets. Your body will love it, and will reward you with myriad superhealthy side effects, from extra energy to smooth, clear skin.

The trick with the Fatburner System is that there *is* no trick. It doesn't cheat or fool your body. Remember: given the right circumstances, your body will go to its ideal weight—and stay there forever.

Overweight or underlean?

We've looked at the crucial role hormones play vis-à-vis your blood sugar balance, and how an imbalance leads to weight gain. As you rev up to start the Holford Diet, I'd like you to understand how we actually lose weight, and to have realistic expectations about the results.

Although I will tell you about some rapid, miraculous weight-loss results, the truth is that the body limits how quickly it can burn off fat without harming you. Many popular diets cheat the body by kicking off with instant weight loss in the first week or two, but after this you pay the price, not only in how you feel, but in weight gain over the long term.

I don't want this to happen to you. I'm more interested in your reaching your ultimate goal and staying there, even if it takes months, not weeks.

At this point we need to look at how much you weigh, and how much you want to lose. But we won't look at poundage alone: we'll be sorting out the relative percentages of fat and lean.

This is because it's not so much being overweight that's the problem, but being underlean. Your body is made of both fat tissue and lean tissue (muscle and organs). A significantly higher proportion of fat increases health risk, so your body fat percentage is actually more important than your overall weight.

Ideally, no more than 15 percent of a man's body and 22 percent of a woman's body should be made up of fat. Yet in the West, the average man has a body fat percentage of a little over 20, and the average woman's is above 30.

Your body fat percentage is a little harder to measure than your weight. With a little patience and a tape measure, you can work it out roughly using the formula in Appendix 1 (see page 324). Some gyms work it out by making a few body measurements with calipers or with a piece of equipment that measures your electrical resistance. Since fat doesn't conduct electricity, the less "electric" you are the more fat you've got.

But how can you measure the fat lost as your fatburning capacity really gets going? Fat is relatively light and bulky, while protein is hard and heavy. So, as you convert fat into lean muscle, you may lose inches more quickly than you lose pounds. This is good news for several reasons. One is obviously that you'll look better. The other is that, when you follow the Holford Diet, you are giving your lean muscle a tune-up so it is ready to burn your excess fat. Exercise is an essential part of the plan (remember, it's for only 15 minutes a day), and the more exercise you do the more efficient your muscles will become at fatburning.

So, as the diet progresses, you'll take a simple measurement with a tape measure once a week, as well as getting on the scales.

Measuring your body mass

The next best measurement to know is your *body mass index* (BMI). To work this out, all you need to know is your weight and height; then look at the graph below. (There's another chart in Appendix 1, on Page 323, that does this for you and shows you the ideal weight range for each height.) If your BMI is between 25 and 30 (Class 1) then you are technically overweight. If it's 30 (Class 2 or 3) or above, you are technically obese.

If you find you are technically obese, it may come as a shock. But you are not alone; the number of overweight and obese people doubled in the 1980s and continued to grow at the same alarming rate in the 1990s. In some parts

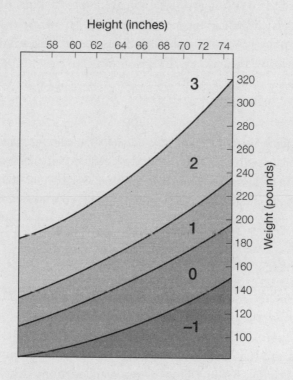

Class 3—severely obese
Class 2—obese
Class 1—overweight
Class 0 —desirable weight
Class –1—underweight

of the United States, as many as 50 percent of women are now obese. By the end of this book you'll understand why. And you will have in hand the best way out of the trap—forever.

Are you overweight?

If you are in Class 1, 2, or 3, then your risk for certain diseases, such as diabetes, is much higher. Weight-related diseases account for about as much of total healthcare cost in the UK as cancer therapy or treatment of heart disease. The closer to your ideal weight you are, the healthier you are and the less risk you have of life-threatening and debilitating diseases.

Statistics show that, if you're over 50, it may be better to be a little on the heavier side of the BMI range of desirable weight.[24] Having a BMI below 23 has been associated with an increased death rate. This is partly because very sick people can lose a lot of weight. But if you are healthy, a BMI of around 20 to 24 is probably the best, whatever your age.

> ### TOP TIP
> Measure your waist. It's the best predictor of insulin resistance. Measure your girth one inch below your belly button. For women, this should be less than 34 inches, for men less than 40 inches. Hip and thigh weight gain is much less harmful for your overall health.

A pound of fat

Go to the butcher and ask for a pound of fat. It's about the size of this book. Now imagine losing twice that amount of fat a week! Sound good? Read on.

The most you can easily lose in a week, without starvation, is between 1 and 2 pounds of fat. If you follow my recommendations strictly you'll lose, on average, 2 pounds of fat a week for the first month. If you follow the general principles loosely, you'll probably lose a pound of fat a week. So, if you're 24 pounds overweight, and you decide to take on board what I've said in essence, you'll lose this weight in 24 weeks—six months, more or less.

Ian W. from Coventry is a typical example:

I bought your book last year in an effort to lose weight. While I was not exactly fat, I was certainly not happy with my size and felt miserable all the time. I tried to stick to the essence of what was in the book. My weight dropped around 1½ stone (21 pounds) over six months and is currently stable. I can now come home from work and feel OK and the evening is mine to do with as I please. I would recommend your approach to anyone for life in general but remember, there is no need for obsession, all you have to do is choose the better option all the time.

Linda H. is a 48-year-old mother of two. For years, she'd tried to lose weight by dieting and painstakingly counting calories. But it was only when she switched to the Fatburner System that the weight came off and her overall energy and health improved. Here's what she has to say:

At 130 pounds and 5 feet 2 inches, I'd tried to diet for six years. I hoped that, if I was very strict, I might get down to 124 pounds, but this never happened. Finally, I decided to try the diet as a "quick fix" for 30 days before I went on vacation. For a month, I followed all the recommendations (except I ate even larger portions than recommended). Amazingly, I lost my craving for sweets! Before starting to eat this way, I'd crave sweets about four times a week, and would binge on cakes, sweets, and biscuits [cookies]. This has completely ended. It's as if I've educated my taste buds into a far healthier eating regimen. The best part? I lost 13 pounds!

I quickly decided to continue eating this way for the rest of my life. Not just because of the weight loss, but because of how wonderful I felt. For instance, an unexpected benefit was that the redness, or rosacea, I'd always noticed on my face, which I thought was a result of aging, disappeared. My energy also increased, so much that I realized I hadn't understood how tired and run-down I was before. I thought being tired was just a normal part of life!

Because I continued following the regimen, for the first time in two years I returned from vacation the same weight as when I left. After the first 30 days, I allowed myself wine on weekends and my weight still remained steady. Today, I have dessert about once a week, but my weight still remains steady. Since my blood sugar levels are stable, one dessert a week is enough. Best of all, it is now a way of life to say no to dessert—not an effort or sacrifice.

Both Linda and Ian achieved their goals easily and are still slim today and experiencing all the health benefits of my diet.

No "miracle" weight loss

Linda lost 13 pounds in 30 days, which is actually a bit more than the maximum average I predict. But, as the weight dropped off, she was never hungry, and her energy levels began to soar. She lost the excess pounds without taxing her body in any way.

Don't be lured by diets that claim amazing weight loss in a couple of weeks. We all feel desperate sometimes—to fit into that outfit, to look good on the beach, just to feel right striding to work. However, you don't want to add insult to injury. Being overweight isn't much fun, and it's bad for our health, but crash diets get rid of a lot of weight that isn't fat, and most of it comes right back afterward. Let me explain why.

We've seen how the body runs on glucose. It's the equivalent of high-octane gas, and it's why athletes rely on glucose drinks, not protein or fat, when they're practicing endurance sports. Your body aims to use a lot of this immediately to power your cells, and you've seen how the excess is laid down as fat.

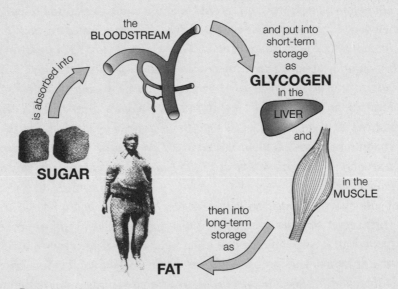

How the body stores energy as fat. The body runs on sugar (glucose), and converts any extra into glycogen, which is stored in muscles and the liver. If glycogen stores are full, the body can convert glucose into fat, our long-term energy storage.

But, before that happens, excess glucose is first put into short-term storage in the liver and muscles in a form known as *glycogen*. It's only when stores of glycogen are full that glucose is converted into fat and laid down for long-term storage. If you have insulin resistance this will happen fast, and the excess fat will be dumped most readily around the belly. So carrying a lot of fat around the middle is a sure sign of insulin resistance.

Conversely, when you run out of glucose, the body breaks glycogen back down into glucose. When glycogen stores are used up, the body burns fat into sugar to stock them up. If it has to, the body can also turn protein into sugar and burn this instead. That's why people on starvation diets lose muscle and possibly even damage body organs.

How losing fast is losing out

Each unit of glucose your body puts into storage as glycogen is bound together with three units of water. So, if you run out of glucose and start burning glycogen, you lose water. This is how you can get rapid short-term weight loss on a very-low-calorie diet, say below 1,000 calories a day, or on a very-low-carbohydrate diet. Since the maximum amount of glycogen in short-term storage in the body is about 2 pounds, you could lose a maximum of 8 pounds—but in reality you'd be more likely to lose 4 pounds. That's why, when you complete the first week of a diet with great gusto and enthusiasm, you may well be rewarded with a 4-pound weight loss. That's 1 pound of fat and 3 pounds of water.

However, the sad truth is that, when you start eating enough for your energy needs again, the glycogen and water stores are replenished, and the water weight comes back.

So the measure of a diet that's actually burning fat is not what happens when you starve yourself during the first week and temporarily run out of glycogen. Instead, it's a regular week-by-week loss of around 1 to 2 pounds, not sudden weight loss over two weeks.

Look at the two charts that follow. The top one shows the average weight loss, week by week, of a group of nine dieters on a regular low-calorie diet. In the first week there's 3 pounds lost, in the second 2 pounds. Things are looking good—5 pounds in two weeks. But most of this is water. By Week 4 there's no loss and, presumably as willpower wanes, the volunteers start eating what they need to eat for energy, restoring glycogen; with that, back comes the water. The end result: an average of 2 pounds lost in 12 weeks.

Weight loss on a low-calorie diet versus the Holford Diet[25]

The bottom graph shows the results of seven Holford dieters. Once again, there's a sudden weight loss in the first week, but then it settles in at an average of a pound a week. After 12 weeks, the average weight loss is 13.7 pounds. This pattern of weight loss indicates fatburning—and where there's fatburning, there's long-term, maintained weight loss.

And it is better not to lose weight faster than this. Ultimately, the amount lost will be about 14 to 28 pounds over three months. Weight loss of over 2 pounds a week will not all be fat loss. The body simply cannot burn off fat that fast. Of course, most of us want to lose 14 pounds in a week, despite having taken a year to put it on!

A good target during the first 30 days is to lose 6 pounds in weight. You'll probably lose more, but it's better to set yourself up for success. Even a weight loss of a pound a week, maintained over a year, equals over 50 pounds.

And this can be achieved, without any suffering, on my diet. After all, Rome wasn't unbuilt in a day.

. . . with one exception

There is, however, one way you can instantly lose weight and never put it back. It's by avoiding a food you are allergic to. One in three people has specific food intolerances, and some of these cause excessive weight gain, probably by triggering excessive fluid retention. Unlike the water that's stored with glycogen, which will come back once you stop starving yourself, this is *excess* water that the body lets go of when you avoid the foods you are intolerant to.

I remember my first overweight patient, Mary, who had struggled with her weight for years. I advised her to cut out wheat, and within two days she had lost 7 pounds! I'm going to tell you how to discover whether you are allergic to certain foods and what to replace them with in Chapter 9.

This step is one of the five simple principles of my diet, which I introduced in Chapter 1. If you want to lose weight forever and turn yourself from a fatmaker into a Fatburner, these form the essential framework for your new life:

1. Eat no more than 40 **ⒼⓁ** of carbohydrate foods a day (I'll show you how easy this is), with protein.
2. Eat essential omega-3 and omega-6 fats, and no saturated, processed, or fried fats.
3. Find the foods you're allergic to, and avoid them.
4. Take the right supplements.
5. Do the equivalent of 15 minutes' exercise a day.

Remember, you're unique

These principles work well for just about everybody—but it's important to remember that you're unique. For one thing, how much you need to eat will vary depending on how tall you are and how much exercise you do. If you are over 6 feet tall or under 5 feet 4 inches, or exercise an hour or more five or more days a week, you'll need to adjust the Holford Diet according to your needs. The principles, however, remain the same.

There's another factor: some people do better on more protein and less carbohydrate than others. Thanks to the excellent research of Dr. Peter D'Adamo, author of *Eat Right for Your Blood Type*, we now know that people with type O blood generally function better on more animal protein, while people with type A blood function better on more carbohydrate and vegetable protein.

If you are blood type O, or simply want to experiment with how you feel eating a little more protein and less carbohydrate, you can do so on the Holford Diet by adding 5 grams of protein a day and subtracting 5 ⓖ. I will make it crystal clear how you do this in practice. It's much simpler than it sounds—you don't need a calculator!

In summary:

- You cannot lose more than 2 pounds of actual fat a week unless you are starving yourself or running for the Olympic team.
- The body loses around 4 pounds in water on a very-low-calorie or very-low-carbohydrate diet when you deplete your body's glycogen stores—but this inevitably comes back.
- You can lose 7 pounds or more fast—and permanently—if you avoid foods you are allergic to.
- Losing inches is more important than losing pounds. Gaining lean body mass and losing fat, measured as your body fat percentage, is the real goal.
- The body will naturally gravitate to its own ideal weight if you give it the right balance and kinds of protein, fat, and carbohydrate.

Why Fatburning Is Easy

The Holford Diet is the state of the art of keeping you satisfied. For a decade, I've been researching exactly what keeps you feeling full—not only which foods, but which foods in combination, and when to eat them.

And you'll be eating plenty of them. If all you've ever heard about weight loss is calorie cutting, this may make you wary. But eating little and often of low-Ⓖ foods will reduce, not increase, the number of calories you consume. And it will be easy and wonderfully satisfying, because you've got three meals and two substantial snacks a day, and no cravings brought on by low blood sugar.

Even better, the process will kick in fast. Most people's blood sugar begins to even out within seven days of starting the Holford Diet, and within 30 days you will no longer be insulin resistant—you'll be reprogrammed to burn fat. That's why I call this a 30-day diet.

Parts Two and Three will get down to the nitty-gritty of the diet. This overview will show you how you can move from being a fatmaker to a Fatburner with real ease.

Seven days to stop cravings

When you're on day one of the diet, chances are you'll feel fantastic right from the start. But, for a few, it may take a few days for that feeling to kick in. This initial hiccup is simply the effect of simultaneously launching a new diet and deciding to go cold turkey on caffeine.

Doing it like this is the quickest way to start the fatburning process, but it does mean that people who drink a lot of coffee or cola, or eat a fair amount of chocolate or sugary snacks, will experience a withdrawal phase. A few people may feel a bit rough for the first three days, and a very small minority can feel bad for the entire first week. The blood sugar dips that go with withdrawal can make you feel sleepy, mentally foggy, anxious, moody, or tired, or can spark cravings and headaches.

If you find yourself experiencing any of these sensations, be aware that it's all caused by resistance. The more insulin, glucagon, adrenaline, and cortisol you've been forcing your body to produce, the more resistant it becomes to their fine-tuning effects. In Chapter 3 I explained about insulin resistance; you can also become adrenaline resistant. Remember that stimulants such as coffee can kick-start the release of adrenaline. If you're downing four or five cups a day or more, you can become increasingly "deaf" to your own adrenaline. You might even find it tough to get out of bed in the morning. You can't hear your own inner adrenaline alarm because you've developed adrenaline resistance.

On the Holford Diet, it takes only a few days to overcome that resistance—on three delicious meals and two snacks a day. I'm also going to be asking you to call in the cavalry—special supplements that work wonders for stabilizing blood sugar and appetite.

If you feel you're very addicted to caffeine or chocolate, however, it is probably best to give yourself two weeks to give it all up before you actually start the diet. You'll see how to do that in Parts Two and Three.

YOU'LL EAT LESS WITHOUT TRYING

After seven days you'll find that your desire to eat high-**GL** foods will rapidly fall away. You won't get the blood sugar dips after meals that lead you to crave the wrong foods. Even though I don't want you to try to eat less, you will naturally do so. Britain's first Fatburner said this: "I lost three stone [42 pounds] and never felt hungry. I know I'll never go back to eating like I used to."

Dr. David Ludwig of the Department of Medicine at the Children's Hospital in Boston decided to put this to the test. He gave children one of two breakfast cereals. One was a low-**GL** cereal made from unadulterated oat flakes. The other was a processed instant oatmeal that sounded good but actually had a high **GL**. Both groups of kids ate the identical calorie amount of each cereal and also had a calorie-identical lunch. In the afternoon and evening they were free to eat as they chose. The children on the low- ⓖⓛ diet ate 47 percent fewer calories in the afternoon: they just weren't hungry.

The same thing will happen to you. That is why Fatburner dieters say that "as far as hunger is concerned it's an easy diet to stick to" (*She* magazine).

The way it works

To get an idea of how the diet tackles hunger, first imagine a plate. Now divide it in half. In any main meal, one of those halves can be chosen from almost a hundred vegetables.

Divide the other half in half. One quarter is protein—fish, chicken, lamb, or vegetarian proteins such as tofu or beans. Later I'll give you portion sizes of, say, a piece of chicken or a piece of fish.

The remaining quarter is a low-ⓖⓛ carbohydrate food serving, equivalent to 10 ⓖⓛ. This could be bread, potatoes, pasta, or any other of the foods that so many high-protein diets forbid. They're firmly part of the Holford Diet, but the serving size will vary depending on the ⓖⓛ of that carbohydrate. For instance, you can eat twice as much boiled as baked potato, or even more corn. You can eat twice as much whole rye bread as white wheat bread. You can eat twice as much whole-meal spaghetti as French fries. Very soon you'll learn which low-ⓖⓛ foods fill you up the best.

This is a sketch of a main meal. You'll roughly follow the same rules for your other two meals, allowing 10 ⓖⓛ per meal—and don't forget, there are two substantial snacks a day, at 5 ⓖⓛ each. So the ⓖⓛ limit for each day is 40, because that's the maximum possible for fatburning.

Dividing up your food

Eating out is easy

I travel around the world, visiting an average of 30 cities in any given year. I've learned that I can follow this diet in every country anywhere in the world. Sure, some countries and types of food are easier than others. It's harder in the United States, where more people are obese, and easier in Thailand, where most people are skinny. The good news is that there are Thai restaurants, Chinese restaurants, Indian restaurants, and many others all around the world that cater perfectly to people on my diet. I'll show you how to make the right choices in Chapter 19.

Effortless shopping

You may have encountered diets for which you had to buy foods by mail order, or hunt out exotic substances in specialty shops. Everything on my diet can be bought in the supermarket—including the organic foods I recommend—or, failing that, in any health food shop. Granted, you may be throwing a few things you've never cooked before into the cart, but I can guarantee it's all going to be delicious—and may even become a culinary adventure. As it's a diet for life, it will never be dull.

Veggie heaven

The diet is a cinch for vegetarians. There's a vast and tasty array of vegetables and good, slow-releasing carbohydrates, as well as recipes for preparing them. On the protein front, vegetarians will just need to ensure they're eating the optimal amount for the diet to work.

Tofu, which comes in a variety of delicious forms, is featured in a number of recipes, or can be substituted for fish or chicken in others. Beans and lentils figure large in the Holford Diet, as they are key to regulating blood sugar. Other vegetarian protein options—Quorn, textured soy protein, yogurt, cottage cheese, eggs—are all well represented. So there's no shunting of vegetarian needs to the sidelines, which can happen with some high-protein diets.

No forbidden foods

Never say never. So I'm not going to tell you never to eat chocolate, bread, pasta or potatoes. But I *am* going to tell you how much of these foods you can eat to keep within your 40-Ⓖ limit for the day. How you do that is up to you.

Let me give you an example. Below are four snacks. Each equals 5 Ⓖ. The choice is yours.

Strawberries	1 large pint
Apple	1 small apple
Peanuts	2 small packets (3 oz.)
Chocolate	Less than a quarter of a bar (1½ oz.)
Oatcake crackers	2 oatcake crackers with third of a container of hummus (8 oz.)

Many people, myself included, like their diets cut and dried. For that reason I have divided carbohydrate foods into low, medium, and high. As you can see, high-Ⓖ foods such as chocolate aren't much fun because you can't eat much of them. Low-Ⓖ foods are the best value because they'll fill you up and stop food cravings.

So my advice is to eat mainly low-Ⓖ foods and food combinations, with occasional medium-Ⓖ foods. High-Ⓖ foods are probably more frustrating than they're worth. All in all, avoiding them is certainly the fastest way to lose weight and gain energy.

And gaining energy is only one of the beneficial side effects of fatburning. In the next chapter we get a taste of many more.

- The Holford Diet reduces your appetite because it stabilizes your blood sugar levels so you don't get hungry.
- Sugar cravings take no more than seven days to cure. After that, you'll find that your food cravings will virtually vanish.
- As long as you don't exceed 40 Ⓖ a day you can eat anything. However, you can eat much more of the best low-Ⓖ foods so you won't go hungry. Either way, you lose weight.

6

Better by Design

With most diets, you will probably experience side effects when you've been following the regime for some time. On very-high-protein diets, you may suffer from constipation or bad breath. On low-fat diets, you may have problems with skin or hair.

The only side effects you'll get on the Holford Diet are extra energy, better memory, clearer skin, and resistance to degenerative diseases such as diabetes and cancer.

As I said at the start, weight loss itself is simply a side effect of optimum nutrition—the only kind the Holford Diet offers. Balancing your blood sugar and ensuring you're getting all the right nutrients will leave you in optimum health, slim, mentally fit, and glowing with vitality.

Here's what you can expect:

- An end to fatigue. You'll never experience that weakened, lowered state that can creep up on you when you follow some low-calorie diets. Instead, you will wake up alert and clear-eyed—and, even better, get through the day without any energy slumps or exhaustion. This is the effect of cutting right back on stimulants and sugar, eating a low-**GL** diet, and supplementing nutrients known to boost energy.
- Younger, smoother skin. You'll discover the six secrets of having great skin, such as eating the right kinds of fruits (berries are tops), vegetables, and omega-3 fats.

- A lowered homocysteine level. Having a high level of this toxic amino acid in the blood can indicate a real vulnerability to many degenerative diseases, from cancer to heart disease. The Holford Diet encourages the best defense: lots of green, leafy vegetables, supplemented with B vitamins and crucial minerals.
- No more blues. Being fat can be depressing, and it's now known that overweight people have lower levels of the "happy" brain chemical serotonin. A low-ⓖⓛ diet emphasizing high-quality carbohydrates will help you beat the blues by raising serotonin levels—and, of course, helping you lose weight.
- A sharper mind. A diet rich in omega-3s, vitamins C and E, and the nutrients and practices that will help balance blood sugar—such as the Holford Diet—will banish mental "fogs," confusion, and poor memory, and significantly reduce any risk of developing Alzheimer's.
- Freedom from stress. Long-term stress causes too much of the hormone cortisol to circulate in the body, and cortisol can damage the brain. But cutting out sugar and stimulants can swiftly lower stress levels, and give your brain a chance to recover and rebuild itself.
- Lowered risk of disease. The Holford Diet, with its emphasis on balancing blood sugar, can clearly reduce your risk of getting diabetes. But it can also significantly decrease your risk of developing heart disease, cancer, and arthritis, and of suffering a stroke.

We'll be looking at all these side benefits in detail in Part Five. For now, get set for the full lowdown on the Holford Diet's five simple principles.

References: Part One

1. MAFF National Food Survey, HMSO (1996); L. Henderson et al., "The National Diet and Nutrition Survey," Trading Standards Office (2003); Department of Health, "Health Survey for England" (data relating to 1995–2002), http://www.publications .doh.gov.uk/stats/trends1.htm.
2. Health Survey for England, National Centre for Social Research (1998).
3. Department of Environment, Food and Rural Affairs (DEFRA) data on http://www .defra.gov.uk/farm/arable/sugar/sugar05.htm#consumption.
4. J. Brand-Miller et al., "Glycemic Index and Obesity," *American Journal of Clinical Nutrition* vol. 76 (2002) (suppl.), 281S–85S.
5. D. B. Pawlak, J. A. Kushner, and D. S. Ludwig, "Effects of Dietary Glycaemic Index on

Adiposity, Glucose Homoeostasis, and Plasma Lipids in Animals," *Lancet,* vol. 364 (9436) (August 2004), pp. 778–85.

6. M. Slabber et al., "Effects of a Low-Insulin-Response, Energy Restricted Diet on Weight Loss and Plasma Insulin Concentrations in Hyperinsulinemic Obese Females," *American Journal of Clinical Nutrition* vol. 60(1) (1994), pp. 48–53.

7. D. S. Ludwig, "The Glycemic Index," *Journal of the American Medical Association,* vol. 287(18) (2002), pp. 2414–23.

8. F. F. Samaha et al., "A Low-Carbohydrate as Compared with a Low-Fat Diet in Severe Obesity," *New England Journal of Medicine,* vol. 348(21) (2003), pp. 2074–81.

9. G. D. Foster et al., "A Randomized Trial of a Low-Carbohydrate Diet for Obesity," *New England Journal of Medicine,* vol. 348(21) (2003), pp. 2082–90.

10. D. M. Bravata et al., "Efficacy and Safety of Low-Carbohydrate Diets: A Systematic Review," *Journal of the American Medical Association,* vol. 289(14) (2003), pp. 1837–50.

11. H. Hull, "The Effect of Food Combining on Weight Loss," ION research project (1997).

12. Pereira M. et al., *Journal of the American Medical Association,* vol. 292 (2004), pp. 2482–90.

13. A. L. Gittleman, *Beyond Pritikin* (New York: Bantam, 1996), revised.

14. M. Appelbaum, "Influences of Level of Energy Intake on Energy Expenditure in Man," reported in *Dieting Makes You Fat,* G. Cannon and H. Einzig (New York: Simon & Schuster, 1985), pp. 56–59.

15. R. Leibel et al., "Changes in Energy Expenditure Resulting from Altered Body Weight," *New England Journal of Medicine,* vol. 332 (1995), pp. 621–28.

16. M. and A. Wynn, "How Dieting Can Damage Your Health," *Which Way to Health?* (February 1995), pp. 22–24.

17. M. H. Pitler et al., "Randomized, Double-Blind Trial of Chitosan for Body Weight Reduction," *European Journal of Clinical Nutrition,* vol. 53 (1999), pp. 379–81.

18. E. Wuolijoki et al., "Decrease in Serum LDL Cholesterol with Microcrystalline Chitosan," *Methods and Findings in Experimental and Clinical Pharmacology,* vol. 21(5) (1999), pp. 357–61.

19. S. C. Ho et al., "In the Absence of Dietary Surveillance, Chitosan Does Not Reduce Plasma Lipids or Obesity in Hypercholesterolaemic Obese Asian Subjects," *Singapore Medical Journal,* vol. 42 (2001), pp. 6–10.

20. W. McArdle, *Medical Aspects of Clinical Nutrition,* Keats (1983).

21. P. Holford et al., ONUK Survey (2004), Institute of Optimum Nutrition, London, www.ion.ac.uk.

22. G. Reaven, "Role of Insulin Resistance in Human Disease," *Diabetes,* vol. 37 (1988), pp. 1595–1607.

23. *Pediatrics,* vol. 112(4) (2003), pp. 900–6.

24. Wynn and Wynn, op. cit.

25. P. Maconaghie, "A Comparison of the Metabolic Diet with the Unislim Diet for Inducing Weight Loss," ION (1988).

Part Two

···················

Five Simple Principles

...............**7**...............

Step 1: Balance Your Blood Sugar

We've seen how the key to losing weight and increasing energy is stabilizing your blood sugar and insulin response to food. Now I'm going to explain the dynamics of this process so it's crystal clear why you are following the rules of this diet. The principles are remarkably simple, and this way of eating will become part of your daily routine very quickly.

There are four ways to stabilize your blood sugar:

- reduce the total amount of carbohydrates in your diet
- choose low-glycemic-load (**GL**) carbohydrates
- combine carbohydrates with protein
- cut back on stimulants and stress

Sounds great, you're thinking, but how do I put it all into practice?

The lowdown on carbohydrates

I'm going to make it really easy. As far as carbohydrates are concerned, there are only two rules:

Rule 1: Eat no more than 40 **GL** a day.
Rule 2: At main meals, eat low-**GL** carbohydrates with protein-rich foods.

We've had a look at **GL** in Part One. If a food is high-**GL**, such as white bread, it will contain a lot of fast-releasing carbohydrate that will contribute to see-sawing blood sugar and all the ills we've seen it leading to, such as weight gain, lethargy, and insulin resistance. (Note that the figure of 40 **GL** a day refers to what we *eat*; there's an extra allowance of 5 **GL** for drinks, or desserts and sweets, discussed in Part Three.)

Everything I'm going to tell you in this chapter is designed to reverse this process, stabilize your blood sugar, lower your insulin release, make you more responsive to the insulin you produce, and turn you into a high-energy Fatburner. You'll feel better and the pounds will fall away. It's a win-win situation for you and your body.

So low-**GL** eating is vital for health. Now we need to find out more about this crucial scoring system.

WHAT DETERMINES **GL**?

How a food is processed, prepared, or cooked is a key element in the **GL** of a food, and therefore in what it will do to your blood sugar.

In the figure below, you can see how blood sugar levels, followed by in-

Glycemic response: spaghetti. Within 40 minutes of a person's eating spaghetti, blood sugar levels are at a maximum. The body releases insulin to help get the glucose out of the blood and into body cells. Two hours later both blood glucose and insulin levels have returned to normal.

Time in minutes

Glycemic response: bread. Within 40 minutes of a person's eating bread, blood sugar levels are almost double those seen with spaghetti. The body produces more than three times as much insulin to bring blood glucose levels under control. The body overreacts and blood glucose goes to low, leading to strong cravings for something sweet or a stimulant such as caffeine. The cravings peak three hours later, when blood glucose and insulin are at their lowest.

sulin, rise and fall after you eat spaghetti. As the blood glucose level rises, the body produces insulin, and down it comes again.

The figure above shows what happens when you eat white bread. Notice that the blood sugar level not only peaks twice as high as with the pasta, but it also dips much lower. It's the peaks that damage your arteries, making them less responsive to insulin, and the troughs that leave you tired, sleepy, and craving carbohydrates or stimulants. Again, you can see a massive increase in insulin release. In fact, compared with levels for spaghetti, four times as much insulin was produced in the first two hours after eating that bread!

What's fascinating is that this particular bread and spaghetti were made from the same flour, using the same amount.[1] So the only difference is in the processing. Bread rises when you feed yeast with sugar, and it is then baked for some time. Pasta is just wheat, and perhaps some egg. It has no yeast or sugar and it isn't cooked so long.

It's obvious that this small difference in preparation makes a big difference in blood sugar response, and hence in how much weight you put on. That's why I recommend that you eat very little bread, but you certainly don't need to give up pasta, especially if it's whole wheat as opposed to refined.

Harking back to Rule 2, it's also important *how* you eat your low-⓬ carbs. I'm going to recommend that you eat some fat and protein with your carbohydrate because this will reduce its low-⓬ score even further.

We'll be looking at the kinds of combinations that work best to lower your blood sugar in a while. But, for now, let's stick to the ⓬ scenario, exploring which carbohydrates you can eat lots of and which you should probably avoid.

ENTER THE GI

It was the discovery that even quite similar foods could have very different effects on blood sugar that led to the classification of foods as slow- or fast-releasing carbohydrates. The fast-releasing foods include white bread, which as we saw above are like rocket fuel, releasing their glucose in a sudden burst. They give a quick shot of energy with a rapid burnout. Slow-releasing carbohydrates such as whole wheat spaghetti supply steadier energy over a longer period of time, and thus help in balancing blood sugar levels.

But how do you know what is fast- and what is slow-releasing? This is where the GI—the glycemic index—comes in. The GI is a scale that compares the levels to which different foods raise your blood sugar with the effect of pure glucose (see below). It is also key in determining a food's ⓬.

To discover a food's GI, a portion of it providing 50 grams of carbohy-

Measuring the glycemic index of a food

drate is eaten, and the effect on the person's blood sugar over a three-hour period is compared with the effect of eating 50 grams of the "reference" food, glucose. Glucose is the fastest-releasing carbohydrate, because it requires no digestion.

In the diagram on the preceding page, the curve created by eating 50 grams of glucose is given a value of 100. If another food raises blood sugar level significantly, and for some time, the area under the curve made by glucose is bigger. Conversely, if a food hardly raises blood glucose levels at all, and only for a short time, the area under the curve is smaller. The amount of food tested obviously affects how high the blood sugar level will go.

Below you can see the GI for a variety of foods. As a general rule, a high GI score indicates the ones to avoid; a low GI score, the ones to eat.

As you can see, apples and oats are slow-releasing, while raisins and puffed-rice cereal are fast.

Glycemic index of common foods

Sugars		Plum	39
Maltose	105	Apple	38
Glucose	100	Pear	38
Honey	55	Grapefruit	25
Sucrose (sugar)	68	Cherries	22
Lactose	46		
Fructose (fruit sugar)	19	*Grains and grain products*	
Xylitol	8	French baguette	95
		White rice	72
Fruit		Bagel	72
Dates	103	Whole-meal bread	71
Watermelon	72	White bread	70
Pineapple	59	Crumpet	69
Melon	65	Ryvita	64
Raisins	64	Pastry	59
Kiwifruit	53	Basmati rice	58
Banana	52	Whole-grain rye bread	58
Grapes	46	Brown rice	55
Orange	42	Brown basmati long-grain rice	47
Strawberries	40	Instant noodles	47
Raspberries	40	Whole-grain wheat bread	46

White spaghetti	40	Skim milk	32
Whole-meal spaghetti	37	Whole milk	27
Barley	26		

Cereals		*Vegetables*	
Puffed rice	82	Parsnip (cooked)	97
Cornflakes	81	Potato (baked)	85
Shredded wheat	75	French fries	75
Weetabix	70	Beet (cooked)	64
Kellogg's Special K	69	Sweet potato	61
Oatmeal	58	Potato (new, boiled)	57
Muesli	55	Corn	54
Kellogg's All-Bran	42	Peas	48
		Carrot	47

Legumes and beans		*Snacks and drinks*	
Baked beans	48	Gatorade	95
Chickpeas	42	Jelly beans	80
Black-eyed beans	42	Fanta	68
Navy beans	38	Fruit-flavored drink	66
Butter beans	36	Corn chips	63
Lentils	29	Granola bar	61
Kidney beans	28	Potato chips	54
Soybeans	14	Orange juice	50
		Mars Bar	49
Dairy products		Chocolate bar	49
Ice cream	61	Apple juice	40
Yogurt	36	Peanuts	14

So much for GI. But what's the inside story on what makes one food fast-releasing and another slow? There are two main factors.

The first is how "complex" the carbohydrate is. On the following page is a diagram of the chemical structures of glucose, regular white sugar, and oats. You don't need to be a scientist to see that oats are more complex than sugar, and sugar is more complex than glucose. All this means is that there's more *to* them.

Since the body can use only glucose for fuel, the sugar pictured—sucrose—has to be chopped in two to release the glucose. When you eat

Glucose   Glucose   Glucose   Fructose

OATS

Glucose   Fructose

SUGAR   GLUCOSE

= slow-releasing   = fast-releasing

Oats are more complex than glucose. Oats need digesting into single glucose units, which takes time and slows down the release of its sugars. This sugar, which is a molecule of glucose and fructose, is slower in turn than a glucose molecule, which needs no digesting and directly enters the bloodstream.

sugar, an enzyme released in the gut does this job for you and before long the glucose is whizzing around your bloodstream.

The carbohydrate in oats, however, needs a lot of digesting into smaller and smaller units in the digestive tract before the glucose is released into the blood. This takes longer, so you don't get such a massive and immediate blood sugar rise.

Cooking some foods affects the release rate by "predigesting" the carbs they contain. That's why the more you cook a carbohydrate food, the faster-releasing it gets. Take potatoes. A baked potato, with a GI score of 85, is worse than a boiled potato, which has a GI of 57. Oats, however, are an exception. There's little difference between cooked oatmeal and uncooked oatmeal. This is largely because the cooking time is very short—you are really rehydrating rather than cooking.

Another factor that slows down the release of carbohydrate in food is fiber. Fiber is an indigestible carbohydrate, and generally, the more fiber a food contains, the slower is the breakdown of carbohydrate. This is doubly true for foods that contain soluble fiber, such as oats. (We'll be looking at fiber in more depth later.)

SUGARS—AND SUGARS

And there's one more important thing you need to know. Not all simple sugars raise your blood sugar level. In the diagram that follows you can see the chemical structure of lactose (milk sugar), sucrose (white sugar), and maltose (grain sugar or malt). The body can use only glucose for energy. Once the glucose is removed from lactose you're left with galactose, and once the glucose is removed from sucrose you're left with fructose. What happens to fructose and galactose, shown in gray? The answer is that they go to your liver, where they can be converted into glucose. But this takes time, so they're classified as slow-releasing.

Now look at the GI scores of glucose, sucrose, and fructose on page 67. As you would expect, glucose is the fastest (100), fructose the slowest (19), while sucrose—a combination of glucose and fructose—is in the middle (68). You'll also notice that maltose is as fast as glucose, and honey isn't far off, at 55. That's because "malt," the sugar, is naturally present in grains and artificially added to things such as cereals and breads—as malted wheat, for example. As you can see from the figure below, malt is just two glucose molecules. It needs virtually no digestion. Most honey is basically glucose (also called dextrose, or grape sugar since it's also found in grapes), especially commercial honey, which is heated to clean out impurities and make it easier to pack into jars.

Lactose (milk sugar) versus sucrose (white sugar) versus maltose (grain sugar or malt). Galactose and fructose (shown in gray) are slow-releasing sugars while glucose is fast. Hence lactose and sucrose are much slower-releasing than maltose, a grain sugar (malt) which is quickly digested into two glucose molecules.

Now have a look at dairy products. You'd expect ice cream to be high-GI. But it isn't that high. It scores 61. This is because lactose is quite slow-releasing. (Be aware, though, that poor-quality ice creams have added glucose.) Milk and yogurt score lower still (27–36).

Looking at fruits, even these can be fast- or slow-releasing. Not all contain fructose. Dates, for example, contain mainly glucose. Grapes and bananas are also high, while apples and berries are mainly fructose. Even better than fructose is a natural sugar called *xylitol,* which is particularly high in plums. This is the reason plums have a low GI score. Xylitol has less than half the GI score of fructose and a seventh of the GI score of sugar, and is highly preferable to any artificial sweetener. Hence 7 teaspoons of xylitol, which tastes just as good, have the same effect on your blood sugar as one teaspoon of regular sugar. I use only xylitol as a sweetener and never use sugar.

The GI score of a food is very useful, but there's one problem. Compare carrots with chocolate, or watermelon with French fries. Why do they have such similar scores? Aren't carrots supposed to be good for you? You'd be absolutely right. Aside from the vitamins and other important nutrients they contain, a carrot or a slice of watermelon contains comparatively little carbohydrate. In fact, you'd have to eat two large carrots to get the same amount of carbohydrate, and the same effect on your weight, as four pieces of chocolate. The chances are you'll eat a lot more than four pieces of chocolate and a lot less than two carrots. Similarly, watermelon has a high GI score but a low ⓖⓛ. This kind of inconsistency is why the GI is a bit misleading.

IT'S THE ⓖⓛ THAT COUNTS

This is where ⓖⓛ comes in—the best way of telling how much weight you'll gain from a food. It's a simple calculation, taking into account both the amount of carbohydrate in a food (the quantity) and its GI (the quality).

To get a food's ⓖⓛ, you just multiply its GI by the amount of carbohydrate it contains (the exact formula is given in Appendix 2). The result will tell you exactly what a given serving of a food does to your blood sugar. I've worked out the ⓖⓛ of hundreds of foods for you and you can find my ⓖⓛ index on pages 330–340.

The chart which follows shows a number of high- and low-ⓖⓛ foods. The ⓖⓛ of the quantities listed is 10 ⓖⓛ—so, for example, two entire pint baskets of strawberries have the same ⓖⓛ as two dates.

ⒼⓁ SCORES OF COMMON FOODS

Low-ⒼⓁ foods	High-ⒼⓁ foods
2 cans tomato juice (5½ oz. each)	1 small can pineapple juice (6 oz.)
2 slices whole-grain rye bread	1 slice white bread
2 pints strawberries	2 dates
Large bowl peanuts	Bag of potato chips
Carton orange juice (1 pint)	Glass of Gatorade
3 bowls muesli (sugar-free)	1 bowl cornflakes

As the golden rule of the Holford Diet is to eat no more than 40 ⒼⓁ a day, it's obvious that if you choose high-ⒼⓁ foods you won't be eating much. You could lose weight this way, but that's not what I want you to do.

It's infinitely more satisfying for you to eat low-ⒼⓁ carbohydrates. You'll be able to eat more, experiment with the recipes more, and generally enjoy your food (remember how that feels?). Let me make this real for you by showing you, on the chart opposite, a standard Fatburner's diet versus a typical diet. ⒼⓁs are shown for each food.

Take a good look at the food on the left. Imagine you ate that breakfast, rather than the one on the right. It would definitely be more filling, wouldn't it? But that's not the only benefit: by eating it, you'd have cut your propensity to turn glucose into fat by almost a third! The great news about eating the ⒼⓁ way is that you can actually eat more food *and* lose more weight. And it's all delicious.

Let's see what that means in real terms. All the meals below have identical ⒼⓁ scores, and identical effects on your blood sugar.

For breakfast you could have:

Either	*Or*
Scrambled egg on rye toast	Fruit and yogurt smoothie

As a snack you could have:

Either	*Or*
Hummus with crudités	Oatcake crackers with peanut butter

For lunch or dinner you could have:

Either	*Or*
Trout with French lentils and roasted tomatoes	Chicken fajitas with salsa and salad

HOLFORD DAILY DIET		AVERAGE DAILY DIET	
	GL		GL
Breakfast		*Breakfast*	
A bowl of oatmeal (1 oz.)	2	A bowl of cornflakes	21
Half a grated apple	3	Banana	12
Small container of yogurt (4 oz.)	2	Milk	2
Milk	2		35
	9		
a.m. snack		*a.m. snack*	
Pint of strawberries	5	Mars Bar	26
Lunch		*Lunch*	
Substantial tuna salad, 3 oatcake crackers	10	Tuna salad sub	15
p.m. snack		*p.m. snack*	
Pear + handful of peanuts	4	Bag of potato chips	11
Dinner		*Dinner*	
Tomato soup, salmon, corn, and green beans	12	Pizza with Parmesan cheese and tomato sauce, plus salad	23
GOOD DAY TOTAL	40 GL	BAD DAY TOTAL	110 GL

It doesn't look much like hard work, does it? And this is a mere sample. I'm going to give you many mouthwatering recipes and menus ranging from the simple to the elegant, all designed to keep you going at 40 🄶🄻 a day. Between these and your own "freestyle" choices using the complete GL food chart on pages 330–340, you'll soon learn which carbohydrates to go for, while your body unlearns how to store glucose as fat.

Before we run through the best low-🄶🄻 foods, I'd like to explain in depth the two important qualities of food that lower 🄶🄻: fiber, and combining protein with carbohydrate.

THE FIBER FACTOR

There's one kind of carbohydrate that's neither slow- nor fast-releasing. This is fiber—all the parts of plants that digestive enzymes cannot break down (although some fiber is digested by bacteria in the colon). While it can't be digested, it does serve a purpose. When you eat a food high in fiber, it tends to slow down the release of sugars in the food. And that, as far as weight control is concerned, is good news.

High-fiber diets are definitely recommended for a variety of general health reasons. People who eat more fiber don't usually suffer from constipation, and have a lower risk of getting bowel cancer, diabetes, or certain kinds of bowel disease. As it is a natural constituent of fruits, vegetables, lentils, beans, and whole grains, there should be no need to add extra fiber if you're eating these foods. Fiber is calorie-free and there is little doubt that a diet high in naturally occurring fiber is more filling. After all, which would you find easier to eat: two cookies or a pound of carrots?

One of the main reasons why high-fiber foods are more satisfying is that fiber absorbs water, so they become bulkier in the gut. About 10 quarts of digestive juices are released every day into the digestive tract, so a food's capability for absorbing this water would make a big difference in how bulky the food would become. Wheat fiber, as in bran, is not very absorbent compared with some vegetable fibers. Placed in water, it will swell to 10 times its original volume. Glucomannan, the fiber from the Japanese konjac plant, however, swells to 100 times its original volume! Glucomannan is given to diabetics in Japan because it helps stabilize blood sugar by "slow-releasing" any eaten carbohydrates.

Soluble or insoluble?

There are two primary kinds of fiber in food: soluble and insoluble. Many foods contain both. Insoluble fiber bulks up fecal content and can "brush" the gut like a broom, preventing constipation. Soluble fiber is different, dissolving in the gut to form a jellylike substance. This kind of fiber slows down the release of glucose into the bloodstream.

Whole cereal grains contain both kinds of fiber and will slow down glucose release the most, whereas ground fiber (which is found in whole-meal bread, for example) has little effect. Fruit and vegetable juices are devoid of fiber, and that's why the sugars they contain are so fast-releasing.

The soluble fiber found in beans, lentils, and oats is particularly effective at slowing down the digestion of food and thus the blood sugar response. Insoluble fiber makes you feel full immediately after eating, while soluble fiber reduces appetite nine or more hours later. This could be because of its effect on glucose in the bloodstream, but, whatever the case, it makes food more satisfying in the longer term.[2] There are quite a few different kinds of fiber in these two categories, but suffice to say that it's important to eat unprocessed whole foods to get the most fiber you possibly can.

King of fibers

Of the fibers in grains, oat fiber is the best at controlling blood sugar and is therefore included in the Holford Diet.[3] Some sources of soluble fiber used therapeutically to help with digestion, diabetes, and weight loss are even better, however. These include psyllium husks (available from health food shops) and glucomannan, which I mentioned above (available by mail order—see page 363 in Resources). The soluble fiber glucomannan has been found to be the most effective at controlling blood sugar.

As such, it's a marvelous aid for healthy weight loss. Two studies, one in Japan[4] and one in the United States,[5] reported an additional 1-pound weight loss a week when patients took 3 grams of glucomannan a day. At ION, we decided to put glucomannan to the test by giving 3 grams a day to 10 overweight people over a three-month period.[6] None made any apparent change to their diet or exercise regime. Nine completed the trial, with an average weight loss of 6 pounds, 10 ounces each, thus confirming the usefulness of this unique fiber.

> ### TOP TIP
> Taking 1 gram of glucomannan before each meal can reduce the ⓰ score and fill you up so you eat less. Always take a capsule with a large glass of water. Glucomannan is at least 50 times more effective than bran.

The power of protein

We've concentrated primarily on carbohydrates so far. But you'll be eating proteins and fats as well, and the balance of these with carbohydrates in each meal makes a big difference to blood sugar balance and fatburning efficiency.

Barry Sears, author of *Enter the Zone,* first made it widely known that combining protein-rich foods with slow-releasing carbohydrates helps to program you to burn fat. Remember how high insulin is bad news, and high glucagon (discussed earlier, on pages 40–42) is good news as far as fatburning is concerned? Well, protein foods tend to trigger a small and equal release of both insulin and glucagon—which happens to be the ideal. Carbohydrates, especially fast-releasing carbohydrates such as cakes and sweets, trigger a substantial release of insulin with little or no glucagon response. Eating fat has little direct effect on either insulin or glucagon. The relative effects of each combination are shown in the chart that follows.

Effects of protein, carbohydrate, and fat on insulin and glucagon

Food eaten	Insulin level	Glucagon level
Carbohydrate only	+++++	No change
Protein only	++	++
Fat only	No change	No change
Carbohydrate and fat	++++	No change
Protein and fat	++	++
High protein and low-ⒼⓁ carbohydrate	++	+
High-ⒼⓁ carbohydrate and low protein	++++++++	+
Low-ⒼⓁ carbohydrate and medium protein	+++	++

From this research, you can see that the best three combinations are protein only, or protein and fat, or low-ⒼⓁ carbohydrates and medium protein. As we've seen, the trouble with a high-protein and high-fat diet is that it isn't good for your health. It's also very restrictive. That's why the best all-around diet for consistent and easily maintained weight loss, with the lowest boredom factor, combines low-ⒼⓁ carbohydrates with protein. It's great for your health and equally effective for your waistline.

HOW MUCH PROTEIN?

Very-high-protein diets have proved effective in weight control, partly because they help to hinder the body in its turning of food into fat and also because you eat less on them. But a lot of the weight loss is water. This is partly because when you starve the body of glucose it breaks down stores of glucose called glycogen, which is stored with water. The other reason is that, when you eat too much protein without enough carbohydrates, ketones are produced. These are toxic, and the body tries hard to get rid of them in urine, which contributes to the fluid weight loss. But any pounds of water lost will come back.

While we all need something in the region of 40 grams of protein a day, eating more than 80 grams a day over the long term will boost your risk of developing osteoporosis, because protein is acidic and can deplete the bones of calcium. It also stresses the kidneys. If the protein source is beef or dairy produce, this may increase the risk of breast or prostate cancer. Also, if a person chooses meat as the main source of protein, his or her diet will inevitably become high in saturated fat, potentially increasing the risk of heart disease. There's not much point being thin and dead!

BEST RATIO FOR FATBURNING

On a short-term basis, such as 30 days up to three months, increasing your protein intake to between 60 and 75 grams a day and focusing on fish, chicken, and vegetarian sources can help restore blood sugar control and boost fatburning.[7] For this reason the Holford Diet provides a greater proportion of calories from protein than the average diet—25 percent of calories, over a norm of 17 percent—to control blood sugar balance and reduce insulin resistance. After that period, protein consumption drops to 20 percent of calories to maintain fatburning. Once you've reached your goal and need only to maintain your weight and blood sugar balance over the long term, the ideal amount of protein would be 15 to 20 percent of calories.

But you won't have to mess around with calorie counting, as this isn't that kind of diet. So what all this means in terms of the food you eat is explained simply and clearly in Part Three. I'll tell you exactly what to do. For now, check out the table that follows, showing the ideal balance of proteins, carbs, and fats.

The perfect balance

	Protein	Carbohydrate	Fat
Average diet	17%	48%	35%
Holford Diet (first 30 days up to three months)	25%	50%	25%
Holford Diet (maintenance)	15–20%	55–60%	25%

Since we all need to eat some protein, some carbohydrates, and the right kind of fats, the best combination is to eat low-GL carbohydrate foods that are also rich in protein. Beans and lentils are an example. People who live in countries whose diets emphasize these foods are consistently thinner and healthier.

The easiest and healthiest way to achieve this perfect balance is to eat the equivalent of 60 grams of protein and 120 grams of low-Ⓖ carbohydrate in a day, and to divide it evenly between each meal—that is, 20 grams of protein and roughly 40 grams of carbohydrate at breakfast, lunch, and dinner. You needn't worry too much about the math: the recipes will do it for you. (Details on the quantity and quality of fats to be eaten are given in the next chapter.) Roughly two thirds of your carbohydrates should come from vegetables and fruit and one third from things such as grains and more "starchy" vegetables.

The simplest way to visualize your meals, as far as lunch and dinner are concerned, is to pair any one of the protein-rich foods shown below with an equivalent-sized serving of any carbohydrate-rich food, plus two servings of vegetables. Remember the plate model from page 55?

To maximize fatburning, you will probably be eating more protein-rich foods in relation to carbohydrate-rich foods than you are used to, as well as more fresh fruit and vegetables. The amount of carbohydrate or protein provided by nonstarchy vegetables (broccoli, kale, cabbage, peas, spinach, carrots, and so on) is small, so these can be eaten relatively freely on the Holford Diet. Aim, too, for two pieces of low-Ⓖ fruit a day.

Fatburning food combinations

(A more comprehensive list of foods is given on pages 161–164.)

Here are a few examples:

Protein	Carbohydrate	Vegetables
Poached salmon	on brown basmati rice	with a green salad
Marinated tofu	on whole wheat pasta	with steam-fried vegetables
Grilled chicken breast	with boiled new potatoes	with steamed green beans
Cottage cheese	on oatcake crackers/ rye bread	with broccoli and tomato salad

The Holford Diet snacks are also great protein/carb combinations. For instance, eating a few almonds or pumpkin seeds, high in essential fats and protein, at the same time as low-Ⓖ fruit can further slow the effect of fruit sugar on your blood sugar. But remember: fruits such as apples and strawberries have a low **GL**, so you are already doing very well.

For breakfast, you can achieve the right balance and amount of protein and low-**GL** carbohydrate by, for example, eating a cup of oat flakes with some seeds, some berries, and skim milk (or soy milk, if you're allergic to milk).

Above all, don't worry about having to calculate all this—the lowdown in Part Three and menus and recipes in Part Four make it remarkably easy.

We've now looked in depth at how to pinpoint the best carbohydrates, and how to combine them, for the most efficient fatburning. But what if you, like millions of others, are in the grip of caffeine and chocolate addictions? Dealing with these very 21st-century addictions is essential to balancing your blood sugar—and, as you'll see, surprisingly painless.

Are you addicted to sugar or stimulants?

Ever had an "I'd kill for a muffin" moment? Or perhaps it was a double espresso, a bar of chocolate, even a piece of toast. Whatever the object of your desire, the urge to get at it probably felt overwhelming. Yet this is a perfectly normal reaction to a blood sugar low.

It is virtually impossible to resist temptation when you're in the middle of a blood sugar crash. One of the reasons sugar is so addictive is that it can cause a release of the body's own feel-good chemicals, opioids and dopamine.

Animals can become addicted to sugar and show all the telltale withdrawal symptoms, including the shakes, when deprived, according to research by Dr. Bartley Hoebel at Princeton University. This is because the more you overstimulate the release of dopamine, the more insensitive you become to its effects. In a sense you are becoming "dopamine resistant," or addicted to your body's own natural highs. This, in turn, upsets your blood sugar levels and ability to control your weight.

Dr. Candace Pert, research professor in the physiology and biophysics department at Georgetown University Medical Center in Washington, D.C., says, "I consider sugar to be a drug, a highly purified plant product that can become addictive. Relying on an artificial form of glucose—sugar—to give us a quick pick-me-up is analogous to, if not as dangerous as, shooting heroin."[8] Dr. Pert is among the chief scientists who discovered the central role endorphins play in addiction. There's certainly plenty of research out there to support her view.[9]

Sugar and high- carbs aren't the only culprits in the case. Stimulants, too, promote the brain's feel-good chemicals. Remember the effect of our in-built fight-or-flight mechanism? It's as if we humans have a fifth gear for emergencies.

In times of stress, the adrenal glands release a combination of hormones, including dopamine and adrenaline, that break down stores of glucose and raise your blood sugar levels, tapping into your energy reserves to provide instant fuel to deal with the apparent danger. Of course, today's emergencies have nothing to do with woolly mammoths on the rampage but take place mainly inside our heads—overdrafts, relationships, parking tickets, and so on. But we still produce adrenaline, and that still raises blood sugar levels.

Stimulants have the same effect, stirring up adrenaline and dopamine. So the nicotine or caffeine in colas, coffee, tea, cigarettes, and chocolate, added to the stresses of 21st-century life, can seriously mess with your blood sugar.

So why do we do it? It's simply because millions of us are caught in the vicious cycle of blood sugar highs and lows already, and feel exhausted much of the time. Stimulants seem to promise instant energy—while, of course, making the problem worse.

We may be eating fast-releasing carbohydrates, devoid of vitamins and minerals. We may be drinking two or three cups of coffee before noon just to deal with our morning weariness. We learn to cope with the rebound blood sugar low after a meal by having a coffee. If we haven't eaten for two hours, we go for another coffee. And, when we drag ourselves home after a hard day's work, we may be drinking still more just to stay awake.

You may feel that coffee, which speeds up the metabolism, is not only keeping you going but helping with weight loss. The irony is that in the not-so-long term it contributes to weight gain by fueling blood sugar imbalance. According to research from Holland by Dr. Paul Smits and colleagues at the University of Nijmegen, a single shot of caffeine can raise adrenaline fivefold, thus raising blood glucose, and decrease insulin sensitivity by 15 percent. This means you become more resistant to insulin and more likely to turn glucose into fat.[10]

A CUP OF CHAOS

Stimulants are addictive. That's why you need more and more to keep you going. Before long, one cup of coffee and the odd cigarette become six or more lattes, mochaccinos, or filter coffees and a pack of cigarettes. By the time you reach this stage, you can't even get going in the morning without a stimulant. The combination of coffee, tea, or nicotine with stress, high-GI foods, and sugar means you lose your blood sugar control and wake up each morning with low blood sugar levels and not enough adrenaline to kick-start your day. So you adopt one of two strategies:

- You reluctantly crawl out of bed on remote control and head for the kettle or coffeepot, make yourself a strong cup of tea or coffee, light up a cigarette or have some fast-releasing sugar in the form of toast, with some sugar on it called jam. Up go your blood sugar and adrenaline levels and you start to feel normal.

Or . . .

- You lie in bed and start to think about all the things that have gone wrong, could go wrong, will go wrong. You start to worry about everything you've got to do, haven't done, and should have done. About 10 minutes of this gets enough adrenaline pumping to get you out of bed.

One of the most seductive aspects of coffee is that it actually seems to make you feel better, more energized and alert. But, wondered Dr. Peter Rogers, a psychologist at Bristol University, does coffee actually increase your energy and mental performance, or just relieve the symptoms of withdrawal? When he researched this he found that, after that sacred morning cup of coffee, coffee drinkers don't feel any better than people who never drink coffee. Coffee drinkers just feel better than they did when they woke up.[11] In other words, drinking coffee relieves the symptoms of withdrawal from coffee. And in the middle sit Starbucks and all the other coffee franchises making a buck or two! It's addictive.

Caffeine blocks the receptors for a brain chemical called *adenosine*, whose function is to stop the release of the motivating neurotransmitters dopamine and adrenaline. With less adenosine activity, levels of dopamine and adrenaline increase, as do alertness and motivation. Peak concentration occurs 30 to 60 minutes after you down that cup.

The more caffeine you consume, the less sensitive your body and brain become to their own natural stimulants, dopamine and adrenaline. You then need more stimulants to feel normal, and keep pushing the body to produce more dopamine and adrenaline. The net result is adrenal exhaustion—an inability to produce these important chemicals of motivation and communication. Apathy, depression, exhaustion, and an inability to cope set in.

Coffee isn't, of course, the only source of caffeine. There's as much in a strong cup of tea as in a regular cup of coffee. Caffeine is also the active ingredient in most colas and energy drinks such as Red Bull, which sold more than 100 million cans in 2003 alone. Chocolate and green tea also contain caffeine, although in much smaller amounts. Have a look at the chart that follows.

How much caffeine?

Product	Caffeine content
Coca-Cola Classic, 12 oz.	46mg
Diet Coke, 12 oz.	46mg
Red Bull	80mg
Hot cocoa, 5 oz.	10mg
Coffee, instant, 5 oz.	40–105mg
Coffee, espresso, cappuccino, latte	30–50mg
Coffee, filter, 5 oz.	110–150mg
Coffee, Starbucks (grande)	500mg
Decaffeinated coffee, 5 oz.	0.3mg
Tea, 5 oz.	20–100mg
Green tea, 5 oz.	20–30mg
Chocolate cake, 1 slice	20–30mg
Bittersweet chocolate, 1 oz.	5–35mg
NoDoz	50–200mg

And, if you add sugar to your coffee or drink a lot of cola, you'll exacerbate the effect of the caffeine on your blood sugar balance, and end up piling on even more weight.

That's why I recommend you cut way back on stimulants, including sugar, right at the start of the diet. If the very thought fills you with dread, and leaves you wildly wondering how you'll get to work without that morning cup, it's pretty certain you're addicted. But by quitting you'll be trading a dispiriting round of fatigue and sudden jolts to the system for feeling energetic all day, every day.

Before you panic, let me say that this is not for life. What I'm asking you to do is go cold turkey: give up stimulants and sugar when you start on the diet and supplement program, and stay off them completely for at least two weeks to a month. This will kick-start your metabolism. After that, you can reintroduce them in moderation if you want to.

Of course, the reason we react with horror to the thought of stopping stimulants is that we "know" we'll feel terrible without them. We know this for a fact because it's the very symptoms of withdrawal—feeling tired, grumpy, and foggy-headed—that make that cup of tea or cappuccino seem like manna from heaven. But, ten minutes later, you want another one.

Once your blood sugar and adrenaline levels are back to normal, however, you can take or leave these stimulants.

So if you follow the Holford Diet and take the supplements I recommend, going cold turkey may well turn out to be much easier than you thought. Nine out of ten people say, two weeks later, that they feel so good they just don't need stimulants anymore. With their energy levels soaring, they can say good-bye to the endless jolts to the system that used to punctuate their days.

The first step is to get real about your use of stimulants. This means completing the "stimulant inventory" that follows, for a week. Write down what you consume every day, and then add up your total at the end of the week. Be honest!

Add up your total number of "units." The ideal is 5 or fewer per week. If you are having more than 10 stimulant units a week, this is going to have an effect on your energy and weight.

Eating slow-releasing energy foods and taking energy-stabilizing vitamins and minerals, which we'll be investigating in Part Three, will give you even energy levels, and the need for stimulants will evaporate. You'll look back on those bleary-eyed mornings and exhausted afternoons with wonder. As one Fatburner volunteer quoted earlier said, "One of the hardest, but best things about it was the insistence on giving up coffee and stimulants." (She also lost 10 pounds in a month.)

KICKING THE HABIT

How does the Holford Diet help you quit? Since all stimulants affect blood sugar levels, you can keep yours even by always having something substantial for breakfast, including an oat-based, not-too-refined cereal; unsweetened yogurt with active cultures, apple, ground sesame seeds, and wheat

	Unit	Sun	Mon	Tue	Wed	Thu	Fri	Sat
Green tea	2 cups							
Tea	1 cup							
Coffee	1 cup							
Cola or caffeinated drinks	1 can							
Caffeine pills such as No-Doz, Excedrin, Dexatrim	1 pill							
Chocolate	2 ounces (approx 1 bar)							
Alcohol (units) Glass of wine is 1 Bottle of beer is ½ Shot of spirits is 1	unit							
Added sugar	1 tsp/5g							
Hidden sugar (see sugar content on ingredients list)	1 tsp/5g							
Cigarettes	1 cigarette							

Add up your total number of "units." The ideal is 5 or fewer per week. If you are having more than 10 stimulant units a week, this is going to have an effect on your energy and weight.

germ; or an egg. You can snack frequently on fresh fruit, and twice a day add in a small handful of nuts or seeds.

Eating a highly alkaline-forming diet can reduce cravings for cigarettes and alcohol, so eat plenty of low-Ⓖ fruit and fresh vegetables. These high-fiber foods also help to keep your blood sugar levels even, and you on an even keel. The worst thing you can do is go for hours without eating—but this isn't something I would ever recommend, anyway.

In this way, going cold turkey at the same time as starting the diet will simply not be the nightmare you imagine. I realize that giving up cigarettes might be a little more difficult than tossing out the beer, wine, and coffee, but even that process will be significantly smoothed once your blood sugar steadies.

My diet will help stabilize your blood sugar and reduce your cravings. Meanwhile, let's look at the culprits.

Coffee contains three stimulants—caffeine, theobromine, and theophylline. Although caffeine is the strongest, theophylline is known to disturb normal sleep patterns and theobromine has an effect similar to caffeine's, although it is present in much smaller amounts than caffeine in coffee. So decaffeinated coffee isn't exactly stimulant-free.

As a nutritionist, I have seen many people cleared of minor health problems such as tiredness and headaches just by cutting out their two or three coffees a day. After you quit, you may get withdrawal symptoms for up to three days. These reflect how addicted you've become. If you begin to feel perky and your health improves afterward, that's a good indication that you're better off without coffee—and, in any case, I recommend having it only as a very occasional treat. The most popular alternatives are Teeccino, Kaffree Roma, or Cafix (made with roasted chicory and malted barley), dandelion coffee, and herbal teas.

Tea is the great British addiction. As we've seen, a strong cup of tea contains as much caffeine as a weak cup of coffee and it is certainly addictive. Tea also contains tannin, which interferes with the absorption of vital minerals such as iron and zinc. Particularly addictive is Earl Grey tea, which contains an extra stimulant, bergamot. If you find you drink more than the occasional weak cuppa, it's time to stop. The best-tasting alternatives are Rooibos tea (red bush tea) with milk, and herbal or fruit teas.

Chocolate bars are usually full of sugar, and cocoa, the active ingredient, provides significant quantities of the stimulant theobromine, also found in coffee. The action of theobromine is similar to caffeine's, though not as strong. Chocolate also contains small amounts of caffeine. Given that array of stimulants, plenty of sugar, and a truly delicious taste and "mouth feel," it's all too easy to become a chocoholic. If you stop eating it for a couple of weeks, substituting fruit, healthy "sweets" from health food shops that are sugar free, and the like, you will find yourself losing the craving.

Cola and **"energy" drinks** contain anything from 46 to 80 milligrams of caffeine per can, as we saw in the chart above. These drinks are also often high in sugar and colorings and their net stimulant effect can be considerable. Check the ingredients list and stay away from drinks containing caffeine and chemical additives or colorings.

Cigarettes raise blood sugar levels by acting as a mild stimulant to the central nervous system. There is also evidence that smoking is linked to an increase in insulin resistance. In addition to disturbing blood sugar balance, cigarette smoking drains the body of vital nutrients and contributes to numerous other diseases such as cancer and heart disease. So, needless to say, cigarettes are a big no-no. If you are addicted to smoking, I can't recommend highly enough the benefits of quitting. Not only will it lower your risk of getting certain kinds of cancer and other diseases, but it will also keep you looking younger and feeling much better overall.

For confirmed smokers, I generally recommend stabilizing blood sugar first with the diet. This will make quitting easier. Also, you will not get the rebound weight gain that often happens if you haven't solved the underlying issue for every smoker, which is blood sugar imbalance. I also recommend increasing your daily exercise during the time you quit smoking, which further boosts your metabolism and stops any rebound weight gain.

There are now a number of successful methods for quitting. On my Web site, you'll find a "How to Quit Smoking" link. Following these steps will dramatically decrease your symptoms of withdrawal and increase your chances of success. (See www.holfordhealth.com and enter "quit smoking" in the search box.)

Alcohol is not strictly a stimulant, but is chemically very similar to sugar, and potentially very addictive. It's also high in calories. Drinking can suppress appetite but lead to cravings for more alcohol, so you can end up quaffing empty calories with no nutritional value. Worse, alcohol also destroys or prevents the absorption of many nutrients, including vitamins C and B complex, calcium, magnesium, and zinc.

Alcohol can also make you fat. It's the most rapidly absorbed sugar, with one fifth being absorbed directly through the stomach. It takes almost two hours to use up 10 grams of alcohol, the amount in half a pint of beer. Alcohol can be rapidly turned to fat by the action of insulin. With chronic use it converts into fat, rather than to glucose or glycogen, and is stored in the liver. Alcohol also interferes with the liver's ability to break down amino acids and turn them into glucose when blood sugar levels are too low.

So, in this sense, alcohol messes up blood sugar and fat control, and regular drinkers tend to put on weight. Habitual drinking can damage the liver, leading to even further inability to control both blood sugar levels and weight. You'll achieve the best results on the Holford Diet by having no more than three small drinks a week, and preferably none at all for the first two weeks to a month.

The stress connection

Sugar and stimulants may not be the only factors playing merry hell with your blood sugar. Serious stress has a very similar effect. If you think you are suffering from it, you're not alone. Many people wake up in a state of anxiety, arrive at work stressed out from commuting, have to contend with a lot of stress at work, and go home in a state of near collapse. Unfortunately, a life of nonstop 21st-century stress takes its toll on your body's chemistry.

We've seen how stimulants trigger the release of adrenaline and cortisol, which prepare the body for action. Stress does this, too. The flood of glucose this then releases for our use stimulates, in its turn, yet more hormones to take the glucose out of circulation. While adrenaline works fast and is gone fast, cortisol lingers. If you're stressed for weeks at a time, your cortisol level stays high, and this is bad news. High cortisol levels, the hallmark of the overstressed, make you even more insulin resistant and even more prone to put on weight. Let me explain why.

Insulin puts glucose into storage, whereas adrenaline and cortisol rapidly raise the glucose supply to cells for fight or flight—partly by blocking insulin's fat-storing effect. That sounds like good news, at least in the short term. And it is. That's why high stress and stimulants, such as coffee, can keep you thin. But when the effect of insulin is blocked, the body simply produces more—and the more it produces, the more insulin resistant you become. So, over the long term, stress can actually lead to weight gain.

HOW STRESSED ARE YOU?

Take a look at the symptoms below. If they sound familiar to you, then you know what I'm talking about. They suggest adrenal stress overload.

- finding it hard to get up in the morning
- feeling tired all the time
- craving certain foods
- anger, irritability, aggressiveness
- mood swings
- restlessness
- energy slump during the day
- regular feelings of weakness
- apathy
- depression
- feeling cold all the time

In a survey of patients visiting ION, 54 percent had a high stress rating at their initial assessment. After six months of improved nutrition, substituting slow-releasing carbohydrates for sugar and stimulants, that figure had dropped to 28 percent.

The amazing thing is that if you balance your blood sugar, it not only affects your weight, but also has wide-reaching benefits for your health, your mood, and your ability to deal with the inevitable challenges of life. When you're stressed, even molehills seem like mountains. When your energy levels are good and your mind is clear, life immediately smooths out and calms down. As Fatburner volunteers from *She* magazine agreed, "Increased alertness was a significant benefit. By the third day, everybody felt well—alert on rising, and three of us (including me) were bounding about full of the joys of spring."

The only way out of the prison of stress, sugar, and stimulants is to reduce or avoid all forms of concentrated sweetness, tea, coffee, alcohol, and cigarettes, and start eating foods that help to keep your blood sugar level stable. By changing to the right foods, backed up with specific nutritional supplements, most people feel an amazing improvement in energy within days.

That's why I recommend that you:

- avoid regular tea and coffee
- stop eating chocolate (you can have some after two weeks to a month!)
- quit smoking
- avoid regular alcohol and reduce your overall intake to three small glasses a week (12 oz. beer, 5 oz. wine, or 1½ oz. 80 proof liquor)
- do what you can to avoid continuously high stress levels

Remember, the very best way is to have *nothing* stimulating when you start the diet. That includes decaf coffee (the continuing taste of coffee doesn't help you break the habit).

After that, but *only if you have to,* you can drink the occasional cup of weak tea. But coffee, as I've indicated, pretty much has to go. Soon you'll find you can sail past coffee shops with not even a twinge of longing—and with a lot more energy than in the days you were chained to a cup.

As far as sugar is concerned, you'll have to be on the lookout. It comes in many disguises. Peruse food labels for glucose, dextrose, and sucrose. Honey is also best avoided for those first two weeks. Fructose (fruit sugar) is somewhat better, but, even so, the emphasis over these two weeks is to get the sweetness you need by having whole foods, such as fruit, instead of sugar on cereals or in desserts.

It's also a good idea to start cutting down on the overall sweetness of what you eat. For example, you can add water to juice. Three oranges may have gone into a large glass of the juice. Would you eat that many whole fruits at one sitting? Even though oranges contain mainly fructose, there's *a lot* of it in pure juice. Dilute it by a third. You'll soon get used to it. After two weeks, you'll find your craving for sweetness is fading—and overall, you'll find it easy to keep going on the Holford Diet.

- Avoid sugar in its many disguises and avoid foods that contain fast-releasing carbohydrates with a high-**GL** score (above 10 per serving).
- Eat foods that contain low-**GL** carbohydrates (below 10 per serving).
- Eat no more than 40 **GL** a day.
- Eat low-**GL** carbohydrates *with* protein-rich foods.

- Eat whole, unadulterated foods high in soluble fiber (beans, lentils, oats).
- Consider supplementing with konjac extract for the glucomannan it contains.
- Cut back on stimulants right at the start of the diet.
- Do what you can to avoid continuously high stress levels.

Part Three shows you how to do all this.

Step 2: Eat Good Fats and Avoid Bad Fats

It may seem counterintuitive, but some kinds of fats boost fatburning. These are the essential fatty acids, or EFAs. So entrenched have we become in fat phobia and the promotion of low-fat diets that the role of EFAs in helping you to burn fat has gone largely unnoticed.

The original idea was that, since 1 gram of fat gives more calories (9 calories) than 1 gram of protein or carbohydrate (approximately 4 calories), the quickest way to cut calories was to cut fat. Theoretically, this should have been the best way to lose weight, if you believe conventional calorie theory. We now know this isn't true. Low- diets work better than low-fat diets, and the of your diet predicts weight gain much more accurately than the fat content of your diet.[12]

Go fish

But then we discovered there were essential fats (polyunsaturates) and nonessential fats (saturates). When you eat 100 grams of saturated fat, all your body can do is burn it for energy or store it as fat. On the other hand, when you eat 100 grams of the polyunsaturated fats from seeds, from their oils, or from fatty fish, the brain and nerves use them, and they boost immunity, balance hormones, reduce inflammation, and promote healthy skin. Only if there's any left will the body use EFAs for energy or to store as fat. In other words, one calorie of saturated fat has an entirely different effect on the body in terms of weight control and health than one calorie of polyunsaturated fat.

And it gets even better. Since you need essential fats, it should come as no surprise to find out that we have "fat receptors" in the mouth. These register whether or not you've eaten what you need. We humans crave fat in the same way we crave sugar or protein. However, only when you eat the right fat—the essential kind—does your body stop craving that smooth, creamy texture. Not only are you satisfied, but you've just consumed a very special substance.

The omega-3 EFAs, found in flax and pumpkin seeds and oily cold-water fish such as mackerel, herring, salmon, and tuna, keep extra weight at bay in a number of ways. They help make hormonelike substances called *prostaglandins,* which help to control metabolism and fatburning. They also help to control and limit the potential damage of insulin resistance, by calming down the inflammatory effects of bursts of high glucose in the blood, which damages the arteries.

The omega-6 EFAs, found in hot-climate seeds such as sunflower and sesame, have similar benefits to the omega-3s, and are especially good for the skin and maintaining hormone balance, for example in combating PMS, but not so important for the brain.

The fat in meat and dairy produce, which is saturated fat, simply doesn't come near EFAs in the health stakes. (Luckily, the Holford Diet helps you reduce the amount of protein—and fat—you get from meat and dairy foods.) Worst of all fats, however, are the kind you find in processed and junk food or in deep-fried foods. These are called trans fats and hydrogenated fats.

There is, however, an "in-between" fat: monounsaturated, or omega-9, fat. Olive oil is a particularly rich source. While this is nowhere near as good for you as food sources of the omega-3 fats, it is also nowhere near as bad for you as saturated fat or trans fats. A number of studies have found that if people switch from saturated to monounsaturated fats, it helps to stabilize blood sugar levels, improve insulin resistance, and control diabetes.[13] This is good news, and a step in the right direction for fatburning.

My diet emphasizes omega-rich foods and avoids trans fats, hydrogenated fats, and saturated fats as much as possible. On the facing page you'll see the common food sources of these different kinds of fats. (Please note that most foods contain a mixture of fats, so some appear more than once, as they're rich in several kinds.)

Fat family	Good dietary sources
Omega-3 family	Fish, especially salmon, mackerel, herring, tuna, and sardines; flaxseeds, pumpkin seeds, and walnuts, and their oils
Omega-6 family	Sunflower, sesame, and pumpkin seeds and their oils; also safflower oil, corn oil, soy oil
Omega-9 family	Olive oil, almonds, walnuts
Saturated fat	Meat, dairy produce, and most eggs (chicken fed flaxseeds have more omega-3 fats in their eggs)
Trans fats and hydrogenated fats	Deep-fried food, burned or browned fat, margarines, most processed meats (such as hamburgers, sausages), and most vegetarian meat substitutes (such as vegetarian sausages)

As you can see from the figure on the following page, modern times have seen big changes in our fat intake. From 1900 to 2000 there was a massive increase in overall fat intake—although we have started to eat less since the late 1980s—as well as a big increase in saturated fat and a decrease in the best fat of all, omega-3s. Consumption of the essential omega-6 fat has gone up, reflecting the switch from butter to margarine. However, this is slightly misleading because a lot of this "polyunsaturated vegetable oil," which is what you find on the label, has been "hydrogenated," a process that makes it at least as bad for you as saturated fat. More on this in a minute.

Say no to saturated fat

To lose weight, it is definitely desirable to cut down on saturated fat. Nowadays even the average child consumes over 700 pounds of saturated fat, the equivalent of 1,314 pats of butter, between the ages of 6 and 16. Eating ex-

How fat intake has changed. In modern times, total fat intake has increased. Saturated fat intake has increased, although it is now leveling off. Omega-6 fat intake has increased but this is slightly misleading because much of it is "hydrogenated" vegetable oils, which act like saturated fats. Consumption of omega-3 fats, in fish and seeds, has gone down, leading to widespread deficiency.

Leaf and Weber, *American Journal of Clinical Nutrition* 1987, 45, pp. 1048–53.

cess fat is associated with obesity, heart disease, cancer, and diabetes, and it puts extra stress on the body's metabolism.[14]

Despite all this evidence, the currently popular high-protein, low-carb diets often kick off with 60 percent of calories from fat! This is double the mainstream recommendations and almost three times what I'd recommend you eat.

Hydrogenated—the "H" word

Just as bad for you as saturated fats are polyunsaturated fats that have been processed, fried, or damaged. Remember, the essential fats are polyunsaturated fats, but once they've been messed around with they're as bad for you as saturated fats, if not worse. When the molecules of these essential fats are

> ## TOP TIP
> All authorities agree that our total fat intake should be less than 30 percent of total calories, but how do you know what percentage of the food you buy is fat? Here is a simple equation that tells you if packaged food is too high in fat.
>
> Look at the number of calories per serving on the label. Now look at the number of grams of fat per serving and multiply it by 10. Is this more than a third of the number of calories per serving? If so, the food is more than 30 percent fat.
>
> For example, a yogurt may provide 160 calories in a 1-cup serving. The fat content per serving is 11 grams. Multiply by 10, giving you 110. Divide 110 by 160, and you get 0.6875. This means that almost 69 percent of the calories in this yogurt come from fat.
>
> Try this simple formula when you next go shopping.

altered by food processing (called *hydrogenation*) or frying, they can no longer benefit the body and are called trans fats. Frying or heating can also make them rancid or oxidized, which means they can set up a chain reaction of oxidation in the body, damaging body cells. Foods rich in trans fats include

- French fries
- hamburgers
- deep-fried fish burgers
- deep-fried chicken nuggets
- candy
- chocolate bars
- potato and corn chips
- cookies
- doughnuts
- margarine
- mayonnaise
- most salad dressings

PG1
Good

PG2
Bad

PG3
Good

Too much insulin, a consequence of insulin resistance, encourages the formation of prostaglandins that promote inflammation, pain, and swelling. Increased intake of omega-3 fats has the opposite effect, reducing pain and inflammation.

Unfortunately, many vegetarian processed foods are also high in these hydrogenated fats. Check the label on the veggie burger or vegetarian sausage packet. If the label lists partially hydrogenated vegetable oil, don't buy it.

Say yes to omega-3 fats

Most of us are deficient in omega-3s already. But, as we've seen, eating them is vital for health—hence the "essential" in "essential fatty acid." And of course they carry a host of healthy benefits, not least of which is their ability to boost fatburning.

Let's take a closer look at how they help in this respect. In the figure above, you can see how the body can make three kinds of prostaglandin—PG1, 2, and 3. PG1 and 3 are good for fatburning. PG2 is not. While omega-3 fats can make only the good PG3, the omega-6 fats can produce either the good PG1 or the bad PG2. People producing a lot of insulin because of blood sugar imbalance tend to produce more PG2. But there's a way to counteract this. Eating more omega-3s, which provide eicosapentaenoic acid or EPA, will help in turning their omega-6 fats into PG1.

I've listed a few of the health benefits of eating omega-3 fats. But there are even more. They reduce the risk of heart disease and of dying from a sudden heart attack by 50 percent and also halve your risk of ever suffering from Alzheimer's disease.[15] The moral of this story is that omega-3s are one of your best friends, not just for fatburning but for overall health. The Holford Diet specifically includes these essential fats in one of four ways:

BREAKFAST—2 teaspoons of seeds (half pumpkin, half flax is excellent, or you can mix in some sesame and sunflower too) with your breakfast cereal, yogurt, or Get Up & Go.

SNACKS—2 teaspoons of pumpkin seeds with fruit.

MAIN MEALS—A small serving of oily fish *or* 2 teaspoons of pumpkin seeds on salad.

SALAD DRESSINGS—2 teaspoons of seed oil.

To obtain enough essential fats you need to pick *two* of any of these options each day.

I realize that, if you've spent years avoiding fat like the plague, this routine might jar at first. Yet the truth is that these essential fats clear up dry skin, stimulate your metabolism, boost brain function, protect your heart, and strengthen your immune system. So in addition to losing weight more efficiently, you'll find that your skin and hair look better than ever, and that your mind and body are in great working order—with a little help from the omegas.

The quantity of fat in the Holford Diet, which amounts to a quarter of overall calories, is lower than that in the average diet, which provides about 35 percent of calories as fat. But the biggest difference between the norm and the Holford Diet is not in the *quantity* but in the *quality* of fat. Eating in this way means that less than a third of the fat you eat is saturated, compared with two thirds in the average diet.

The recipes in Part Four will take care of all this for you. The way you cook foods is also important. The best method is actually leaving the food raw, but steaming, boiling, poaching, steam-frying, baking, and grilling are all good too, in that order of preference. Avoid all deep-fried food and, as much as possible, anything fried.

> ### TOP TIP
> A great way to cut calories is to have a substantial breakfast and dinner and a light snack lunch, with one small snack at midmorning and another in midafternoon.

- Eat foods high in the essential omega-3 and omega-6 fats, with an emphasis on omega-3 fats from fish, and from flax and pumpkin seeds and their oils.
- Avoid foods high in saturated, hydrogenated, or processed fats.
- Avoid fried, burned, or browned food.

Part Three shows you how you do all this.

Step 3: Eliminate Your Hidden Allergies

Not all the weight you want to lose is fat. You might be holding as much as 15 pounds of extra fluid, or even more, without knowing it. And it could all be because of a food allergy.

One in three people has hidden food allergies, which cause the weight to pile on. If you are one of them, I'd like to help you find out what your bad foods are and which foods to eat instead. I'd also like to show you how to "desensitize" yourself to foods you're allergic to so you can eat them once more. This normally takes about three months.

Rebecca S. is a case in point. In her twenties Rebecca had stable weight and good skin, and used to exercise three or four times a week. But in her thirties she started to pile on the pounds. Over three years her weight drifted from 140 pounds up to more than 180 pounds and her dress size went up to 14. She also developed itchy patches on her face and had a lot of colds and sinus trouble. She didn't exercise because she didn't feel good.

"I started feeling tired and lethargic and generally unwell," she said. "I didn't have the energy to go to the gym anymore."

For breakfast she'd have toast, then a main meal of meat and potatoes with gravy for lunch, and a sandwich for dinner. "But it seemed like the foods I ate were blowing me up, which is why I thought I could have a food allergy." She decided to test herself for a food allergy, which nowadays you can do with a home test kit, involving a pinprick of blood. The results showed that she was reacting to milk, egg white, and gluten—the protein found in wheat, barley, and rye. Within a week of excluding these foods she found that her skin and mood improved and the weight started to fall away. After six months she had lost 45 pounds.

After three months of strictly avoiding the foods she'd become allergic to, she reintroduced egg whites and then milk to see if there was a reaction. Now she's fine on both foods, but still reacts to wheat.

"I can't tell you how much better I feel. I'm 100 percent," she said. "It has transformed my health. Having the food intolerance test has been the best thing I've done. I wish I'd done it sooner." In the end, Rebecca shed all the weight she'd gained during the previous three years.

But first, let's explore why losing control of water balance can cause considerable weight gain and see whether this may be part of your problem.

Water retention, allergies, and bingeing

More than two thirds of your body is water. If you dehydrate the body by not drinking enough water or by drinking lots of coffee or tea, which are diuretic and cause a loss of body fluid, you could lose weight. But this is neither healthy nor lasting weight loss.

Another way to lose water is to eat very few calories or very little carbohydrate. Then, as we've seen, the body will use up your glycogen, which is stored with water—and thus you'll lose water, too. However, this weight will come piling back on, unless you wish to live your entire life on a high-protein, low-carb diet, or a very-low-calorie diet, guzzling coffee, dehydrating, and aging rapidly. It is excess body fat, not water, that is associated with the long-term problem of obesity.

Just in case you wondered, drinking plenty of water doesn't lead to weight gain (unless you were seriously dehydrated in the first place). In fact, the opposite is true. The more water you drink, the less likely you are to be overweight, according to the MyNutrition survey we conducted on 37,000 people.

It's a good idea to drink, at the very least, a quart of water every day because it helps the body to eliminate toxins released from fatty tissue as you burn it up. It also helps to dilute the bloodstream to prevent an overconcentration of sugar or protein. (This is why you become thirsty after eating a large dinner or sweets.) Some people have reported tremendous weight loss and health improvements simply by drinking 2 quarts of water a day. I rec-

> **TOP TIP**
> Press the tip of your finger into the inside of your shinbone. Does your finger make a dent? If it does, you are probably waterlogged.

ommend you drink the equivalent of eight glasses of water every day, which includes any hot drinks such as herbal teas.

However, the body can sometimes retain too much water, creating unnecessary weight gain. This is not a consequence of drinking too much, but indicates instead a loss of the body's ability to control water balance, leading to edema or water retention. Breast tenderness, experienced by many women before their periods, is caused by water retention. In fact, you can easily gain 7 to 14 pounds in body weight this way—and lose it in as little as 48 hours if you eliminate the cause.

ARE YOU WATERLOGGED?

- ☐ Does your face look puffy, especially around the eyes?
- ☐ Does your abdomen, on pressing, feel waterlogged and bloated?
- ☐ Do your arms feel puffy rather than like pure fat and muscle?
- ☐ Do your ankles ever swell up?
- ☐ Do your fingers ever swell up so it's hard to get your rings off?
- ☐ Do you have dry skin or dandruff?
- ☐ Do you ever experience sudden fluctuations in your weight?
- ☐ Do you suffer from breast tenderness?
- ☐ Are you prone to allergies?

If you answer yes to three or more of the questions above, chances are that water retention is partly to blame for your weight problem. There are four reasons why retention of excess fluid in the body can occur, the most common of which is allergy. But let's look at the other three culprits first.

Are you fat deficient?

The first of these is fat deficiency. Of course, for many people "fat" is a dirty word. Yet, as we learned in Chapter 8, you can't live without essential fats.

Have you ever wondered how the body could possibly be something like two thirds water? How do we keep it all in? The answer is fat. The body holds its water within cells encased in a membrane that's made mainly of essential fats. If you lack them in your diet, you lose the ability to maintain the right water balance. Your skin dries up and you may get dandruffy and sweaty. At the same time, your cells become waterlogged and you look puffy and gain weight.

As we've seen, essential fats are used in the body to make hormonelike substances called prostaglandins, which help control the body's water balance. In women, these fats also balance hormones throughout the menstrual cycle. Without them, the body is more likely to retain excess fluid, especially premenstrually or during menopause. So one way that consuming enough essential fats can help you to lose weight is through water loss, if you're suffering from water retention.

Are you "sugarlogged"?

You'll also retain excess fluid if your diet is full of sugar. There are two reasons for this. First, every molecule of sugar holds water wherever it is in the body and in whatever form it is in—glucose, glycogen, or fat. If a person is "sugarlogged" from eating too much sugar, he or she will retain excess fluid. While it is good to maintain proper glycogen stores, there is no need to have excess fat or excess circulating glucose. By balancing your blood sugar, you also help to prevent excess weight being stored as water.

Secondly, too much sugar and too much insulin lead to sodium (salt) retention. Normally the kidneys get rid of the right amount of sodium. However, when you lose control of your blood sugar, the kidneys don't filter out enough, so your body's sodium levels rise. Salt attracts water, and gradually your whole body becomes a little more waterlogged. In due course, blood sugar problems can lead to kidney problems, including kidney stone formation. This is one of the reasons why high-protein diets, which also tax the kidneys, are not advisable for those with blood sugar problems.

How are your kidneys?

Your kidneys filter your blood and regulate how much water to keep in your system and how much to excrete. This filtration happens through over a million clusters of tiny blood-vessel masses known as *glomeruli*, which collectively create a surface area about the size of your living room. Through the glomeruli you filter about 48 gallons of blood every day. Your ability to do this decreases with age so, especially if you are over 50, your kidneys may not be working 100 percent. This needn't be a problem, but there is a point at which it becomes one.

One of the telltale signs of decreasing kidney function is swollen ankles, especially after you've drunk a lot. This means the kidneys can't work fast enough to get rid of the excess fluid. One of the major reasons kidney function decreases is continual damage caused by peaks in blood sugar. The glucose damages the glomeruli. That's why people with diabetes are especially prone to kidney problems. If you do suspect you have poor kidney function, it's best to get this checked by your doctor and to stay away from high-protein diets (see page 342).

Another way you can give your kidneys a break, and help reduce excess water retention, is to take in more potassium and magnesium and less sodium. On average, a person in the United States is eating at least 4 to 5 grams of sodium a day, which is at least 5 times more than we need. The worst-offending foods are meat and processed foods.

Potassium and the mineral magnesium, both very abundant in fruits and vegetables, help balance out sodium in the body. Potassium works together with sodium in maintaining water balance and proper nerve and muscle impulses. The more sodium you eat, the more potassium you need, and few of us eat enough of the latter. Fruits, vegetables, and whole grains are rich in potassium. You need five servings of fruits and vegetables a day to get the right amount of it. Magnesium also helps balance hormones and helps solve premenstrual problems, especially breast tenderness.

A high-meat diet tends to be high in sodium, while a largely plant-based diet, with more vegetarian food, tends to be high in potassium and low in sodium. The Holford Diet is therefore naturally low in salt.

Salt content of foods

Food	Amount	Sodium contained
Bacon	2 slices	2g
Typical pizza	Large slice (11 oz.)	1.6g
BLT sandwich	1 (8 oz.)	1.6g
Cornflakes	1 bowl	1g
Cheddar cheese	1 oz.—a sandwich	0.5g
Instant soups	1 serving	1g or more
Potato chips	3 oz.	2.7g
Bread	3 oz.	1.3g
Hamburger and bun	1	1–2g
Sausages	3 oz.	5g

NOT ALL SALTS ARE CREATED EQUAL

Much sodium is hidden in the form of baking powder, brine, and monosodium glutamate. As we've seen, the net result of too much sodium is water retention and weight gain, and possibly high blood pressure and muscle cramps. While there is no need to add salt to food, since there's more than enough in natural foods, not all salts are created equal.

	Sodium	Potassium	Magnesium	Other trace minerals
Solo sea salt	41%	41%	17%	✓
Nu-Salt	0%	99%	0	0
Sea salt	<99%	0.2%	<1%	✓
Table salt	<100%	0	0	0

Table salt, the stuff you might sprinkle on your dinner, is pure sodium chloride. Sea salt isn't much better on the sodium front, although it does have tiny amounts of other beneficial minerals. Nu-Salt is okay on the sodium front, but doesn't contain any other minerals.

My favorite is Solo sea salt, which has also been shown to actually lower high blood pressure, according to research published in the *British Medical Journal*.[16] Since blood pressure and water retention are caused by the same dynamics, it's a good bet that sea salt will reduce the risk of water retention, and hence weight gain. This is because it has 60 percent less sodium and much more of the beneficial minerals potassium and magnesium.

Also check the foods you buy. Most processed foods use sodium chloride.

THE LOWDOWN ON REDUCING WATER RETENTION

In a nutshell, here's what you have to do to reduce the risk of excess water retention:

- balance your blood sugar
- eat five servings of fruits and vegetables every day
- eat seeds (rich in essential fats, plus magnesium and potassium)
- eat whole foods and whole grains such as beans, lentils, brown rice, and brown bread
- eat more oily fish (rich in essential fats) and less meat
- don't add salt to your food, unless it's sea salt
- choose "low sodium" processed foods
- drink the equivalent of eight glasses of water, including herbal teas, a day.

This alone may cause you to lose weight if water retention is part of your problem. But the real gold, in terms of weight loss, is to find out which foods you are allergic to and stay off them.

Is a hidden allergy leaving you waterlogged?

The most common reason for weight gain caused by fluid retention is allergy. The word "allergy" simply means an intolerance that causes a reaction in the immune system.

Your body is like a tube. The digestive tract, which has a surface area the size of a small soccer field, is the gateway between the outside world and your body. It's guarded ferociously by your immune system. If a substance that isn't on the guest list, so to speak, tries to gate-crash and get through your digestive tract and into the bloodstream, your immune system goes haywire.

But why does this lead to waterlogging and weight gain? The reason is twofold. First, histamine, the stuff that makes you sneeze when it's in your nose, makes the tiny blood vessels called capillaries more leaky. This allows the immune system's army of white blood cells to move into the battlefield. At the same time, more fluid passes into your tissues. If this is happening several times a day, you literally become waterlogged. Allergic reactions also mess up the balance of prostaglandins, and this too can lead to water retention as well as abdominal bloating.

Take the case of Joanne M., who is 36. She didn't have just weight to lose, but girth.

> *I used to stand in front of the mirror, grab a handful of my tummy—and despair. After a big meal I looked five months pregnant! It wasn't just my weight, which hovered around 154 pounds, it was the bloating (I'd gone up to a size 14) and the physical symptoms. I'd have to undo my trousers every time I had a big meal and I was often constipated.*
>
> *When I was in my late teens, I was diagnosed with irritable bowel syndrome [IBS]. Instead of looking for the cause, doctors simply prescribed drugs to ease the symptoms. Reading up about the problem, I got the impression a high-fiber diet would help the constipation and stop my tummy bloating. But my health regime of whole-meal bread, baked potatoes, and beans was actually making it worse.*
>
> *I felt exhausted all the time and usually fell asleep by 9:30 in the evening. My husband, Steve, kept telling me I had to do something about it. So in September 2002 I sent away for a food-intolerance blood test. The results told me I was sensitive to all dairy products, yeast, salmon, trout, haricot beans, and string beans. Within a week I was going to the loo [to have a bowel movement] every two days (instead of weekly), my tummy was gone and I was down to a size 10. My lethargy was caused by the yeasty foods I ate. I've gone from 156 pounds to 129 pounds and look so much trimmer now.*

The more often you are reacting allergically, the more resistant you become to insulin. This is because the body releases masses of immune messengers called *cytokines* to deal with the allergy, and cytokines make you less responsive to insulin. Also, repeated allergic reactions mean that more garbage ends up in your bloodstream as your immune cells fight off the invaders.

All this has to be cleaned up by your liver, your body's detoxifying organ. Eventually, the liver's detox capacity gets overloaded. When this happens, your body dumps the toxins in the least harmful place—your fat cells. The more full of toxins your fat cells become, the more weight you gain and the harder it becomes to take off those extra pounds. This is why people with allergies find it harder and harder to lose weight. Also, this continual process of toxin overload can turn a mild allergy into something more severe.

Many people don't find out about their allergies until it's really obvious.

Lori D., for instance, didn't think about testing herself for allergies until she nearly died at the age of 54 simply from drinking a glass of pineapple juice.

> *I weighed 119 pounds until 10 years ago when I suddenly went up to 210 pounds and size 18. One fateful evening I had a sore throat and drank a quart of pineapple juice throughout the night. By morning my throat had closed up, I could hardly breathe, and I'd turned purple. I drove to my GP, where I collapsed on the step.*
>
> *Because of this I decided to have proper food tests done, which proved that I was intolerant not only to milk and yeast, but also to pineapple [and to] cranberry and kidney beans. Now that I've cut out those foods, I feel really good. My once-stubby fingers are now slim and I've lost more than 7 pounds in two weeks. Knowing I'm food-intolerant helps as it makes me think about what I should be eating and helps me stick to my diet.*

DISCOVERING WHETHER YOU'RE ALLERGIC

Allergies can be responsible for many symptoms, especially digestive problems, from bloating to constipation, and from diarrhea to abdominal cramps. These are almost always accompanied by mental and physical symptoms, such as mood changes, chronic tiredness, depression, increased appetite, sleepiness after meals, inability to concentrate, and a host of minor ailments from itches and rashes to asthma and sinus problems. Check yourself out with the questionnaire below.

YOUR INSTANT ALLERGY CHECK

- ☐ Can you gain weight in hours?
- ☐ Do you get bloated after eating?
- ☐ Do you suffer from diarrhea or constipation?
- ☐ Do you suffer from abdominal pain?
- ☐ Do you sometimes get really sleepy after eating?
- ☐ Do you suffer from hay fever?
- ☐ Do you suffer from rashes, itches, asthma, or shortness of breath?
- ☐ Do you suffer from water retention (see the "Are you waterlogged?" questionnaire on page 101)?

- ☐ Do you suffer from headaches?
- ☐ Do you suffer from other aches or pains, from time to time, possibly after certain foods?
- ☐ Do you get better on vacations abroad, when your diet is completely different?

Any yes answer to these questions means there's a real possibility that you have an allergy. If you score four or more yeses, it's pretty much guaranteed.

As we've seen, bloating, pain, diarrhea, and constipation are often indicators of an allergy. Lisa M. is a classic case. She had suffered for six years with abdominal bloating before she figured out that the cause might be an allergy.

> My bloating was so bad that my boyfriend David measured round my waist and found I'd ballooned by 5 inches in one day. Anything I ate seemed to go straight through me—but despite that, I remained 5 stone [70 pounds] overweight. My doctor reckoned my body had gone into starvation mode, making the most of anything I fed it because of my tummy upsets.

Lisa then took a food-intolerance test, which revealed she was sensitive to eggs, milk, wheat, yeast, rye, and beef. "I'd been practically living on these foods," she said. "I had eggs for breakfast most days, and for lunch I'd often choose cottage cheese and egg sandwiches, thinking they were a healthy option. Little did I know I was poisoning myself."

Within three days of dropping the culprit foods, Lisa began to feel much better. "I've now gone six months without a tummy upset and I've lost nearly three stone [42 pounds]!" she said. "I feel like I have my life back."

PINPOINTING THE ALLERGEN

It may seem odd, but more often than not the foods people are allergic to are also the foods they really crave. If you're craving and eating something fre-

---

TOP TIP

Do you get bloated after eating and have to undo a button or two? If so, the chances are you are eating something you are allergic to.

quently, as though you're mildly addicted, there is a chance you're allergic to that food. Through my work with a number of allergic and overweight clients, it became clear to me that they were bingeing only on certain food groups. When they were instructed to eat as much as they liked of anything *except* the suspected allergen (the food provoking an allergic reaction), they often ceased bingeing. And when they avoided the allergen completely, they often lost 3 to 4 pounds and occasionally as much as 7 pounds, almost overnight.

This sort of short-term weight loss can only be the result of excess fluid retention, and nothing to do with fat. You can't burn *one* pound of fat in 24 hours, even if you are starving—much less 7!

One of the physical symptoms of an allergic reaction can be a sudden fluctuation in blood sugar level which, in turn, affects appetite. So could allergic reactions trigger bingeing? In honesty, nobody has a definite answer to this question, but my observations of a number of clients certainly show that sometimes allergies do play a role in overweight problems, and there's a one-in-three chance they play a role in yours.

There are two ways to find out what you are allergic to. The first we could call educated trial and error: avoid suspect foods for 14 days and note what happens by taking the pulse test, explained below.

The pulse test

Most people are free of symptoms within 14 days of avoiding an allergy-provoking food. And most will react on reintroducing the food within 48 hours, although some may have a reaction delayed by up to 10 days. Delayed reactions are much harder to test. For some, symptoms improve considerably when they leave out offending foods. For others, noticeable changes are slight.

One simple way to help identify possible suspects is the pulse test. The pulse test demands that you avoid all suspect foods for 14 days, then reintroduce them one by one, with a 48-hour gap between each item to be tested. Take your resting pulse, sitting down, before you eat the food, then take it again after 10 minutes, 30 minutes, and 60 minutes. Mark all this down on a chart like the

(continued on next page)

one on page 111. If you have a marked increase in pulse rate—more than 10 points—or have any symptoms of ill health within 24 hours, including immediate weight gain, bloating, fatigue, headache, or joint ache, for example, avoid the food and wait 24 hours before testing the next food.

The avoidance/reintroduction test for allergies. If you avoid a food you are allergic to, you may notice an improvement in how you feel within 14 days. If you then reintroduce the food, you may notice a return of symptoms.

While day-to-day changes in symptoms are hard to pin down to specific causes, avoidance of suspect foods for 14 days often lessens symptoms, which then increase significantly on reintroduction. So you'll be able to pinpoint which foods or drinks make you worse. It is very important to observe symptoms accurately because you may have preconceived ideas about what you do or don't react to, perhaps because of what somebody has told you, or because you dread being allergic to certain foods that you're addicted to.

(If you have ever had a severe or life-threatening allergic reaction, do this avoidance/reintroduction test *only* under the supervision of a suitably qualified practitioner.)

Suspect food	Pulse		Pulse and symptoms	
	Before	10 minutes	30 mins	60 mins
Milk	_____	_____	_____	_____
Yeast	_____	_____	_____	_____
Egg	_____	_____	_____	_____
Wheat	_____	_____	_____	_____
_____	_____	_____	_____	_____
_____	_____	_____	_____	_____

IGG ALLERGY TESTING—THE GOLD STANDARD

Because the body sometimes delays its allergic reaction to a food, avoidance/reintroduction tests don't always pick up the allergy. This happens because you may not suspect the food, and so do not test it. Or you may suspect only one food, yet be allergic to a range of them, so you'll continue to have a background of allergic reactions and may thus have difficulty losing weight.

The best and truly accurate way to find out what you are allergic to is to have what's called a *quantitative IgG ELISA test*. This is the gold standard of allergy testing. "Quantitative" means the test shows not only whether you are allergic, but also how strong your allergic reaction is. Many of us live quite healthily with minor allergies. But stronger allergies can create all sorts of problems, including weight gain. ELISA is the technology used. You don't need to know all the details but, trust me, it's the most accurate system and it's used by almost all the best allergy laboratories in the world.

To convey why the quantitative IgG ELISA test is so good, I need to explain a bit about the human immune system.

Your immune system can produce tailor-made weapons that latch onto specific substances to help escort them out of your body. They are like bouncers on the lookout for troublemakers. The bouncers are called *immunoglobulins,* or Ig for short. There are different types. The real heavies are called IgE, although most allergies involve IgG reactions. IgE reactions tend to be more immediate and severe, like Lori's reaction to pineapple. However, most "hidden" allergies that may be insidiously causing weight gain are IgG-based. In an ideal world you test for both, but I normally start by testing a person for IgG sensitivity to food.

All that's needed for testing is a pinprick of blood, which is absorbed into a tiny tube and sent to a laboratory. The lab then sends back an accurate read-out of exactly what you are allergic to. Your body doesn't lie. Either you have IgG bouncers tagged for wheat (for example) or you don't. Your diluted blood is introduced to a panel of liquid food "testers," and if you've got IgG for that food, a reaction takes place.

A number of laboratories do IgG testing (see page 366 in Resources), and one offers a handy test kit you can use at home. YorkTest has devised a clever procedure that involves a painless pinprick device and an absorbent material that you place against the pinprick. This material is then sent to the laboratory for testing (see page 366).

The good news about IgG-based allergies is that if you avoid the offending food strictly for three to six months, the body forgets that it is allergic to it. The reason is that there will no longer be any IgG antibodies to that food in your system. This doesn't hold for IgE-based reactions, however.

To give you an example, I have an IgE allergy to milk. I react within 15 minutes. Even if I avoid dairy products for a year, I still react if I consume it. I used to have an IgG to wheat. I avoided wheat for three months and now I no longer react. In my case, weight gain wasn't the problem: it was migraine headaches. I had them every other week from the age of 6 until I was 20, when I discovered that wheat and milk were triggering them.

Fenton R., like me, had regular headaches, sinusitis, and fatigue and had been plagued by acid indigestion for 20 years. He was also gaining weight year after year. Doctors were unable to help him, suggesting he drank too much soda and should exercise more. Indigestion tablets helped for only about 20 minutes before the problem returned with redoubled force.

He decided to have a food-intolerance test. The results came back showing he was intolerant of eggs, cow's milk, yeast, and wheat. He took all the rogue foods out of his diet, for example by switching to soy milk, and within two days the indigestion began to ease. Now it has gone completely, along with all the other health problems that had dogged him—including an excess 28 pounds in weight.

It feels as though a shroud has been lifted from me. Not only have I lost the weight, I have 100 percent more energy. It used to be an effort to go up the stairs. I used to get headaches most days, and they have gone. I used to get sinus twinges almost every day, and they have cleared up. I used to sweat a lot, and thought I was just a sweaty person. But now I can walk and run and just don't sweat. My skin used to be cold all the time, but now it's nice and warm. I feel more relaxed as well. It got to the stage where I couldn't even think clearly, but now I can do so once again.

THE USUAL SUSPECTS

The ten most common foods or food groups that people are allergic to are shown in the box that follows, in order. Of all these foods, by far the most common allergy-provoking substances are cow's milk, followed by yeast, eggs, and wheat. This doesn't necessarily mean that these foods are bad for you; that depends on whether you are allergic to them.

> ## The Top Ten common food allergies
> cow's milk
> yeast
> eggs
> wheat
> gliadin grains
> oats
> nuts
> beans
> white fish
> shellfish

COW'S MILK

This provides the most common food allergy. It's present in most cheeses, cream, yogurt, and butter and is hidden in all sorts of food; sometimes it's called *casein,* which is milk protein.

Logically, its status as an allergen isn't surprising, since it is a highly specific food, containing all sorts of hormones designed for the first few months of a *calf's* life. It's also a relatively recent addition to the human diet. Our ancestors, after all, weren't milking buffalo. Approximately 75 percent of people (25 percent of people of Caucasian origin and 80 percent of Asian, Native American, or African origin) stop producing lactase, the enzyme that's needed to digest milk sugar, once they've been weaned. Is nature trying to tell us something? However, it's not the lactose, the sugar in milk, that causes the allergic reaction. It's the protein.

If you react to cow's milk, you won't necessarily react to goat's milk or sheep's milk. However, many people do react to all dairy products. Because of this, you'll find that there is very little dairy in the recipes in Part Four. In most cases, if you strictly avoid your allergy-provoking foods for three months, your body can "unlearn" the allergy. So avoidance doesn't have to be a life sentence.

There are many alternatives to dairy now, including soy and quinoa "milks." Try them out and find one you like (but avoid rice milk, due to its high ⓖⓛ). Use the ⓖⓛ chart on pages 330–340 for your guide to quantity.

YEAST

After milk, yeast is the most common culprit in allergies. Yeast is not only in bread, as baker's yeast, it's also in beer and, to a lesser extent, wine. If you have been allergy tested, you'll know whether you are allergic to brewer's or baker's yeast. Most people who are allergic to yeast at all are allergic to both. Beer is fermented with brewer's yeast. If you've noticed that you feel worse after beer or wine than after spirits—the "cleanest" being vodka—then you may be yeast sensitive. Does this mean you can't drink? Not at all. Just stick to spirits and champagne! Champagne is made by a double-fermentation process that means there's much less yeast in it.

(A word about alcohol. As well as causing allergies in some, alcohol irritates the digestive tract, making it more permeable to undigested food proteins. This increases your chances of developing an allergic reaction to anything, and it's why some people feel worst when they both eat foods they are allergic to and drink alcohol. For example, you might be mildly allergic to wheat and milk and feel fine after either. But when you have both, plus alcohol, you don't feel great.)

Some people think they are allergic to wheat because they feel worse after eating bread. If you've noticed this—perhaps feeling sluggish, tired, or blocked up—but feel fine after pasta, you may not be allergic to wheat, but to the yeast in the bread.

Take Janette B., who is 45. Noticing her weight creeping up, Janette didn't link it with food sensitivity:

Over seven years my weight soared by 3 stone [42 pounds] to 13 and a half stone [189 pounds] and although I was a member of a slimming club, stuck strictly to a low-calorie diet, and took regular exercise, I could never lose more than about a stone [14 pounds].

Not only was Janette heavier than before, but also she felt constantly tired and uncomfortably bloated after meals, particularly when she'd eaten bread. "I was so frustrated by my weight and so fed up with feeling exhausted that I decided to have a food-intolerance test," she said. The results showed she was intolerant of yeast and milk and also sensitive to corn and soy, as well as navy and kidney beans. Simply by avoiding her "bad" foods, Janette lost 28 pounds in 5 months!

If you're allergic to yeast, you've got to be on the lookout for hidden yeast in stock cubes and processed food. As the Holford Diet features whole foods and fresh ingredients, and avoids yeasted breads, this should be far less of a problem for you. I also recommend using yeast-free vegetable stock cubes if they are available.

EGGS

Some people are allergic to egg white, but not egg yolk. If you are sensitive to eggs, when you come to reintroduce them, it's best to start by reintroducing egg yolk. If you don't react within five days, then reintroduce egg white. Eggs are in quite a lot of processed foods and bakery items, so check the label carefully.

WHEAT, GLIADIN GRAINS, AND OATS

Wheat is the grain that more people react to than any other. It contains gluten, a sticky protein also found in rye, barley, and oats. Gluten sensitivity occurs in about 1 in 100 people, but is medically diagnosed in fewer than 1 in 1,000.[17] However, it is a specific type of gluten, *gliadin*, which most people react to. The only way to know for sure exactly what you are allergic to is to have a food-intolerance test. If you have had an allergy test you'll know whether you are sensitive to gluten, gliadin, or wheat.

If you are gluten sensitive, then you cannot eat wheat, rye, barley, or oats. Excellent alternatives are rice, quinoa, buckwheat, millet, and corn (although some gluten-sensitive people do react to corn). Quinoa and millet cook in 15 minutes, in much the same way as rice. From the **GL** point of view, quinoa is the best. These days, you can find rice, corn, and buckwheat breads and pastas in bigger supermarkets and good health food stores.

However, there's no gliadin in oats. If you are gliadin sensitive, then you can eat oats, but not wheat, rye, or barley.

If you are sensitive only to wheat, the "fix" is relatively easy. Just eat rye, barley, or oats. For example, you can eat rye bread, oatcake crackers, oatmeal, and oat-flake cereals, but not Weetabix or wheat bread.

In the big scheme of things, wheat's prominence as an allergen shouldn't be surprising. Grains are the second-most-recent addition into the human diet, and weren't eaten by hunter-gatherers. They have been eaten by farmers for something like the last 10,000 years, but only in certain parts of the world. For example, no gluten grain naturally grows in North America, so Native Americans have been exposed to gluten for only about the last 200 years at most.

A worrisome trend in the United States, where low-carb diets are the craze, is to remove the carbohydrates from wheat products so you're eating just the protein portion. As the protein is principally gluten, it's a recipe for disaster for anyone with a hidden gluten allergy.

NUTS AND BEANS

These are part of the same food family, along with fruit seeds. In essence, they're all seeds. The most common individual allergens in this group are, in descending order, cashews, Brazil nuts, almonds, peanuts, navy beans, and soybeans. You can react to one and no others, but if you do react to one member of this family there's a greater chance that you'll react to another member of the seed/bean/nut family. Coffee, from the coffee bean, and chocolate, from the cocoa bean, are also members of this family.

WHITEFISH AND SHELLFISH

This is another major allergen, but most people who are allergic to it react to whitefish, not to oily fish such as salmon, mackerel, and herring, which are so rich in omega-3s. If you're also allergic to those kinds, have a tablespoon of ground seeds with breakfast every day (see page 153), together with a good-quality supplement, to keep your essential fatty acids topped up.

Shellfish allergies are very common, with prawns and abalone two of the worst villains. You may be allergic to mussels, scallops, whelks, oysters, and squid, which are all mollusks, or to lobsters, crayfish, prawns, and shrimp, which are all crustaceans. Octopus is in a world of its own! Be careful here, though. If you're allergic to squid but not to octopus, be aware that some people sell squid as octopus to make a bigger profit, because they can buy it more cheaply.

If you suffer from food allergies, you don't have to feel deprived on the Holford Diet. It is always sensible to vary your diet as much as possible, and the menu plans and recipes in Chapters 27 and 28 are designed to include a wide range of ingredients. Such a varied diet, together with the introduction of exciting new foods such as quinoa, soy products, and legumes such as flageolet and cannellini beans, ensures that there is plenty to tempt your taste buds, even if you do have to avoid certain items.

When you have an allergy test, the best laboratories give you clear instructions on what not to eat and what you can eat, as well as giving you the backup of a nutritionist to answer any of your questions. If you avoid foods that cause symptoms, you will probably find that your health improves in ways that you didn't ever imagine. I can't count the times I've heard people say, "I didn't even know I could feel this good." The Holford Diet and supplements will also help to reduce your allergic potential further.

After three months of abstaining from the allergen, you may then find that you can tolerate it in small periodic "doses." For some people, the allergy disappears completely. Others have to be careful about certain foods for life. Once you have more than a sneaking suspicion that you are allergic, it is best to have an allergy test.

- Find out whether you are allergic to something you're eating, and if so, avoid it. You can do an avoidance/reintroduction test but, quite frankly, it's better to have a proper quantitative IgG ELISA test.
- After three months, you can reintroduce the foods you tested positive for, although ideally you should not eat them every day.
- Even if you are not allergic to it, reduce the amount of cow's milk you eat and drink, substituting goat cheeses, soy products, and the like.
- Even if you are not allergic to it, reduce the amount of wheat you eat, substituting other grains such as oats, rye, and rice.
- Limit alcohol. Ideally, drink no more than three small glasses of wine, half-pints of beer, or measures of spirits a week.
- Drink the equivalent of eight glasses of water a day.

Part Three shows you how to do all this.

10

Step 4: Take the Right Supplements

So far, you've learned that by changing the quality of the big guys—fats, carbohydrates, and proteins—you can lose weight because your body's metabolism finally starts working properly. Now, I'd like to take a look at the little guys: vitamins and minerals.

Your body's daily functions depend on a myriad of chemical reactions which, in turn, depend on vitamins and minerals. Your fatburning capability, for instance, relies on your getting optimal amounts of certain micronutrients. For example, to make insulin, you need zinc and vitamin B_6. Insulin's ability to control blood sugar levels is helped by the mineral chromium. To turn glucose into energy, rather than fat, you need B vitamins, magnesium, and vitamin C. And to burn fat you need all these, plus the B vitamin biotin.

No doubt you've heard the mantra "As long as you eat a balanced diet, you get all the vitamins and minerals you need" from someone, sometime. As I've said, this is the greatest lie in nutrition today. Why? Because there's only a slim chance that your diet meets even the full range of RDAs—and also because it all hangs on your definition of "need" as well as what you want from life.

RDAs, or *recommended daily allowances,* of vitamins and minerals are in any case misleading at best. Governments the world over have worked these out by starting from the bottom—that is, looking merely at preventing the obvious vitamin-deficiency diseases. These range from scurvy (vitamin C deficiency) and beriberi (vitamin B_1) to pellagra (niacin). But, as we learn more and more about the health-promoting properties of vitamins and minerals, RDAs have crept up and up. In the UK, for instance, the RDA for vitamin C has moved up from 30 milligrams to 45 milligrams to 60 milligrams, and in the United States it's now 85 milligrams.

The problems with RDAs go further than this, though. They are mere averages, and you are far from average. You are unique. According to Dr. Roger Williams, a pioneer in nutrition who discovered vitamin B_5 (pantothenic acid) and helped discover folic acid, even identical twins can have twentyfold differences in their nutritional needs![18] Where you live, how much exercise you get, your gender, and your genes can easily alter your needs for various nutrients by a factor of 10. That's why I call the RDAs "ridiculous dietary arbitraries." So, if you are happy with average poor health, go for the RDAs.

Optimum nutrition, maximum weight loss

Let's say, though, that you want the most out of life. You want to be the right weight and stay there, and you see your health not just as an absence of ill health, but as total well-being. If this is you, you need *optimum* nutrition.

At ION, we worked out micronutrient needs by starting from the top. We sought the intake of a vitamin that would promote optimal health, not just prevent scurvy. We asked the question "What amount of vitamin X equates to the maximum possible well-being and the smallest possible risk of disease?" For the past 20 years, we've been investigating the effects of vitamins, minerals, and essential fats on weight, IQ, memory, mood, energy, immunity, infections, life span, pregnancy, and disease risk. From this we established the ODAs, or *optimum daily allowances*. These are the amounts of nutrients that will tune up your body's metabolism, making it easier for you to lose weight, and keep it off for good.

Have a look at the chart on p. 120. You'll notice that the ODAs are often 10 times the RDAs. You'll also see what the average diet provides—and what you could be achieving if you were eating a healthier diet, with plenty of whole foods, fruit, and vegetables. But there's still a shortfall between what we've researched as optimum and what you are likely to get in food.

And that's where supplements come in. They make up the difference—the difference between how you feel now and how you *could* feel if you were optimally nourished, losing weight steadily, and feeling fantastic.

NUTRIENTS	RDA	Average diet (100% RDA)	Good diet	Shortfall	ODA
Vitamin A (mcg)	800	900	1500	Shortfall 1000	2,500
Vitamin D (mcg)	5	4	7	Shortfall 4	11
Vitamin E (mg)	10	14	50	Shortfall 250	300
Vitamin C (mg)	60	100	200	Shortfall 1800	2,000
Vitamin B₁ (mg)	1.4	2	5	Shortfall 30	35
Vitamin B₂ (mg)	1.6	2.18	5	Shortfall 30	35
Vitamin B₃ (mg)	18	39.6	50	Shortfall 35	85
Vitamin B₅ (mg)	6	2.175	20	Shortfall 80	100
Vitamin B₆ (mg)	2	3.1	5	Shortfall 70	75
Folic Acid (mcg)	200	325.5	400	Shortfall 400	800
Vitamin B₁₂ (mcg)	1	5.95	10	Shortfall 15	25
Biotin (mcg)	150	36.50	120	Shortfall 105	225
GLA* (Omega-6) (mg)	–	20	40	Shortfall 110	150
EPA/DHA* (Omega-3) (mg)	–	60	100	Shortfall 600	700
Calcium (mg)	800	(800:good diet)	912.5	Shortfall 200	1,000
Iron (mg)	14	12.8	15	Shortfall 5	20
Magnesium (mg)	300	272	350	Shortfall 150	500
Zinc (mg)	15	9.3 / 10		Shortfall 10	20
Iodine (mcg)	150	193.5	240	Shortfall 60	300
Selenium (mcg)*	–	40	50	Shortfall 50	100
Chromium (mcg)*	–	50	75	Shortfall 50	125
Manganese (mcg)*	–	3	6	Shortfall 4	10

Key

■ Average diet
▨ Good diet

RDA = Recommended daily allowance
ODA = Optimum daily allowance (diet plus supplements)
* items marked with an asterisk have no RDA

RDAs versus ODAs and dietary intakes. This chart shows the differences between the RDA, our average intake, and our ideal intake. The gray amounts are the levels we could reach if we ate a good variety of fruit and vegetables daily—i.e., a good diet.

Using vitamin C as an example, the RDA is 60mg. The average intake is 100mg. If you eat plenty of fruit and vegetables you could achieve 200mg. The optimal intake is somewhere between 1,000 and 3,000mg. The ODA is set at the midpoint of 2,000mg. The shortfall between a good diet (200mg) and the ODA (2,000 mg) is 1,800mg. This is the kind of level worth supplementing.

Turning glucose into fuel, not fat

To understand how vitamins and minerals help with the crucial job of fat-burning, let's take a close look at what happens to glucose in the body.

The brain, muscles, liver, skin, immune system, heart, and arteries are all simply collections of cells that do different jobs for the body, whether it's digesting, thinking, or moving. The fuel that keeps them going is, as we've found, glucose. So maintaining an even level of blood sugar—the cells' fuel reserve—is the first step in making energy.

Within each of our 30 trillion or so cells exist tiny energy factories called *mitochondria*. These turn glucose into another chemical, *pyruvic acid,* a process that releases a small amount of energy, which can be used by the cell to carry out its work. If there isn't enough oxygen around while this is happening, a by-product called *lactic acid* builds up. That's why, when you do strenuous exercise after a relatively sedentary period, your muscles ache the next day. The more you exercise, developing larger muscles, the less strain you put on them and the more oxygen they can use. This is what aerobic exercise is all about—providing muscle cells with enough oxygen so they can work properly.

Next, pyruvic acid is turned into *acetyl-coenzyme A,* or AcoA. This substance is perhaps the most vital in fueling our body, because if you're starved of glucose, as when for example a marathon runner "hits the wall," you can break down fat or protein to make AcoA and use this for energy. But, because this method is relatively inefficient, your body prefers to rely on carbohydrates, and glucose, for fuel.

From this point on, oxygen is needed every step of the way. AcoA enters a series of chemical reactions known as the *Krebs cycle* (named after its discoverer, Ernst Krebs). During this cycle, hydrogen molecules split off, meet oxygen—and *bang!* Energy is released. In fact over 90 percent of all our energy is derived from this final stage. The waste products from this process are carbon dioxide (which we exhale), water (which goes to form urine), and heat. That's why you get hot when you exercise. Muscle cells make lots of energy, creating heat.

Best vitamins for fatburning

Complex carbohydrates and oxygen are only half the story. All these chemical reactions are carefully controlled by enzymes, which are themselves dependent on no fewer than nine vitamins and six minerals (see the figure on the facing page). Any shortage of these critical catalysts and your energy factories, the mitochondria, go out of tune. The result is inefficient energy production, a loss of stamina, and highs and lows—or just lows. These lead to cravings. And whatever your body can't easily turn into energy, it turns into fat. So part of the weight-control equation is making energy efficiently.

The important vitamins here are the B-complex vitamins, a family of eight different substances. Every one is essential for making energy. Glucose can't be turned into pyruvic acid without B_1 and B_2 (niacin). AcoA won't work properly without B_1, B_2, B_3, and, most important of all, B_5 (pantothenic acid). The Krebs cycle needs B_1, B_2, and B_3 to do its job properly, along with vitamin C. Fats and proteins can't be used to make energy without B_1, B_2, B_6, B_{12}, folic acid, and biotin.

It used to be thought that as long as you ate a reasonable diet you'd get enough B vitamins. But studies have shown that, over the long term, slight deficiencies—which are all too easy to develop—result in depletion of these vitamins within cells. The results can be serious. Early warning signs are poor skin condition, anxiety, depression, mental confusion and irritability, fatigue, and excessive weight in particular. Health and diet surveys, including our own, consistently show that people who take multivitamins containing B vitamins are less overweight.

Most people's diets fall short of the optimal requirements for these vital vitamins, and few even achieve the basic RDAs. In one ION study a group of 82 volunteers, many of whom already had a "well-balanced diet," were assessed to calculate their optimal nutritional needs.[19] All 82 were given extra B vitamins in supplement form, often in doses 20 times as high as the RDAs. After six months, 79 percent of participants reported a definite improvement in energy, 61 percent felt physically fitter, and 60 percent had noticed an improvement in their mental alertness and memory.

Being water-soluble and extremely sensitive to heat, B vitamins are easily lost when foods are boiled. The best natural sources are therefore fresh fruit, raw vegetables, and wheat germ. Seeds, nuts, and whole grains contain reasonable amounts, as do meat, fish, eggs, and dairy products. But these levels are reduced when the food is cooked or stored for a long time.

As well as eating these foods—and Part Three will give you the details— I strongly recommend that you use a high-strength multivitamin supplement to guarantee an optimal intake of all the B vitamins, plus at least 1,000 milligrams of vitamin C.

Turning food into energy. The glucose we eat is converted within our cells to release and give us energy. This is done by enzymes that, in turn, depend on vitamins and minerals. Consuming enough vitamins and minerals helps turn food into energy instead of fat.

Best minerals for fatburning

The minerals iron, calcium, magnesium, chromium, and zinc are also vital for making energy. Calcium and magnesium are perhaps the most important because all muscle cells need an adequate supply of these to be able to contract and relax. A shortage of magnesium, which is very common in people who don't eat a lot of fruit or vegetables, often results in cramps, as muscles are unable to relax. Magnesium is involved in 75 percent of the enzymes in your body—and it is absolutely vital for blood sugar control and burning carbohydrate for energy, rather than storing it as fat.[20] While most diets provide enough calcium, few provide enough magnesium. Good multivitamins will give you an additional 150 milligrams of magnesium and calcium. It is well worth taking a supplement.

Zinc, together with vitamin B_6, is needed to make the enzymes that digest food.[21] Zinc and B_6 are also essential in the production of insulin. A lack of zinc disturbs appetite control and causes a loss of taste or smell, a combination that often leads to overeating of meat, cheese, and other strong-tasting foods. Zinc deficiency is very widespread. The optimal intake is 20 milligrams a day, while the average intake is 9 milligrams.

It's well worth correcting this shortfall by taking a daily multivitamin/mineral that gives you 10 milligrams of zinc, as well as eating zinc-rich foods such as seeds and "seed" foods, meaning anything you could plant in the ground that would grow. This includes beans, lentils, and peas. Broccoli, including the "Tenderstem" variety (also known as broccolini), is also a good source. And oysters are the very best. If you ate an oyster a day, you wouldn't need to supplement with zinc!

CHROMIUM—THE SECRET OF BALANCING BLOOD SUGAR

The older you are, the less likely you are to be getting enough chromium—an essential mineral that helps stabilize blood sugar levels and, hence, weight.[22] The average daily intake is below 50 micrograms, while an optimal intake, certainly for those with a weight and blood sugar problem, is around 200 micrograms. Chromium is found in whole foods and is therefore higher in whole-wheat flour, bread, or pasta than in refined products. (Flour has 98 percent of its chromium removed in the refining process—another reason to stay away from overprocessed products.) Beans, nuts, and seeds are other good sources, and asparagus and mushrooms are especially rich in chromium.

Since chromium works with insulin to help stabilize your blood sugar level, appetite, and weight, the more uneven your blood sugar level, the more chromium you use up. Hence a sugar and stimulant addict, eating refined foods, is most at risk of deficiency.

Two studies carried out at Bemidji State University in Minnesota have shown that chromium supplementation helps to build muscle and burn fat.[23] Because it helps to lower cholesterol as well as stabilize blood sugar levels, it is especially helpful for people at a high risk of developing diabetes.[24] And, in trials where it was taken by people who made no change to their diets, chromium had a small effect on weight loss compared with placebos.[25] The real benefit of chromium supplementation is that it reduces sugar cravings and hence your appetite for the wrong foods. So, all in all, taking chromium, following the Holford Diet, and getting exercise are a winning formula.

Whether or not you can achieve an optimal intake of chromium from diet alone is debatable. It is therefore wise to take supplements of this fat-burning mineral as well as to eat whole foods. The best form of chromium is chromium polynicotinate, which means it's bound with vitamin B_3 (also called *nicotinic acid*). Most good multivitamins will contain 30 micrograms of chromium, but you can help balance your blood sugar and reduce sugar cravings more quickly by taking 200–400 micrograms a day for the first three months of the Holford Diet. Chromium supplements, usually in 200-microgram amounts, are readily available in any health food store.

Diet pills—the next generation

I'm hardly a fan of diet pills. Few actually work, and those that do often act like stimulants, speeding up your metabolism and giving you short-term weight loss—and potential *long-term* problems. Over time, some may end up slowing down your metabolism, and may even promote weight gain. This category includes ephedra (now banned), guarana, and other sources of caffeine. Others, such as conjugated linolenic acid (CLA for short), promised great results in animal studies, but failed to deliver significant weight loss in human trials.[26]

There are two, however, that I like and recommend: hydroxycitric acid (HCA for short) and 5-hydroxytryptophan, or 5-HTP.

HCA CURBS YOUR APPETITE
HCA is extracted from the dried rind of the tamarind fruit *(Garcinia cambogia),* which you may know from Indian and other Eastern cuisine. HCA is not a vitamin, but it will help you lose weight. Originally developed by the pharmaceutical giant Hoffmann-LaRoche, it has been proved to slow down the production of fat and reduce appetite. It has been extensively tested and found to have no toxicity or safety concerns.

HCA works by inhibiting the enzyme that converts sugar into fat. The carbohydrate in a meal is first used to provide fuel and short-term energy stores as glycogen. Any excess is then converted to fat by the enzyme ATP-citrate lyase. HCA dampens down the activity of this enzyme. Evidence of HCA's fatburning properties has been accumulating since 1965.[27] For example, participants in one eight-week, double-blind trial reported an average weight loss of 11 pounds, 2 ounces per person, compared with 4 pounds, 3 ounces on a dummy pill.

HCA also reduces the synthesis of fat and cholesterol. Animal studies have confirmed this, and it may be that HCA has a role to play in helping those with high triglyceride (fat) or blood cholesterol levels. There is also evidence that HCA may enhance the burning of calories and increase energy levels. According to John Sterling, whose company BioCare was among the first to introduce HCA in the UK, "People are reporting very positive results. HCA doesn't help everybody, but it is helping about 50 percent of those who've tried it."

A recent trial conducted by the University of Maastricht in the Netherlands confirms that HCA acts as a powerful appetite suppressant, reducing weight with no harmful effects. In the study—which was the best kind, a so-called double-blind, placebo-controlled, randomized, crossover trial—12 men and women were given a tomato juice drink three times a day for two weeks. They then had a two-week break. Following this, the group were divided up, unbeknownst to them. Some participants drank tomato juice with a placebo, others one containing 300 milligrams of HCA, three times a day for the next two weeks.

Only those taking the HCA-loaded drink ate less—a total of 15 to 30 percent fewer calories. However, they didn't report that they tried to eat less, tried to restrict their diet, or experienced any loss of enjoyment regarding their food. They just happened to eat less. They also lost more weight, averaging 1 pound of extra weight loss a week.[28]

I recommend taking HCA, especially during the first three months of the Holford Diet. Most supplements provide 450 milligrams per capsule. You need twice this amount to make a difference, so take one capsule up to half an hour before two meals each day. It is widely available as a supplement.

5-HTP HELPS YOU "THINK THIN"

Have you ever thought about why you get hungry? You might think the obvious answer is because you haven't eaten. But that isn't always true, is it? And don't you often find yourself craving something sweet even though you've just eaten more than enough food?

The two most powerful controllers of your appetite are your blood sugar level and your brain's level of serotonin, the "happy" neurotransmitter. Serotonin is made from an amino acid, or building block of protein, called *tryptophan.* Many people have low levels of this vital brain chemical and feel depressed as a result. This is especially true of people on weight-loss diets, most of which are notoriously low in tryptophan.

But that isn't all. Serotonin controls appetite. The more you have, the less you eat—and the less you have, the more you eat (most people eat more when they are depressed, and low in serotonin).

If you are low in serotonin, one of the quickest ways to restore normal levels, and normal mood, is to supplement your diet with a special form of tryptophan called 5-hydroxytryptophan, or 5-HTP for short. It's found in meat, fish, and beans, although in rather small amounts. But one, the African Griffonia bean, contains significant amounts, and extracts of Griffonia are sold as 5-HTP supplements.

It's not just speculation that 5-HTP works: it's been proven to make you feel happier and want to eat less. While it's been known for some time that giving 5-HTP to animals causes a reduction in appetite, followed by a loss in weight, two recent studies, conducted by Dr. C. Cangiano and colleagues at the Department of Clinical Medicine, University of Rome (La Sapienza), in Italy, show that 5-HTP does the same thing in overweight people.[29]

In the first study, 20 obese volunteers took either 5-HTP (900 milligrams) or a placebo for 12 weeks. During the first six weeks, volunteers could eat what they liked. During the second six weeks the volunteers were recommended a low-calorie diet. In both phases those taking 5-HTP consistently ate less, felt more satisfied, and consequently lost weight.[30] What was particularly interesting was that they ate less carbohydrate.

The second study gave 25 overweight non-insulin-dependent diabetic volunteers either 5-HTP or a placebo for two weeks, with no dietary restriction. They could eat what they liked. In the words of the researchers, "Patients receiving 5-HTP significantly decreased their daily energy intake, by reducing carbohydrate and fat intake, and reduced their body weight."[31]

Why the reduced craving for carbohydrates? Imagine two breakfasts. One is an Atkins-style bacon and eggs, high in protein. The other is cornflakes with chopped banana and a muffin. Which will give your serotonin a boost, thereby satisfying you more? If you think about it logically, you'd say the

> **TOP TIP**
>
> Have one low-**GL** carbohydrate-only snack a day. This raises the brain's level of serotonin, which makes you happier and reduces sugar and carbohydrate cravings.

protein-rich, hence tryptophan-rich, breakfast. But you'd be wrong. It's the cornflakes, banana, and muffin breakfast.

Why? Even though the bacon and eggs do contain tryptophan, it has a hard time getting from your blood into your brain—it just doesn't compete well with all the other amino acids in these high-protein foods. However, it does get into the bloodstream. So what drives it into your brain? The answer is insulin. Insulin, which is released by a high-carbohydrate breakfast, carries tryptophan into the brain, and gives you a mood boost. What this means is that when you are feeling tired, hungry, and a little blue you crave something sweet, not a sausage. Sound familiar?

One big secret of successful weight loss is to (a) ensure you have enough serotonin so you have less desire to eat in excess and (b) keep your blood sugar level, and insulin release, even, so you don't have increased appetite due to blood sugar dips. Remember, too much insulin drives blood sugar into body fat, while too little means low serotonin levels and increased carbohydrate cravings. It's a careful balancing act and one that the Holford Diet takes into account. Here's what I recommend to maximize weight loss.

Fatburning supplements—the basics

I recommend that you supplement your well-balanced diet with fatburning vitamins and minerals, to ensure your metabolism is working at peak efficiency. The ideal intake is different for every individual and can be personalized for you by a nutritional therapist (see page 362). However, the chart below gives a good approximation of the optimal supplement levels for an average person, given that he or she is eating a healthful, balanced diet.

Vitamins	Optimum daily intake
Vitamin A	1,500mcg
Vitamin B$_1$ (thiamine)	25mg
Vitamin B$_2$ (riboflavin)	25mg

Vitamin B$_3$ (niacin)	50mg
Vitamin B$_5$ (pantothenate)	50mg
Vitamin B$_6$ (pyridoxine)	50mg
Vitamin B$_{12}$ (cobalamine)	10mcg
Folic acid	200mcg
Biotin	50mcg
Vitamin C	1,000mg
Vitamin D	5mcg
Vitamin E (d-alpha tocopherol)	100mg

Minerals	Optimum daily intake
Calcium	200mg
Magnesium	150mg
Iron	10mg
Zinc	10mg
Manganese	3mg
Chromium	30mcg

In summary, what this means is taking, on a daily basis:

DAILY SUPPLEMENTS
2 × multivitamin/mineral
1 × vitamin C 1,000mg

Most health food stores can help you find supplements to meet these levels in the simplest and least expensive way, choosing from a variety of good brands. Decent, high-strength multivitamin/mineral supplements will tell you to take two a day—you just can't get these optimum levels in one tablet. Supplements should be taken with food, preferably with breakfast, or spread throughout the day, since it is during the day that we make most energy and hence need a good supply of these nutrients.

Fatburning supplements—pulling out the stops

During the first three months, if you want all the help you can get in stabilizing your appetite and sugar cravings, I recommend the combination of HCA, 5-HTP, and chromium. These are the daily levels you need for maximum effect:

	Optimum daily intake
Hydroxycitric acid (HCA)	900mg
5-hydroxytryptophan (5-HTP)	100–200mg
Chromium	200–400mcg

Bear in mind that 5-HTP is much more effective at normalizing the brain's serotonin levels if taken with some carbohydrate, such as a piece of fruit. This will also help prevent the slight abdominal discomfort that a small minority of people get when they take 5-HTP. My advice, therefore, is to supplement both your morning and afternoon snacks with 50 milligrams of 5-HTP.

A word of caution: Don't take 5-HTP if you are on selective serotonin reuptake inhibitor drugs (SSRIs) such as Prozac (fluoxetine), Paxil (paroxetine), or Zoloft (sertraline), to name just a few. These drugs block the reuptake of serotonin, while 5-HTP provides the brain with the raw material to make enough in the first place. (Logically, 5-HTP should be a more effective antidepressant with fewer side effects. It is—and if you want the proof, see my book *Optimum Nutrition for the Mind*.) Theoretically, taking both could overload you with serotonin. Although I know of no case as such, I don't recommend taking both antidepressant drugs and 5-HTP.

Also take 200 micrograms of chromium twice a day, with your mid-morning and afternoon snack. Both these supplements tend to reduce sugar cravings and make you feel less hungry and more satiated.

HCA works best before meals. Most supplements supply 450 milligrams per tablet or capsule. You need twice this amount to make a difference, so take one capsule up to half an hour before two meals each day.

All these supplements are easy to find in most health food stores.

- Supplement with a high-strength multivitamin and mineral, plus vitamin C every day.
- Supplement with additional chromium, HCA and 5-HTP, especially if you are prone to sugar cravings and have poor appetite control, for the first three months.

Part Three shows you how to do all this, too.

11

Step 5: Do 15 Minutes
of Exercise a Day

The body is designed to be active. If you've ever truly enjoyed exercise—anything from a brisk walk in the park to trekking in the Himalayas—you'll know that wonderful feeling of being at ease and at one with your body. But, even if you've hated exercise, were "bad at sports" as a child, and wouldn't touch an activity vacation with a barge pole, you'll find that the kind of exercise I advocate is amazingly easy to get into, and enjoy.

Exercise is the final puzzle piece in the fatburning picture. Let's take a look at why, and how, it works.

Why exercise?

If you haven't led a very active life, or did once but have gradually become more sedentary, it's not surprising. Life in the West conspires against it. Cars, remote controls, food processors, home-delivery restaurants, "home entertainment centers," escalators, elevators . . . every year, there are more gadgets and conveniences that do away with the need to expend energy. Ultimately, all roads here lead straight to the sofa, and, if you give in, couch-potato syndrome awaits.

Once that happens, it's all too easy to pile on the pounds. There is no doubt that part of the reason for the massive increase in the number of overweight people is that we are becoming less active.[32] And not only does less activity mean fewer calories burned, but also it interferes with the body's appetite mechanisms, rate of metabolism, and ability to keep blood glucose levels stable. In other words, some exercise is essential for the body's chemistry to stay "tuned up."

Now, according to calorie theory, exercise is a poor method of losing weight. After all, running a mile burns up only 300 calories. That's equivalent to two slices of toast or a piece of apple pie. But this argument misses three key points.

1. **The effects of exercise are cumulative.** Okay, so running a mile a day burns up only 300 calories. But if you do that three days a week for a year, that's 22,000 calories, theoretically equivalent to a weight loss of 11 pounds! Also, the number of calories you burn up depends on how fat or fit you are to start with. The fatter and less fit you are, the more benefit you'll derive from small bouts of exercise.

2. **Moderate exercise decreases your appetite.** A degree of physical activity is necessary for appetite mechanisms to work properly. Those who do not exercise have exaggerated appetites and hence the pounds gradually creep on.

3. **Exercise boosts your metabolic rate.** The most important reason exercise is a key to weight loss is its effect on your metabolic rate. According to Professor William McArdle, an exercise physiologist at City University of New York, "Most people can generate metabolic rates that are 8 to 10 times above their resting value during sustained cycling, running, or swimming. Complementing this increased metabolic rate is the observation that vigorous exercise will raise metabolic rate for up to 15 hours after exercise." [33]

Dynamic duo—diet and exercise

Combining diet and exercise is the best way to lose weight. Weight lost through restrictive dieting is often half fat and half lean tissue, such as muscle. Since muscle burns up more energy (calories) than fat, the less muscle you have, the slower your metabolism is. Combining the Holford Diet with a good exercise program ensures you lose fat, not lean muscle. The best kinds of exercises to help to burn fat efficiently are brisk walking, jogging, cycling, swimming, aerobic dance, stepping, cross-country skiing, circuit training, or any aerobic exercise that is steady, continuous, and of a certain intensity.

Such exercises also tone the body, reduce the risk of osteoporosis, increase muscle tissue, and reduce one's body fat percentage (high ratios of body fat to lean tissue have been linked to heart disease, diabetes, and some cancers). They will strengthen your heart and lungs, reduce your risk of heart disease, help control stress, and improve circulation.

Exercise improves insulin sensitivity

But exercise does more than make you leaner. It also helps regulate body chemistry that's essential for fatburning. According to Vanessa Hebditch of the British Diabetic Association, "Being overweight reduces insulin sensitivity so the risk of developing diabetes is higher. However, there is proof that exercise increases insulin sensitivity, thereby reducing risk." A 24-year study of nearly 6,000 men found that increased physical activity was linked to a reduction in the risk of diabetes, regardless of the level of obesity.

Exercise is especially important in middle age because we are less likely to be able to maintain an even blood sugar level as we age.[34] Unsurprisingly, our sensitivity to insulin decreases with age, along with our control of blood sugar. But physical activity in middle and old age improves insulin sensitivity, therefore helping to stabilize blood sugar levels and weight.[35] Athletes have vastly improved blood sugar control, enhanced insulin sensitivity, and faster metabolic rates.[36]

And there's more. High-intensity exercises such as aerobics reduce insulin levels and raise glucagon levels. This means you improve your production of good prostaglandins, boost circulation (and thus the supply of oxygen and nutrients to cells), and increase your ability to burn fat.

Anaerobic exercise such as lifting weights doesn't burn fat in the same way, or to the same extent. If it is intense enough, though, it may release human growth hormone (controlled by good prostaglandins), which builds muscle and burns fat.

In short, exercise offers a huge array of benefits. If you haven't really gotten into it before, it opens up an undiscovered world of vitality, health—and sheer enjoyment.

> **TOP TIP**
> Go for a stroll after a meal, especially if you tend to get sleepy after you eat. It helps to stabilize your blood sugar and insulin level.

How much exercise?

Exercise shouldn't mean a fanatical struggle for some mythical level of fitness. The important thing is merely to stay within the "training heart rate zone" for your age. Appendix 5 shows you how to work this out (see page 355).

The most traditional formula for calculating your "training heart rate zone" is to subtract your age from 220. This allows you to estimate your maximum heart rate. This is not the level at which you need to work; it is the predicted maximum your heart can perform at. Once you have calculated your maximum then it is one small step to calculating your training zone.

An overweight, out-of-condition person may reach his or her training heart rate zone by walking just a few hundred yards. A fitter, leaner person may have to walk briskly for at least five minutes to push his or her pulse up to the training zone. This is why you need to monitor your pulse while exercising to make sure that you do not over- or underexercise, and that you achieve the best fatburning benefits. As you get fitter and leaner, you'll find that you will have to push harder—perhaps by walking faster or adding more hill walking to your program—to reach your training zone.

According to surveys, the best benefits in terms of longevity come from expending more than 2,000 calories a week in exercise. Walking uses up 300 calories an hour, so you'd need to walk for six hours a week. Jogging is twice as efficient, so you'd need to do only three hours a week. The more overweight you are, the more calories you burn up, so you may need to do only two hours.

If you are doing the right kind of exercise, all you need to do is 15 minutes a day. And this will be enough both for losing weight and for trimming your figure. If you want to confine your exercising to the working week, you can do 21 minutes Monday to Friday and leave the weekend free. Alternatively, you may choose to double up and exercise three times a week for 35 minutes. It doesn't sound that difficult, does it? And it isn't.

When to exercise

The best time to exercise is two hours after eating. If you exercise first thing in the morning, make sure you have breakfast right after. Even better, if you aim to eat some fruit, perhaps an apple, with your breakfast, have half before you exercise, then the other half with the meal.

Don't exercise late at night. Exercise promotes adrenal hormones including cortisol. Cortisol should be lowest at night and too much can make it hard to sleep. Also, if possible, exercise in natural daylight because you'll make vitamin D in your skin, which means stronger bones.

One great way to up your general level of exercise is to simply get more active generally. Use the stairs instead of the elevator. Walk or cycle instead of driving everywhere. Run around with your kids, or take up a sport. There are many ways in a day to develop fitness, and soon, this way of living becomes a habit.

The Fat Way	The Fit Way
Take an elevator	Use the stairs
Use a cart when shopping	Use a hand basket
Drive to work	Walk or cycle some of the way
Drive to the store	Walk to the store
Spend the night watching TV	Take up an active hobby
Get other people to make you a cup of tea	Get up and make yourself a cup of tea
Use power tools for gardening or DIY work	Use manual tools when it's just as quick
Go upstairs as little as possible at home	Run upstairs as often as possible
Use automatic car washes	Wash the car yourself
Stick children in front of TV	Actively play with them
Have business meetings inside	Go for a walk where possible

The more you exercise, the less you eat

Contrary to popular belief, moderate exercise actually decreases your appetite. According to new evidence on appetite research, both animals and humans consistently show decreased appetite with small increases in physical activity. One study looked at an industrial population in West Bengal, India.

Those doing sedentary work ate more and consequently weighed more than those doing light work. As the level of work increased from light to heavy, workers ate more, but not relative to their energy output. The result was that the heavier the work, the lighter the worker.

Job classification	Daily caloric intake (kcal)	Body weight (lb)
Sedentary	3,300	148
Light work	2,600	118
Medium work	2,800	114
Heavy work	3,400	113
Very heavy work	3,600	113

Building muscle, burning fat

Having the right balance of hormones, especially insulin—the fat-storage hormone—helps the body to use protein and, if you're exercising, to turn the protein you eat into muscle. And muscle, in its turn, burns fat. Thus the exercise plan I've outlined above works marvelously with the Holford Diet to turn you into a lean and healthy Fatburner.

A word of warning for the scale watchers, though: when you start a committed exercise program, and lose fat and gain lean muscle, you will lose inches faster than pounds. In the first month you'll look trimmer and feel fitter but may lose less weight than you wished. This is because muscle is denser and hence heavier than fat. In other words, a pound of muscle takes up less space than a pound of fat.

Remember, the enemy is not so much your weight, but having too high a body fat percentage. So check this every month using the chart in Appendix 1 (page 325), rather than only jumping on the scales. The more lean muscle you gain, the more ability you'll have to burn fat—and that's what counts.

How do you fit the food around your exercise? Generally, as I've said above, it's good to eat a balanced meal one to two hours before training. Or you can have a light snack half an hour before. Drink plenty of water while you're exercising, and eat either a balanced snack or a light meal within an hour of finishing a hard workout. Don't let yourself get so hungry that you eat the wrong food. Glucose drinks, energy bars, and the like abound, but by now you'll realize that they're not the way to go for fatburning.

Now we're ready to look in depth at how you're going to put all the pieces together, in Part Three.

- Exercise at least 15 minutes a day, or 35 minutes three times a week.
- Choose aerobic types of exercise that raise your heart rate into the training zone.
- Choose exercise that helps you to build more muscle, which, in turn, burns fat.

References: Part Two

1. Y. Granfeldt, I. Byorck, and B. Hagander, "On the Importance of Processing Conditions, Product Thickness and Egg Addition for the Glycaemic and Hormonal Responses to Pasta: A Comparison of Bread Made with 'Pasta Ingredients,' " *European Journal of Clinical Nutrition*, vol. 45 (1991), pp. 489–99.
2. H. Delargy et al., "Effects of Amount and Type of Dietary Fibre (Soluble and Insoluble) on Short-term Control of Appetite," *International Journal of Food Sciences and Nutrition*, vol. 48 (1997), pp. 67–77.
3. H. Kissilef, *American Journal of Physiology*, vol. 238 (1980), pp. 14–22; S. Konnyyaku, *Agricultural Biological Chemistry*, vol. 34(4) (1970), pp. 641–43; M. Matsuura, *Japanese Diabetic Association*, vol. 23(3) (1980), pp. 209–17.
4. A. Mito, data held in ION library, source unknown.
5. D. Walsh, unpublished study at GNC Research Center, Fargo, North Dakota (1982).
6. P. Holford, "The Effects of Glucomannan on Weight Loss," ION (1983).
7. D. Jenkins et al., "Glycemic Index of Foods: A Physiological Basis for Carbohydrate Exchange," *American Journal of Clinical Nutrition*, vol. 34 (1980), pp. 362–66.
8. C. B. Pert, *The Molecules of Emotion* (New York: Pocket Books, 1999).
9. J. Cleary et al., "Naloxone Effects of Sugar-Motivated Behaviour," *Psychopharmacology*, vol. 176 (1996), pp. 110–14; S. A. Czirr and Reid, "Demonstrating Morphine's Potentiating Effects on Sucrose Intake," *Brain Research Bulletin*, vol. 17 (1986), pp. 639 12; E. Blass et al., "Interactions Between Sucrose, Pain, Isolation Distress," *Pharmacology, Biochemistry of Behaviour*, vol. 26 (1986), pp. 483–89; L. Leventhal et al., "Selective Actions of Central Mu and Kappa Opioid Antagonists upon Sucrose Intake in Sham-fed Rats," *Brain Research*, vol. 685 (1995), pp. 205–10; A. Moles and S. Cooper, "Opioid Modulation of Sucrose Intake in CD-1 Mice," *Physiology and Behaviour*, vol. 58 (1995), pp. 791–96; E. Cheraskin and W. M. Ringsdorf, "A Biochemical Denominator in the Primary Prevention of Alcoholism," *Journal of Orthomolecular Psychiatry*, vol. 9(3) (1980), pp. 158–63.
10. G. B. Keijzers et al., "Caffeine Can Decrease Insulin Sensitivity in Humans," *Diabetes Care*, vol. 25(2) (2002), pp. 364–69.
11. N. J. Richardson et al., "Mood and Performance Effects of Caffeine in Relation to Acute and Chronic Caffeine Deprivation," *Pharmacology, Biochemistry and Behavior*, vol. 52(2) (1995), pp. 313–20.
12. C. Ebbeling et al., "A Reduced-Glycemic Load Diet in the Treatment of Obesity," *Archives of Pediatrics and Adolescent Medicine*, vol. 157(8) (2003), pp. 773–79.
13. A. Garg, "High Mono-unsaturated Fat Diets for Patients with Diabetes Mellitus: A Meta-analysis," *American Journal of Clinical Nutrition*, vol. 67 (1998) (suppl.), pp.

577S–82S; T. Hung et al., "Fat Versus Carbohydrate in Insulin Resistance, Obesity, Diabetes and Cardiovascular Disease," *Current Opinion in Clinical Nutrition and Metabolic Care,* vol. 6(2) (2003), pp. 165–76.

14. C. Bolton-Smith et al., "Dietary Composition and Fat to Sugar Ratios in Relation to Obesity," *International Journal of Obesity,* vol. 18 (1994), pp. 820–28.

15. C. M. Albert et al., "Blood Levels of Long-Chain n-3 Fatty Acids and the Risk of Sudden Death," *New England Journal of Medicine,* vol. 346(15) (2002), pp. 1113–18; M. Morris et al., *Archives of Neurology,* vol. 60 (2003), pp. 940–46.

16. J. Geleijnse et al., "Reduction in Blood Pressure with a Low Sodium, High Potassium, High Magnesium Salt in Older Subjects with Mild to Moderate Hypertension," *British Medical Journal,* vol. 309 (1994), pp. 436–40.

17. T. Gerarduzzi et al., *Journal of Pediatric Gastroenterology and Nutrition,* vol. 31 (2000) (suppl.), S29, Abst. 104.

18. R. Williams, *The Wonderful World Within You* (City: BioCommunications Press, 1998).

19. "The Vitamin Controversy," ION (1988).

20. R. Wunderlich, *Sugar and Your Health,* Good Health Publications (1982).

21. S. Davies, "Zinc, Nutrition and Health," in *1984/5 Yearbook of Nutritional Medicine* (1985).

22. S. Davies et al., "Age-Related Decreases in Chromium Levels in 51,665 Hair, Sweat and Serum Samples from 40,872 Patients—Implications for the Prevention of Cardiovascular Disease and Type II Diabetes Mellitus," *Metabolism,* vol. 46(5) (1997), pp. 1–4.

23. G. Evans, "The Effect of Chromium Picolinate on Insulin Controlled Parameters in Humans," *International Journal of Biosocial and Medical Research,* vol. 11(2) (1989), pp. 163–80.

24. R. Riales et al., "Effects of Chromium Chloride Supplementation on Glucose Tolerance and Serum Lipids Including High Density Lipoprotein of Adult Men," *American Journal of Clinical Nutrition,* vol. 34 (1981), pp. 2670–78; A. Abraham et al., "The Effects of Chromium Supplementation on Serum Glucose and Lipids in Patients with and without Non-insulin-dependent Diabetes," *Metabolism,* vol. 41 (1992), p. 768; W. Glinsmann et al., "Effects of Trivalent Chromium on Glucose Tolerance," *Metabolism,* vol. 15 (1966), pp. 510–15; R. Levine et al., "Effects of Oral Chromium Supplementation on the Glucose Tolerance of Elderly Human Subjects," *Metabolism,* vol. 17 (1968), pp. 114–24; K. Hambidge, "Chromium: A Review," in *Disorders of Mineral Metabolism, vol. 1: Trace Minerals,* Academic Press (1981), pp. 272–94.

25. M. H. Pittler, C. Stevinson, and E. Ernst, "Chromium Picolinate for Reducing Body Weight: Meta-analysis of Randomized Trials," *International Journal of Obesity and Related Metabolic Disorders,* vol. 27(4) (2003), pp. 522–29.

26. T. Larsen, S. Toubro, and A. Astrup, "Efficacy and Safety of Dietary Supplements Containing CLA for the Treatment of Obesity; Evidence from Animal and Human Studies," *Journal of Lipid Research,* vol. 44(12) 2003, pp. 2234–41.

27. D. Clouatre and M. Rosenbaum, *The Diet and Health Benefits of HCA,* Keats Publishing (1994).

28. M. S. Westerterp-Plantenga and E. M. Kovacs, "The Effect of Hydroxycitrate on Energy Intake and Satiety in Overweight Humans," *International Journal of Obesity and Related Metabolic Disorders,* vol. 26(6) (2002), pp. 870–72.

29. A. Amer et al., "5-Hydroxy-L-tryptophan Suppresses Food Intake in Food-Deprived

and Stressed Rats," *Pharmacological Biochemical Behaviour,* vol. 77(1) (2004), pp. 137–43.

30. C. Cangiano et al., "Eating Behavior and Adherence to Dietary Prescriptions in Obese Adult Subjects Treated with 5-hydroxytryptophan," *American Journal of Clinical Nutrition,* vol. 56(5) (1992), pp. 863–67.

31. C. Cangiano et al., "Effects of Oral 5-hydroxy-tryptophan on Energy Intake and Macronutrient Selection in Non-insulin-dependent Diabetic Patients," *International Journal of Obesity and Related Metabolic Disorders,* vol. 22(7) (1998), pp. 648–54.

32. A. Prentice and S. Jebb, "Obesity in Britain: Gluttony or Sloth?," *British Medical Journal,* vol. 311 (1995), pp. 437–39.

33. W. McArdle, chapter in *Medical Aspects of Clinical Nutrition,* Keats Publishing (1983).

34. D. Broughton et al., "Review: Deterioration of Glucose Tolerance with Age: The Role of Insulin Resistance," *Age and Ageing,* vol. 20 (1991), pp. 221–25.

35. C. Hollenbeck et al., "Effect of Habitual Exercise on Regulation of Insulin Stimulated Glucose Disposal in Older Males," *Journal of the American Geriatric Society,* vol. 33 (1986), pp. 273–77.

36. P. Ebelin et al., "Mechanism of Enhanced Insulin Sensitivity in Athletes," *American Society for Clinical Investigations,* vol. 92 (1993), pp. 1623–31.

Part Three

....

The Action Plan

In a Nutshell

The Holford Diet is not a gimmick. It has been tested over 20 years of clinical experience, and is backed by hundreds of scientific trials. It is the best way of helping you lose weight and gain health, easily and enjoyably, because it works with your body's natural design. All you have to do is get your blood sugar balance back to normal, to kick-start your body's own formidable fatburning ability. And in this section I'll show you how—every step of the way.

The key principles behind the Holford Diet are explained in Part Two. Make sure you understand these before you start.

If you're ready—here are the ground rules:

Food

OUT

- **Avoid sugar** in its many disguises, and avoid foods that contain fast-releasing carbohydrates with a high-Ⓖ score—that is, above 10 Ⓖ per serving.
- **Avoid foods high in saturated, hydrogenated, or processed fats, or high in damaged fats;** examples are sausages, fried food, and junk food.
- **Eliminate any foods you're allergic to.** You can do an avoidance/reintroduction test, but in the long run it's better to have a proper quantitative IgG ELISA test. (After three months you can reintroduce the foods you tested positive for, ideally not eating them every day.)

IN

- **Eat no more than 40 ⓖ a day,** choosing foods that contain low-ⓖ carbohydrates, below 10 per serving.
- **Eat low-ⓖ carbohydrates with protein-rich foods.**
- **Eat whole, unadulterated food, high in soluble fiber** (beans, lentils, oats).
- **Eat foods high in the essential fats** omega-3 and omega-6, with an emphasis on omega-3 fats from fatty cold-water fish, seeds, and seed oils.

Drink

OUT

- **Limit or avoid alcohol.** Ideally, drink no more than three small glasses of wine, half-pints of beer, or shots of spirits a week.
- **Limit or avoid caffeinated drinks.** Ideally, drink no more than one regular coffee or two weak teas a day. Avoid all caffeinated carbonated drinks.

IN

- **Drink the equivalent of eight glasses of water a day,** including uncaffeinated herbal teas or diluted juices.

Supplements

IN

- **Supplement your diet with a high-strength multivitamin and mineral, plus vitamin C, every day.**
- **Supplement your diet with additional chromium, HCA, 5-HTP or konjac extract (glucomannan fiber)** if you are prone to sugar cravings and have poor appetite control, for the first three months.

Exercise

IN

- **Exercise at least 15 minutes a day,** or 35 minutes three times a week.

Each one of these makes a difference in its own right. Put them all together and amazing things can happen, because the whole is far greater than the sum of its parts. This is the most effective way to reduce body fat percentage, lose excess weight, and gain health without a rebound effect. Do all this for 30 days and you will switch your body's metabolism from storing fat to burning fat. You will be a Fatburner.

Putting all this into practice is even simpler than it sounds. In essence, all you have to do is this:

- **Eat any recommended breakfast, lunch, or dinner, plus two of the snacks.**
- **Take the recommended supplements every day.**
- **Do fatburning exercise on a regular basis.**

There are two ways to do this. Either follow the four weeks of sample menus, together with recipes, in Part Four. Or, for the more independent Fatburner or any time you're eating out (including working lunches), you can devise your own plan, using the chart on pages 330–340. Simply follow the golden rules, and you'll be following the Holford Diet.

Whichever way you choose, it's a good idea to stick to the Week 1 menu. This will give you a good idea about quantities, and how to prepare some of the fatburning foods that may be new to you.

Exercise is important for everybody. Combining the Holford Diet with a regular exercise program (at least three times a week) will undoubtedly give you top results.

It's as simple as that!

One of the first things you'll feel is the satisfaction—you won't have that starved feeling some diets give you. According to Hilary Evans, the first-ever Fatburner, "I have never felt hungry on this diet." She lost over 20 pounds.

Chances are you'll also feel more energized and alert within days of starting the Holford Diet. Beyond that, it just gets better.

Now let's look at what you need to do before you start.

Getting Ready

Getting ready for the diet is a bit like a warm-up before you exercise. You need a week to prepare—restock your fridge with fatburning foods, find the best alternative foods and drinks and your nearest suppliers, and get used to some of the new foods.

As I said in Part Two, if you're addicted to coffee, tea, chocolate, alcohol, and/or cigarettes, you'll need to cut them all out of your life when you start the diet. I realize that cigarettes might take a bit more time, although you'll be surprised how a combination of resolve, modern techniques for quitting, and getting into the fatburning way of life will help cut the cravings. This is also a great time to try out your exercise options (see Chapter 22) and fit them into your weekly routine.

Remove temptations

You'll need to remove any edible temptations. Start by using up or throwing away the foods you'll need to avoid (see the following chapters). This is a great time to have people over for dinner! Restock your kitchen with the recommended foods and drinks. Do the same at work.

Some of the foods on this diet may be new to you, but all of them are readily available in your local health food store or supermarket. There's a shopping list for you, as well as guidance on how to prepare foods that may be new to you, in Chapter 18.

Setting your targets

Most people start diets hoping to lose in a month what they gained in a year. They vow never to eat chocolate again and to exercise every day. This approach usually ends in failure.

Remember, the purpose of the Holford Diet is to reprogram your body to burn fat. While it is specifically designed for you to lose weight, equally important is changing your body's chemistry so that you become more inclined to burn unwanted fat than to store it. This takes about 30 days. Once this is achieved, losing weight becomes much easier.

In the meantime, you don't want to start out like a rookie in diet boot camp. So here's my advice on easing into this new way of eating and exercising.

BE REALISTIC

Be realistic, and take it one step at a time. Set yourself targets for changing your diet and getting exercise that you know you will reach. The weight will look after itself. It is far better to take one step toward permanently changing your lifestyle than to take four steps forward and four steps back because you were overambitious to start with.

After all, we often eat because we are under pressure or stressed. Boredom, frustration, anger, or a lack of direction all lead to feelings that can be temporarily suppressed with food. Even making small dietary changes is, to begin with, stressful. It takes time to adjust. So don't add to your stress by expecting too much from yourself and then failing to meet your targets.

BE PATIENT

It took years to get that fat. Does it really matter if you take months, rather than weeks, to lose it? Our impatience drives us toward the countless get-slim-quick diets that have been shown, time and time again, not to produce long-term results.

It is very hard for the body to lose more than 2 pounds of actual fat in a week, although you can also lose a lot of excess fluid when you stop eating something you're allergic to. Anything more rapid is likely to be mainly the short-term loss of fluid caused when you eat too little carbohydrate for energy production, leaving the body to break down stores of glycogen. Glycogen is stored with water—hence the apparent loss of fat that's really loss of water.

Obviously, this won't be happening with the Holford Diet: good-quality, low-🕒 carbs are an important part of it, as is sure and steady weight loss.

WHAT RESULTS CAN I EXPECT?

According to studies on the Holford Diet, the average weight loss achieved is 1–2 pounds a week over a 12-week period. That's 14–28 pounds in less than three months. It is better not to lose weight faster than this. Weight loss of over 2 pounds a week will not be all fat loss.

Generally speaking, a good target during the first 30 days is to lose 6 pounds. This is easily achievable on the Holford Diet. But don't forget that your body fat percentage is far more important than your weight, so don't rely on your scales as the only means for checking your progress. As you begin to make more lean muscle you won't lose so much weight, because lean muscle is heavier than the fat you burn off. But you will lose inches, since muscle is more compact than fat.

Making muscle is good news, and not only because you'll look leaner. Muscle cells are more metabolically active and therefore have the capacity to burn off fat, while fat cells don't. So, as you make more lean muscle, your ability to burn fat increases. Therefore, with the Fatburner System, you'll be able to lose weight and inches consistently, month after month, as well as gain health and vitality.

How do you measure your body fat percentage? You can do this roughly on a week-by-week basis using the equation in Appendix 1. If you do have access to the equipment for measuring it, perhaps at your gym, aim to reduce it by 10 percent each month until you reach the optimal level of not more than 15 percent for a man and 22 percent for a woman.

The chart in Appendix 1 shows the ideal weight range for your height. These figures are calculated from life insurance figures. If you're within your ideal range, but still want to trim a few pounds, I recommend that you don't aim to lose more than 4 pounds a month until you reach your target. If you are above the ideal range your target should be no more than 8 pounds a month.

WEEK-BY-WEEK PLANNING

When you're setting your target, it is good to have long-term and short-term objectives. Let's call your long-term objective your goal. What weight would you like to be, ideally? The following questions help to give you a realistic yardstick to go by. What do you weigh now? What, in your opinion, is your ideal weight? How does that compare with the chart in Appendix 1? When were you last that weight? What is the most you've ever lost on a diet?

When you've answered these questions, you'll have a good idea of your ultimate goal. Once you've set it, you can work out your target, week by week, and fill it in on the chart on page 348. For example, if you want to lose 15 pounds, your target after one week would be to weigh 1½ pounds less and so on for 10 weeks, after which you'll have achieved your goal.

Now you are ready to get fatburning! The next three chapters tell you what to eat for breakfast, lunch, dinner, and snacks.

14

What to Eat for Breakfast

First of all, don't skip breakfast. It's the most important meal of your day. There's an old saying in England, "Breakfast like a king, lunch like a prince, dine like a pauper," and it's absolutely true. Here's why.

When you wake up, your blood sugar is low because you haven't eaten. So you need to eat. But many people in the grip of a firm resolve to lose weight make the fatal mistake of trying not to eat anything for as long as possible. Unless propped up with liquid stimulants (coffee or tea), nicotine, or instant sugar in the form of a piece of toast or a croissant, that resolve becomes weaker and weaker as your blood sugar level dips lower and lower, until the chances of making the right food choices become smaller and smaller. So you buckle under the strain and end up bingeing on high-**GL** foods. Sound familiar?

That's why you must eat breakfast. The only question is what and how much. Nutritionists at Oxford Brookes University set out to test this by giving children either a low-**GL** breakfast or a high-**GL** breakfast, then measuring who ate the most as the children helped themselves to a buffet lunch. While both breakfasts were rated as equally satisfying by the children immediately after eating, by lunchtime those who'd had the high-**GL** breakfast were more hungry and ate more food.[1] Exactly the same thing has been shown in adults, too.[2]

The message is clear. Eat a low-**GL** breakfast. It will satisfy you for longer so you'll eat less later.

Breakfast

1 Always have breakfast

2 Choose any one of the following combinations of protein-rich and carbohydrate-rich food

CARBOHYDRATE-RICH

A cup of oatmeal plus an apple or pear

A banana, pear, or peach

2 slices whole-grain rye bread

Apple, pear, banana, kiwifruit, peach, apricot, orange, or grapefruit

PROTEIN-RICH

Skim milk or soy milk

Get Up & Go, plus skim milk or soy milk

1 free-range egg (boiled or poached)

Yogurt (natural, live, low-fat)

2 teaspoons of seeds (half pumpkin, half flax—ground)

ESSENTIAL FATS

4 Add 2 teaspoons of ground seeds (half flax, half pumpkin seeds)

3 Have a cup of herb tea, coffee alternative, or glass of water with your breakfast

The Holford Diet: breakfast

There are two ways to do this. The simplest is to choose from any of the Fatburner breakfasts listed on page 231. These are already calculated to give you no more than 10 Ⓖ, plus the right amount of protein and essential fats.

Or you can do it yourself. The DIY Fatburner breakfast is also very straightforward. The fundamental rules are shown in the diagram above.

There are five fundamental breakfasts that give you the right balance of both carbohydrate and protein. Here they are:

Carbohydrates		Protein
Cereal/fruit	+	seeds/yogurt/milk
Fruit	+	yogurt/seeds
Bread/toast	+	egg
Bread/toast	+	fish (e.g., kippers)

The question is which and how much cereal, fruit, toast, and so on. Let's kick off with the cereal-based breakfast, sweetened with fruit rather than sugar.

The best cereal-based breakfasts

A good cereal-based breakfast needs to include a low-🄶🄻 cereal, a low-🄶🄻 fruit as a sweetener, and a source of protein and essential fats. The goal, remember, is no more than 10 🄶🄻.

In the chart below you'll see how much of the following six cereals you can have to total 5 🄶🄻. As you can see, the best value in terms of your appetite are rolled oats, either cooked as in oatmeal or eaten raw, just as you would cornflakes. Basically, you could eat as much as you like, given that two servings will fill anybody up.

CEREAL	5 🄶🄻
Rolled oats	2 servings
All-Bran	1 serving
Unsweetened muesli	1 small serving
Alpen	half a serving
Raisin Bran	half a serving
Weetabix	1 biscuit

Below, on the right-hand side you can see how much of these six fruits you could eat to equal 5 🄶🄻.

FRUIT	5 🄶🄻
Strawberries	1 pint
Pear	1
Grapefruit	1
Apple	1 small
Peach	1 small
Banana	less than half

TOP TIP

Smart animals—from parrots to people—eat seeds. Seeds are incredibly rich in essential fats, minerals, vitamin E, protein, and fiber. You need a tablespoon a day for 100 percent health. Here's the magic formula:

1. Fill a glass jar that has a sealing lid half with flax seeds (rich in omega-3), and half with sesame, sunflower, or pumpkin seeds (rich in omega-6).
2. Keep the jar sealed and in the fridge to minimize damage from light, heat, and oxygen.
3. Put a handful in a coffee/seed grinder, grind up, and put a tablespoon on your cereal. Store the remainder in the fridge and use over the next few days.

So your best bet out of these would be to have oatmeal, hot or cold, or raw rolled oats with as many strawberries as you could eat. Alternatively, you could have a bowl of All-Bran and a grapefruit, or a bowl of unsweetened muesli with a small grated apple. Or you can build your own breakfast using the full ⓖ chart in Appendix 2 on pages 330–340.

As far as protein is concerned, there's some in milk (or in soy milk, if you're allergic to dairy). Rice milk is high-**GL** and best avoided. Yogurt (unsweetened) is also high in protein. So, have a spoonful of yogurt, some milk, or some soy milk on your cereal if you'd like.

Another source of protein, as well as countless vitamins, minerals, essential fats, and fiber, is seeds. I recommend you have a tablespoon of ground seeds on your cereal as well. This really adds flavor and, because it gives you the essential fats you need, you won't crave less desirable food sources of fat.

The best cereal-based breakfast is Fatburner Muesli, made by mixing oatmeal flakes, oat bran, ground seeds, fresh berries, and yogurt. See the recipe on page 232. A serving has a **GL** of 8 and is completely satisfying.

THE BEST YOGURT-BASED BREAKFASTS

If you are fond of yogurt, you could dispense with the cereal altogether and have yogurt, fruit, and seeds. Let's take a look at how this adds up. In the chart below you'll see how much yogurt you can eat for 5 **GL**. (A small container of yogurt is 6 ounces.)

YOGURT	5 **GL**
Plain yogurt	2 small containers (12 oz.)
Nonfat yogurt	2 small containers
Low-fat yogurt with fruit and sugar	less than 1 small container (<4 oz.)

So provided you choose a yogurt that doesn't have added sugar, you can eat two small containers, sweetened with any of the fruits you like from the fruit chart on page 152, plus a tablespoon of ground seeds.

Get Up & Go–based breakfasts

Get Up & Go is a powder that you blend with a piece of fruit, choosing from any of the 5-**GL** servings of fruit shown above, and half a pint of skim milk (or sugar-free soy milk).

Get Up & Go is made from a special blend of quinoa, brown rice, and soy flour, giving an excellent quality of protein balanced with carbohydrate, mainly from whole apple powder, together with oat bran, rice bran, and psyllium husks for added soluble fiber, plus sesame, sunflower, and pumpkin seeds and some almond meal, cinnamon, and natural vanilla for flavor. In addition, it has added vitamins and minerals, including 50 micrograms of chromium and 1,000 milligrams of vitamin C, plus all the B vitamins.

When it's made up, it's guaranteed to keep you feeling full till lunchtime, and yet has only 283 calories. The best fruits to use in Get Up & Go are strawberries, raspberries, a soft pear, blackcurrants, and banana. If you use banana, use only half. Get Up & Go provides about 5 **ⒼⓁ**, so you're looking for no more than another 5 from the fruit you blend with it.

The best egg-based breakfasts

While it is true that more than half the calories in an egg come from fat, the kind of fat depends on what you feed the chicken. Most eggs come from battery chickens. If you know how unhealthy they are, you don't eat their eggs, which are high in saturated fat.

However, some egg producers give their chickens feed rich in fatty acids, for example flaxseeds. These are both free-range and rich in omega-3 fats, and much better for you than ordinary eggs. I recommend that you have no more than four eggs a week on the Holford Diet—and only this kind of egg. Have either two small eggs, or one large egg, per meal. Poach, boil, or scramble them, but don't fry them, since the high heat damages the essential fats.

As eggs are pure protein and fat, what carbohydrate can you have with them? If this is your entire breakfast, you can use up your entire 10-**ⒼⓁ** quota by having any of the following bread servings.

BREAD	10 **ⒼⓁ**
Oatcake crackers	1
Pumpernickel bread	2 thin slices
Sourdough rye bread	2 thin slices
Rye whole-meal bread (yeasted)	1 slice
Wheat whole-meal bread (yeasted)	1 slice
White, high-fiber bread (yeasted)	less than 1 slice

As you can see, your best-value breads are oatcake crackers, which are a Scottish favorite, or European-style pumpernickel breads, or sourdough rye bread, made without yeast. Unlike the light, white, fluffy "fake" breads we've been conditioned to eat, which are full of air, superrefined, and nutritionally inferior, sourdough and the like are real breads, substantial, fiber-rich, and delicious. You may find the change a bit of a shock at first, but you'll find that they are very satisfying.

Real breads are better for two reasons. One is the way they're processed, which I discussed in Part Two. They have far fewer additives, use coarsely ground flours, and, in the case of sourdough, contain much less yeast. All this keeps the Ⓖ score lower.

Also, some grains are better than others because of the type of carbohydrate, or sugar, they contain. Wheat and corn are high in a fast-releasing sugar called *amylopectin*, while barley, rye, and quinoa are higher in one called *amylose*, which is slower-releasing. Most rice, by the way, has a high Ⓖ score because it contains a large proportion of amylopectin. Basmati rice, however, has more amylose and is therefore slower-releasing. Brown basmati is best.

Of the grains, oats are among the best. While the Ⓖ of wheat varies depending on what's done to it, oats are the same in any shape or form. Whole oat flakes, rolled oats, or oatmeal, as used in oatcakes, all have a low glycemic effect.[3]

Kippers, anyone?

Kippers (smoked herring) may seem an unusual choice, but they make a fabulous fatburning breakfast—tasty and highly nutritious. Rich in protein and omega-3 fats, one kipper and any of the bread portions shown above will meet your needs for a fatburning breakfast.

Now let's move on to snacks, since that's the next thing you are going to eat.

15

What to Eat for Snacks

The Holford Diet is all about enjoying your food while losing weight and boosting health, and snacks give you even more scope for enjoyment. But what to eat? Those with sugar sensitivity are likely to reach for snacks that compensate for changes in blood sugar levels and hormonal responses. Most commercial snacks are incredibly high in sugar or fat. It won't surprise you that a Mars Bar is almost two thirds sugar with the rest mainly fat; but even some so-called granola bars are deceptively unhealthy, made with refined sugar and masses of hydrogenated fat.

However, research shows clearly that "grazing" (eating little and often) is healthier for you than "gorging" (having one or two big meals a day).[4] Grazing helps keep your blood sugar level even and this makes overeating far less likely, as you'll never experience any between-meal hunger pangs. For this reason, I recommend you have a midmorning and a midafternoon snack. The ideal snack is one that provides no more than 5 ⓖⓛs and also some protein, and the simplest snack food is fruit. Let's see what you could eat to stay within 5 ⓖⓛ for your snack.

FRUIT	5 ⓖⓛ
Strawberries	1 large basket
Plums	4
Cherries	1 small basket
Pear	1
Grapefruit	1

FRUIT (*cont.*)	5 ⒼⓁ
Orange	1
Apple	1 small (can fit in the palm of your hand)
Peach	1 small
Melon/watermelon	1 slice

Berries, plums, and cherries are your best-"value" fruit snacks. Berries include raspberries, blueberries, blackberries, and any others that you can get your hands on in season. You can further slow down the ⒼⓁ score of these fruits by eating them with five almonds or two teaspoons of pumpkin seeds. Other than chestnuts, almonds are the best nut because they have the most protein compared with calories. Pumpkin seeds are also high in protein and in omega-3 fats. Flaxseeds are the highest for omega-3 but are too small to make good snacks, and need to be ground up because they have a hard outer coating.

Another snack option would be some kind of bread with a protein-based spread. Cottage cheese, hummus, and peanut butter are good examples. Hummus, if you haven't encountered it before, is a Middle Eastern chickpea spread or dip, deliciously rich-tasting although low in ⒼⓁ. It tastes great with oatcakes, on rye bread, or with a raw carrot (see recipe on page 248). (A large carrot is still less than 5 ⒼⓁ.) If you like peanut butter, buy the kind with no added sugar or hydrogenated oils. A slice of any of the bread servings below with either hummus or peanut butter gives you the right kind of low-ⒼⓁ carbohydrate with some protein to keep your blood sugar level even.

Oatcake crackers, and oats in general, are excellent as far as weight and blood sugar are concerned. Oats contain *beta-glucans,* a type of fiber that helps to slow down the release of glucose into the blood, lessen insulin response, and also lower cholesterol and heart disease risk. Of all the grains, it's the best for losing weight, and for controlling your blood sugar.[5]

Watch out when buying oatcake crackers, though. Many contain sugar. The best are Nairn's, since not only do they have sugar-free, organic types, but also they use palm fruit oil, which contains unsaturated fat, as opposed to palm oil, which is higher in saturated fat.

BREAD	5 ⒼⓁ
Oatcake crackers	2 crackers
Pumpernickel bread	1 thin slice
Sourdough rye bread	1 thin slice

Rye whole-meal bread (yeasted)	half a slice
Wheat whole-meal bread (yeasted)	half a slice
White, high-fiber bread (yeasted)	less than half a slice

So here are a selection of 5-Ⓛ snacks to choose from:

- a piece of fruit, plus five almonds or two teaspoons of pumpkin seeds
- a thin slice of rye bread or two oatcake crackers, 5 ounces of cottage cheese
- a thin slice of rye bread/two oatcake crackers, and 5 ounces of hummus
- a thin slice of rye bread/two oatcake crackers, and peanut butter
- crudités (a carrot, pepper, cucumber, or celery) and hummus
- crudités and cottage cheese
- 5 ounces of yogurt, no sugar, plus berries
- cottage cheese plus berries

As you can see, you won't be bored between meals, as there's lots of scope for mixing and matching. These suggestions are only to give you an idea of what to expect. You'll find an array of snack recipes in Chapter 28, including Flageolet Bean Dip, Smoked Salmon Pâté with oatcake crackers and crudités, and Quinoa Tabbouleh.

............16.............

What to Eat for Lunch and Dinner

Main meals are really something to look forward to on the Holford Diet, as you'll see from the recipes and menus in Part Four. But how do you put it all together? The easiest way to get the right nutritional balance is to imagine all the different foods on a plate. I showed you this method in Part Two, and you'll find it described again below.

Half the plate will consist of very-low-**ⓖ** vegetables. This includes peas, broccoli, carrots, Italian flat beans, zucchini, and kale, among many others. These vegetables, listed on page 164, will account for no more than 4 **ⓖ**, and I'm going to show you how to prepare them in minutes. If you haven't been all that interested in vegetables before, you'll be amazed by how fresh and zingy they can taste when they're cooked in these ways.

The other half of your plate is divided into two, one for protein-based food such as meat, fish, or tofu, and the other for more "starchy" vegetables, which account for 6 to 7 **ⓖ**. There's a chart showing this on page 162. So, a quarter of what's on your plate is protein-rich, a quarter is carbohydrate-rich, and half is made up of very low-**ⓖ** vegetables. You'll soon get the hang of it. It's ridiculously simple.

More fish, less meat

Let's kick off with the protein serving on your plate. Remember from Part Two that the overall amount of protein—by which I mean the protein contained in the various foods, not protein-rich foods—at each meal will be 20 grams. The protein-rich food on your plate will provide 15 grams of this, and the table below tells you how much you need to eat of each of these to get that 15 grams. (The one serving of carbohydrate-rich starchy vegetables and two servings of very-low-ⓖⓛ vegetables will provide the remaining 5 grams.)

In the table I've listed a lot of fish options and fewer meat options. In fact, red meat is missing entirely. White meat tends to be much lower in fat, and fish is much higher in the essential omega-3 fats, so, becoming a "fishichicketarian" is a great way to lose weight and gain health.

Does this mean you can never eat red meat again? Certainly not. Once you've attained your target weight you can have lean red meat once a week.

How big is a protein serving?

Food	Weight	Serving
Tofu and tempeh	5½ oz.	¾ pack
Textured vegetable protein	3½ oz.	3 tbsp.
Chicken (no skin)	2 oz.	1 very small breast
Turkey (no skin)	2 oz.	½ small breast
Quorn	4 oz.	⅓ box
Salmon and trout	2 oz.	1 very small fillet
Tuna (canned in water)	2 oz.	⅓ of a 6-oz. can
Sardines (canned in water)	2½ oz.	⅔ tin
Cod	2 oz.	1 very small fillet
Clams	2 oz.	¼ can
Prawns	3 oz.	6 large prawns
Mackerel	3 oz.	1 medium fillet
Oysters	—	15
Yogurt (natural, low-fat)	8 oz.	1 cup
Cottage cheese	4 oz.	½ cup
Hummus	8 oz.	1 small container
Skim milk	—	2 cups
Soy milk	—	2 cups
Eggs (boiled)	—	2
Quinoa	4½ oz.	large bowl
Baked beans	11 oz.	1 can
Kidney beans	6 oz.	½ can
Black-eyed peas	6 oz.	½ can
Lentils	6 oz.	½ can

Starchy vegetables

As we see on the plate on page 55, carbohydrate-rich "starchy vegetable" servings should be roughly the same size or weight as protein servings. But this depends on how each food weighs up. For example, if you are eating chicken with rice, the serving size of rice is somewhat larger than the piece of chicken for each to be roughly the same weight, because chicken is dense and heavy and rice is relatively light.

Remember, starchy vegetables will account for a maximum 7 ⓖⓛ of your meal (out of a total of 10 ⓖⓛ). Let's take a look at what quantities of different starchy vegetables you can eat to keep within that limit, leaving 3 ⓖⓛ for the very-low-ⓖⓛ veggies that occupy half the plate.

STARCHY VEGETABLES	7 ⓖⓛ
Pumpkin/squash	a big serving (6½ oz.)
Carrot	one large (5½ oz.)
Rutabaga	a big serving (5½ oz.)
Quinoa	a big serving (4½ oz.)
Beets	a big serving (4 oz.)
Polenta	a serving (4 oz.)
Pearl barley	a small serving (3½ oz.)
Whole-meal pasta	half a serving (3 oz.)
White pasta	a third of a serving (2½ oz.)
Brown rice	a small serving (2½ oz.)
White rice	a third of a serving (1½ oz.)
Couscous	a third of a serving (1½ oz.)
Broad beans	a serving (1 oz.)
Corn on the cob	half a cob (2 oz.)
Boiled potato	three small potatoes (2½ oz.)
Baked potato	half (2 oz.)
French fries	tiny portion (1½ oz.)
Sweet potato	half (2 oz.)

As you can see, there are some obvious winners. Whole-meal pasta and brown rice are much better than white pasta and white rice. (As we saw earlier, brown basmati rice has the lowest ⓖⓛ score of all the different types of rice.) Rutabaga, carrots, and squash are much better than potato. Boiled potato is better than baked potato, which is in turn better than French fries.

> **TOP TIP**
>
> Try a new food every week. For example, have you ever eaten barley or quinoa? Barley can be cooked like rice and is very tasty in soups and casseroles. So is quinoa—actually a seed rather than a grain—which takes only 13 minutes to cook and is packed with extra protein, iron, and vitamins.

Some of these foods may be new to you. If so, you'll be bowled over by, say, the nutty flavor of quinoa and the smooth, rich savor of the squashes. If you love pasta, switching to the whole-meal variety is painless. It cooks the same way, but you can eat more of the unrefined variety and stay slim.

Beans and lentils

It's telling that beans and lentils are no longer widely eaten in many of the world's fattest nations. These are the best foods for both balancing your blood sugar and giving the right mix of protein and carbohydrate. It's this rare double whammy that keeps their Ⓖ score low. (Another reason why lentils and soybeans are so low is that they contain a substance that prevents the digestion of amylose, therefore slowing down its release further.) Soy also keeps your arteries healthy by lowering the "bad" LDL cholesterol. A serving a day, as either soy milk or tofu, can lower your LDL cholesterol by over 10 percent.

Any meal containing beans and lentils can be quite generous with the portion size because you are getting both the protein and the carbohydrate from the same food. However, when you are eating these foods as your source of protein, combine with only *half* the serving size of a carbohydrate-rich food, instead of an equal serving. For example, if you were making Dal (Lentil Curry) (see page 266), you'd have a cup of lentils and half a cup of rice. This is, of course, because you're already getting a significant amount of carbohydrate in the lentils.

This is how much you can eat, assuming you are not eating another starchy vegetable, to stay within 7 Ⓖ. (Most regular cans of beans provide around 8 ounces.)

BEANS AND LENTILS	7 ⓖⓛ
Soybeans	2 cans
Pinto/cranberry beans	¾ can
Lentils	¾ can
Baked beans	½ can
Butter beans	½ can
Split peas	½ can
Kidney beans	½ can
Chickpeas	⅓ can

If you're not vegetarian, you may be relatively unfamiliar with beans and lentils. You may have encountered dal, baked beans, hummus, or cassoulet, but never actually thrown a bag or can of lentils or beans into your shopping cart. These are great foods, immensely satisfying in flavor and texture, and they feature in all of the world's great cuisines. You'll be making mouthwatering dishes with them, from hummus and Flageolet Bean Dip to Lentil and Lemon Soup, Dal, and a fiery chili, to name just a few.

Unlimited vegetables

Now it's time to move on to the other half of your plate. This is made up of what I call the unlimited vegetables. Of course, there are limits, but these are vegetables for which a serving is less than 2 ⓖⓛ. A serving of peas, for instance, is a cup.

UNLIMITED VEGETABLES		
Arugula	Eggplant	Peas
Asparagus	Endive	Peppers
Bean sprouts	Fennel	Radish
Broccoli	Garlic	Scallions
Broccolini	Green beans	Snow peas
Brussels sprouts	Italian flat beans	Spinach
Cabbage	Kale	Tomato
Cauliflower	Lettuce	Watercress
Celery	Mushrooms	Zucchini
Cucumber	Onions	

If the word "cabbage" makes you think of watery soup, and Italian flat beans have always been something you pushed around on your plate, be prepared:

> **TOP TIP**
> Eat your food slowly. Chew each mouthful 20 times, as this will
> further slow the release of the carbohydrate in your food.

I have some seriously delicious recipes for these. You'll end up eager to find new ways of eating them—and looking amazing, thanks to the vitamins, minerals, and other phytonutrients they're brimming with.

So, to recap: I want you to eat two servings of "unlimited" vegetables, one serving of "starchy" vegetables, and one serving of protein-based food. Together, they'll help you feel full at the end of every meal.

Vegetarians

If you're a strict vegetarian, you'll need to eat more tofu, beans, lentils, soy products, and Quorn than usual to achieve the target for protein intake. A serving size of tofu for a main meal is 5½ oz., which is almost a whole package. Part Four contains a number of recipes and ways to use tofu—the vegetarian Fatburner's best friend—along with recipes using a variety of beans and lentils. And many of the recipes containing chicken or fish can be adapted by substituting tofu or a tofu steak, and I make a point of mentioning this. (For more detailed general advice for vegetarians, see Chapter 20.)

Fats and oils

This diet is not low-fat; you'll be able to eat enough to keep you satisfied. As far as fats and oils go, what's important is which fats you use, and how you use them.

Creams: If you want to make a savory dish creamier, try adding a teaspoon of tahini (sesame spread) or a tablespoon of coconut milk or coconut cream.

Salad dressings: When using seed oils for salad dressings, pick either flaxseed oil or a blend of oils that gives at least one part of omega-3 fats to one part of omega-6 fats. These seed oils need to be cold-pressed and stored in a lightproof container.

Two good seed-oil blends are Essential Balance and Udo's Choice, available in health food stores. Also good is walnut oil. You can lightly drizzle these oils onto vegetables instead of using butter.

Cooking oils: For steam-frying (see below) and sautéing, use a small amount of butter, coconut butter, or olive oil. Coconut butter adds a great flavor to steam-fries.

Cooking methods

All carbohydrate foods release their carbohydrate somewhat faster once cooked. The longer you cook something and the higher the temperature, the faster-releasing the food becomes. It's therefore best to eat food as close to raw as possible.

This doesn't mean endless salads. You can steam, steam-fry, boil, and poach food without cooking it to death. Next best are baking, grilling, sautéing, and stir-frying. Worst are frying and deep-frying.

Steaming is the best way of cooking green, leafy, less starchy vegetables, since it preserves a lot of their vitamins and minimizes any raising of ⓖⓛ. This method can be used with any food and is very successful with fish—but perhaps not ideal with starchy vegetables, which require longer cooking, or with red meat. Many different kinds of steamers are available, or you can improvise with a colander, pot, and lid.

Boiling raises the ⓖⓛ of foods more than steaming, but less than baking. Changes can be kept to a minimum by using as little water as possible, keeping the lid on, and cooking the food as whole as possible. Also, eat all vegetables al dente—a little crisp, not soft.

Steam-frying figures large in the Holford Diet because it adds loads of taste without compromising on health. The great advantage of this style of cooking is that the lower temperature of steaming doesn't destroy nutrients to anything like the extent that frying does, and you use only a small amount of oil, if any. As with boiling and ordinary steaming, aim to keep vegetables al dente.

To steam-fry, use a shallow pan or a deep frying pan with a thick base and a lid that seals well. You can steam-fry without oil by first adding two tablespoons of liquid to the pan—water, vegetable stock, soy sauce, or a watered-down bit of the sauce you'll use for the dish. Once it boils, immediately add some vegetables, "sauté" rapidly for a minute or two, turn the heat up, add a tablespoon or two more of the liquid, and clamp the lid on tightly. After a minute, add the rest of the ingredients. Turn the heat down after a couple of minutes and steam in this way until cooked.

Or you can add between a teaspoon and a tablespoon of olive oil, butter, or coconut oil to the pan, warm it, add the ingredients, and sauté. After a couple of minutes, add two tablespoons of liquid as above and clamp the lid on. Steam ingredients till done.

Poaching is like steam-frying without the sautéing. You can make delicious water-based sauces. For example, you could cook fish in vegetable broth flavored with ginger, garlic, lemongrass, spices, and wine (the alcohol boils off).

Waterless cooking requires specially designed pans in which you can "boil" foods by steaming them in their own juice and "fry" foods with no oil. Both methods are excellent for preserving both nutrients and flavor.

Baking is useful, especially if the food is large and has a thick skin (such as a whole or half pumpkin). Avoid coating food with oil, because the oil will oxidize with cooking, which creates free radicals (highly reactive, harmful molecules). You can roast a potato without adding oil. The higher the temperature and the longer you cook something, the higher the ⓖⓛ becomes.

Frying should be kept to a minimum, and deep-frying avoided altogether. When you do fry, use butter, coconut oil (saturated fat), or olive oil (mono-unsaturated) rather than other vegetable oils (polyunsaturated oils), since these are much more prone to oxidation.

Grilling foods that contain fat is less damaging than frying, but browning or burning a food does create free radicals. Try to avoid barbecued food, or at least ensure what you eat is not charred.

Microwaving is a problematic cooking method, although admittedly fast. Because the food cooks in its own water, it seems better than most cooking methods for preserving the water-soluble vitamins B and C. A Spanish study, however, found that microwaved broccoli lost vast amounts of major antioxidants (nutrients working to rid the body of free radicals) compared with steaming.

Moreover, the temperatures reached in fat particles are very high, so avoid microwaving oily fish: it will destroy the essential fats that the fish contains. And remember that microwave ovens do give off electromagnetic radiation, even six feet away.

If you must microwave, it is better to use lower-voltage/heat settings for longer. Cover dishes to encourage steaming, although you do need to leave some room for steam to escape.

What to limit and avoid

The trick with any diet is to fill yourself up with the good stuff so there's little room left for less desirable foods. Some of the goodies, however, such as oily fish, still need to be limited because, although they contain valuable fats, too much of any fat is bad for you.

FOODS TO LIMIT

The chart opposite shows you which foods to limit and how much to limit them to. Some of these are included in the recipes in specific amounts be-

---

TOP TIPS

- Buy foods as fresh and unprocessed as possible and eat them soon afterward.
- Eat more raw food. Be adventurous. Try raw beets and carrot tops in salad.
- Cook foods as whole as possible, slicing or blending before serving.
- Use as little water as possible, preferably steaming, poaching, or steam-frying.
- Fry foods as infrequently as possible.
- Favor slow-cook methods that introduce less heat.
- Don't overcook, burn, or brown food.

cause they contain important nutrients. Some are high in fat, while others are high in sugar, so do not have more than the recommended amounts.

Dried fruit	choose fresh fruit or soak dried fruit
Coconut	can be used in small amounts to flavor dishes
Seeds	limit to four teaspoons a day, maximum, or one heaping tablespoon
Nuts	same as seeds (don't have both, and seeds are better)
Salad dressings	stick to the measures given in Part Four
Avocados	twice a week, maximum
Vegetable oil and butter	use sparingly, as in the recipes
Tahini (sesame spread)	use a small amount instead of butter
Fatty fish such as herring, mackerel, tuna, kippers	three times a week, maximum
Chicken (no skin), game	twice a week, maximum
Milk and yogurt	stick to skim milk and low-fat yogurt
Eggs	three a week, maximum

FOODS TO AVOID

These foods are high in fat and/or fast-releasing sugar, or are devoid of nutrients, so they're best strictly avoided. Once you have attained your target weight, they may be eaten on rare occasions.

High-fat meats including beef, pork, lamb, sausages, and processed meats
Lard, drippings, suet, and gravy
Deep-fried foods
Cream and store-bought ice cream
High-fat spreads and mayonnaises
All cheeses except cottage cheese, low-fat Quark or fromage frais, and half-fat Cheddar cheese
Rich sauces made with cream, cheese, or eggs
Sugar, sugar-laden sweets, and foods with added sugar
Pastries, cakes, and cookies
White bread
Snack foods such as chips

Main Meals

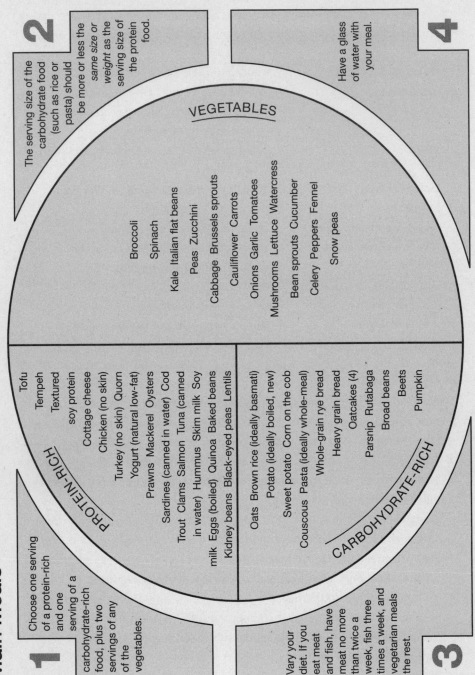

1 Choose one serving of a protein-rich and one serving of a carbohydrate-rich food, plus two servings of any of the vegetables.

2 The serving size of the carbohydrate food (such as rice or pasta) should be more or less the *same size or weight* as the serving size of the protein food.

3 Vary your diet. If you eat meat and fish, have meat no more than twice a week, fish three times a week, and vegetarian meals the rest.

4 Have a glass of water with your meal.

VEGETABLES

Broccoli
Spinach
Kale Italian flat beans
Peas Zucchini
Cabbage Brussels sprouts
Cauliflower Carrots
Onions Garlic Tomatoes
Mushrooms Lettuce Watercress
Bean sprouts Cucumber
Celery Peppers Fennel
Snow peas

PROTEIN-RICH

Tofu
Tempeh
Textured soy protein
Cottage cheese
Chicken (no skin)
Turkey (no skin) Quorn
Yogurt (natural low-fat)
Prawns Mackerel Oysters
Sardines (canned in water) Cod
Trout Clams Salmon Tuna (canned in water) Hummus Skim milk Soy milk Eggs (boiled) Quinoa Baked beans
Kidney beans Black-eyed peas Lentils

CARBOHYDRATE-RICH

Oats Brown rice (ideally basmati)
Potato (ideally boiled, new)
Sweet potato Corn on the cob
Couscous Pasta (ideally whole-meal)
Whole-grain rye bread
Heavy grain bread
Oatcakes (4)
Parsnip Rutabaga
Broad beans
Beets
Pumpkin

The Holford Diet: main meals

17

Drinks, Desserts, and Sweets

So far, we've looked only at food. But what about drinks—including al-cohol? You'll have a broad choice of hot drinks and juices, and will be able to have a few convivial glasses of wine a week. And there are plenty of mouthwatering desserts in Part Four to choose from, as well as sweets that won't overshoot your **GL** allowance by a mile and that are available at your local health food store.

As you now know by heart, the food you eat will have 40 **GL** a day. On top of this, the **GL** allowance for drinks, desserts, and sweets is 5 **GL**. Your 5 daily **GL** could come from a glass of juice or wine, a Fatburner dessert, or even some chocolate—just not all four in the same day.

As before, if you're drinking a lot of coffee or tea, getting through a fair amount of chocolate, drinking alcohol fairly frequently—or doing all three—you will need to stop all of them for at least two weeks to a month when you start the Holford Diet. Thus any withdrawal symptoms will be short-lived: the nutrients and supplements you're taking in will be getting to grips with the bottoming out of your blood sugar. You could feel a bit rough for several days, but this will dissipate fast.

Gradually, you should see any cravings for supersweetness or alcohol begin to disappear. By the time you're ready to reintroduce the odd piece of chocolate, cup of tea, or glass of Sancerre, the switchover to fatburning will have begun and you'll be able to handle the occasional treat without encouraging any imbalance in blood sugar.

Cold drinks

The best drink for fatburning is water—and you need to drink the equivalent of 2 quarts, or 8 glasses, a day. If that seems an enormous amount, be aware that you can factor in any herbal teas, coffee substitutes, and juices you drink. Leaving a bottle on your desk at work makes it easier to remember to keep it topped up. When you're thoroughly hydrated, you'll feel much better in every way. This is a habit that will—like the rest of the Holford Diet— become second nature.

Fruit juices, whether concentrated or fresh, have a relatively high ⓖⓛ because the fibers have been removed. The best is apple juice, although even this should be drunk diluted—half juice, half water, or, even better, two-thirds water, one-third juice.

Here's how much you can drink for 5 ⓖⓛ points.

DRINK	5 ⓖⓛ
Tomato juice	1 pint
Carrot juice	small glass (6 oz.)
Grapefruit juice, unsweetened	small glass (6 oz.)
Apple juice, unsweetened	small glass (6 oz.), diluted 50:50 with water
Orange juice, unsweetened	small glass (6 oz.), diluted 50:50 with water; or juice of one orange
Pineapple juice	half a small glass (3 oz.), diluted 50:50 with water
Cranberry juice drink	half a small glass (3 oz.), diluted 50:50 with water
Grape juice	an inch's worth of liquid!

Stay away from all carbonated, sweetened, caffeinated drinks and sugar-sweetened fruit drinks. You should also abstain from so-called diet sodas, which often contain caffeine and/or artificial sweeteners. You can use fruit-flavored drinks sweetened with apple juice concentrate, which contains more slow-releasing fructose, rather than grape juice concentrate, which has a much higher score.

A good rule of thumb is to have no more than one glass of juice a day, diluting it as you need to in order to have no more than 5 ⓖⓛ a day. So have, say, either a glass of carrot juice, or a glass of diluted apple juice.

> **TOP TIP**
> Drink slowly. Sip rather than gulp your drinks. This helps to slow-release the sugars in fruit juice, as does diluting them.

Alcohol

The effect of alcohol is similar to that of sugar, and if you want to burn fat fast it is best avoided during the first two weeks to a month of the Holford Diet. Amé and other soft drinks made of natural ingredients with no added sugar are good alternatives if you remember to keep within the 5 Ⓖ rule.

After the initial "cold turkey" period of two weeks to a month, you can start drinking again, in moderation. That means three drinks a week, either a small glass of good-quality wine, half a pint of beer or lager, or a small shot of spirits. Of these, the best is neat spirits, then white wine, red wine, and finally beer. Beer has the highest carbohydrate content, double that of red wine and eight times that of white wine.

Hot drinks

Refer to pages 80–85 for a full discussion of coffee, tea, and all their permutations. By now you'll know that, whether you're addicted to endless cups of tea or are a real espresso fiend, you'll need to abstain completely for two weeks to a month on the diet. Luckily, there are many wonderful, nonaddictive alternatives around—really delicious and inventive herbal teas, excellent coffee substitutes—so it should be positively enjoyable to do so. After all, when you're fizzing with energy from diet alone, stimulants lose their sparkle pretty fast.

> **TOP TIP**
> If you're addicted to coffee try a Teeccino with some frothed milk and a touch of cinnamon. If you're addicted to tea try Rooibos (red bush) tea with milk.

That said, when the time comes, you can reintroduce weak tea. Drinking it from time to time shouldn't be a problem. Coffee has several addictive substances in it, however, and should be reserved for an occasional treat.

Sugar and sweets

Sugar is perhaps a greater addiction than many people realize, and kicking the habit could prove a little tough (see page 79). But your taste buds will become acclimatized. Fruit will help when you crave something sweet (see the list on pages 157–158 for the low-Ⓖ fruits). Also, get used to diluting fruit juices with water, as outlined above. Once you're sugar-free, the odd sweet food is no big deal.

Many "sugar-free" foods use grape juice concentrate as a sweetener. They might as well use glucose. Some use apple juice concentrate and, as it's high in fructose, it is much better for you. Some health-conscious drinks use blue agave cactus nectar, which is better still.

The best sugar-free alternative is xylitol (see page 364 in Resources). It is a natural sweetener found in many fruits and vegetables, but has a much lower Ⓖ score—a seventh that of sugar and half that of fructose. Plums, for example, are naturally high in xylitol and hence taste sweet but have a very low Ⓖ score. So, if you are addicted to having three teaspoons of sugar in your tea, cutting to one teaspoon of xylitol will have cut your Ⓖ load by 14.

SUGAR	5 Ⓖ
Xylitol	10 tsp.
Blue agave cactus nectar	10 tsp.
Fructose	5 tsp.
Lactose	2 tsp.
Sucrose	1 tsp.
Honey	1 tsp.
Glucose	1 tsp.
Malt	1 tsp.

Chocolate

As we've seen, chocolate is full of sugar and cocoa, which contains stimulating substances including caffeine, theobromine, and theophylline. Higher-quality dark chocolate tends to have less sugar, but obviously more of the stimulants. Some chocolates even use some of the "healthier" sugars described above. But the fact is that, whichever way you cut it, chocolate is addictive and contributes to blood sugar problems and hence weight. When you're two weeks to a month into the diet, you may well find you've lost any cravings for it. But, if you still fancy some here and there, limit it, like desserts, to once a week.

So, how much equals 5 **GL**?

SWEETS	5 **GL**
GoodCarb Real Belgian Chocolate Brownie (all varieties)	1½ bars
Fruitus oat and fruit bar	1 bar
Rebar fruit and vegetable bar	½ bar
Granola bar	less than ½ bar
Regular chocolate bar, milk or dark	less than ¼ bar
Mars Bar	⅕ bar

One way of quitting the chocolate or sweets habit is to find good alternatives, which luckily abound in good health food stores. My favorites are Organic Food Bars and CocoChia Snack Bars, which contain healthy high-quality ingredients.

But you can't munch on these all the time, either: they'll simply keep your sweet tooth going. And be aware, too, that many so-called health bars are packed with sugar, hydrogenated fat, and other not-so-healthy ingredients—so always check labels.

Desserts

It's the same story with desserts. If you eat a lot of desserts, or if you are insulin resistant, you will probably crave something sweet at the end of each meal. It is very important to break this habit because, if you don't, it will keep your blood sugar level seesawing. It takes only three days in most cases to stop the craving. So, after your initial stimulant- and sugar-free period, limit desserts to one a week, perhaps on the weekend.

You'll find wonderful recipes for Fatburner desserts in Chapter 28, including Chocolate Ice Cream and Kiwi and Coconut Pudding. These don't exceed 5 🌀 and aren't loaded with saturated fats. Don't have desserts when you are eating out (see Chapter 19), because almost all restaurant desserts are heavily loaded with sugar and saturated fat.

You can have a 5-🌀 dessert with your meal and leave out one of your snacks, but having the snack is better because you are grazing more than gorging. This helps to keep your blood sugar level even, which as we've seen prevents weight gain.

So, in summary, once you've started the diet, you can be drinking unlimited hot drinks such as Teeccino, Rooibos tea, or herbal teas, and one glass of diluted juice a day. After you've gone through two weeks to a month with no coffee, tea, sweets, or alcohol, you can have, taking the place of juice on that day, a small glass of wine, a half-pint of beer, or a shot of spirits up to a maximum of three times a week; or six pieces of chocolate or a Fatburner dessert, once a week. And don't forget your 2 quarts of water a day.

But, whichever option you choose, the goal for your drinks, sweets, and desserts is to keep within 5 🌀 a day. Enjoy!

...................**18**...................

Shopping

Everything you need for the Holford Diet is easily available in the supermarket or, for a few specialty items, your local health food store.

Some of the ingredients may be new to you, so this chapter will tell you where to get them and give you some guidance on what to do with them. The following shopping list includes all you need to get stocked up and ready for fatburning.

The cupboard staples list includes anything that keeps for a week or more. Fresh fruits and vegetables form a large part of what you eat and need to be restocked on a regular basis, but you may want to check the recipes and menus in Part Four first to see what you'll need. The same holds true for fresh fish—just buy what you need for that week. As for supplies from health food stores, these are becoming far cheaper than they once were as demand is growing. And some items once available exclusively from such stores, such as whole-meal pasta, are now widely available from supermarkets. So scout around for products, and prices, that suit you.

Your shopping list

From the supermarket

Foods for the fridge
Apples, pears, oranges, raspberries (fresh or frozen), strawberries, blueberries, melon, peaches, kiwifruit

Mushrooms, celery, green onions, avocado, parsley, carrots, bean sprouts,
    peppers, zucchini, eggplant, cucumber, lettuce, frozen peas, tomatoes
Fresh root ginger
Flat-leaf parsley and basil
Skim milk
Very-low-fat, live natural yogurt (with no additives)
Cottage cheese, low-fat Quark or fromage frais, half-fat Cheddar cheese
Very-low-fat mayonnaise
Free-range eggs
Tofu—plain, smoked, and marinated pieces
Tahini
Cod, haddock, mackerel, herring, salmon (go for wild salmon if possible)

Cupboard staples
Lemons
Potatoes and sweet potatoes, onions, garlic
Rolled oats and oat flakes
Wheat germ
100 percent rye bread, pumpernickel bread
Oatcake crackers (the best are Nairn's sugar-free variety)
Brown rice
Soba noodles
Bulgur (cracked wheat)
Couscous
Millet
Whole-meal spaghetti and other whole-meal pasta
Whole-meal flour
Chickpeas, various dried beans, lentils
Cooked chestnuts
Raw (unroasted/unsalted) mixed nuts, cashews, almonds, walnuts
Sunflower, sesame, pumpkin, and flax seeds
Raisins, dried apricots
Canned pineapple chunks (unsweetened, in juice)
Canned tomatoes, tomato paste
Tuna in water
Anchovies in olive oil (drain on paper towel before use)
Sardines in water
Olive oil (cold-pressed, extra-virgin)

Cider vinegar

Balsamic vinegar

Dried herbs and spices (turmeric, cumin, paprika, cayenne pepper, coriander)

Honey

Vanilla essence

Herbal teas

Sugar-free sparkling fruit drinks

From the health food store

Foods for the fridge

Alfalfa seeds or sprouts

Lentil or bean sprouts

Seed-oil blends, such as Udo's Choice

Cupboard staples

Kallo, Pacific, Imagine, and similar brands (instant vegetable stocks)

Tamari (an alternative to soy sauce)

Whole-wheat lasagna and macaroni, and whole-wheat or buckwheat spaghetti

Millet

Quinoa

Pear and apple butter (a sugar-free alternative to jam)

Whole Earth sugar-free jam

Get Up & Go

Dandelion coffee

Roma, Cafix, Teeccino

How to use the new foods

In Part Four, you'll be discovering how to cook with all these foods. For now, here's a bit of background on some that may be new to you.

Quinoa is actually a seed rather than a grain, and looks much like millet. It was once eaten by the Inca and was reputed to be the source of their empire's strength; it is still eaten widely in the Andes. Quinoa tastes slightly nutty and something like rice, and it's an excellent source of protein, as well as slow-releasing carbohydrate.

You cook quinoa like rice, adding up to three times as much water as quinoa and cooking it for about 13 minutes. It's best eaten as an accompaniment to, for example, a steam-fry or a casserole. You could also add it to a soup to thicken it up or eat it cold as part of a salad, much like couscous, and it makes a tasty pilaf cooked with onions, brown rice, and peas.

Tofu is, in terms of protein quality, second only to quinoa—and is also an excellent source of both protein and slow-releasing carbohydrate. Both tofu and quinoa, when eaten with carbohydrate-rich foods, slow down the release of their sugars.

Tofu is made from soybeans and is something like a bland cheese. It comes in different textures: soft (good for desserts or making things "creamy") or hard (better for steam-fries and main meals). While rather flavorless itself, it rapidly absorbs the flavor of any sauce. So if you are cooking a Chinese steam-fry flavored with soy sauce, garlic, and ginger, the tofu will readily soak up these flavors and taste delicious. With plain tofu, you need to drain the liquid off first.

You can also buy tofu smoked, marinated, or braised (but avoid fried tofu). These varieties, which are firmer than plain tofu and already delectable-tasting, make an excellent substitute for meat or chicken in steam-fries, stews, and casseroles. You can also add flavor to tofu by marinating it for 20 minutes before you cook with it. You can even make a tofu steak, or include tofu in sandwiches. I recommend suppliers who guarantee that their soybeans have not been genetically modified.

Lentils and beans are excellent and inexpensive foods. Both lentils and beans need to be boiled in plenty of water. Lentils, depending on the type, take between 15 and 25 minutes. Beans need to be soaked overnight, then boiled, usually for up to two hours. You can buy presoaked, cooked beans in cans, which you can simply drain and add to recipes.

Even if your bean experience is limited to Boston baked beans, you'll soon become an enthusiast. Their taste and texture are very satisfying, and, as they're such a big part of cuisine around the world—from India, Mexico, and South America to the Far East—the range of dishes you can make from them is huge. Hummus and other dips, chili, casseroles, lentil roast, and soups are only part of the story, as you'll see in Part Four.

Salad ingredients can be used much more imaginatively than most people think. With a few exceptions, most vegetables can be eaten raw. Raw, uncooked, and grated beets, cabbage, broccoli, zucchini, and carrot tops can all be used along with peppers, tomatoes, grated carrots, baby corn, and a variety of leafy vegetables such as watercress, arugula, lettuce, chicory, red cabbage, and spinach. You can also add marinated tofu pieces, almonds, and, less frequently, avocados, to increase the protein content. There are plenty of salad and salad dressing recipes to choose from in Part Four.

Tahini is a spread made from sesame seeds and their oil. As it's high in essential fats, it's a lot better for you and more flavorful than butter. I use tahini on bread and toast instead of butter, and often add some to savory dishes at the end for a creamier texture and added flavor. Use in moderation, as instructed in the recipes, and keep in the fridge.

Seeds contain vitamins, minerals, protein, fiber, and essential fats. They are therefore a superfood, yet many people shy away from them because of fat phobia or simply ignorance about how to use them. Flax seeds (linseeds) and pumpkin seeds are the best for the essential omega-3 fats, while sesame and sunflower are the best for the omega-6 fats. A combination of all four, stored in a glass jar in the fridge to minimize oxidation, then ground in a coffee grinder, makes a great addition to any cereal. Four teaspoons give you a good daily intake of essential fats plus lots of other key nutrients, including bone-building calcium, magnesium, and zinc. Seeds are best uncooked or thrown in at the last moment of cooking, such as in a steam-fry, since heating lowers the quality of their essential fats.

Seed-oil blends should be cold-pressed and preferably organic, stored in a lightproof container and kept refrigerated. The best blends of oils are those that provide roughly equal proportions of omega-3 and omega-6 fats, usually by combining flaxseed oil, pumpkin seed oil, sesame oils, sunflower oil, or borage oil. Two such oils are Omega Nutrition's Essential Balance and Udo's Choice, available from health food stores. These can't be cooked, so they're for adding to soups at the end of cooking, or to cereals, vegetables, and salad dressings.

Eating Out

You don't need to stay in every night, slaving over a hot stove (or a salad bowl) on the Holford Diet. But when it comes to eating out you will need to be choosy. As I've said, I travel the world on lecture tours and I always find excellent restaurants as I go, simply by choosing Chinese, Japanese, Malaysian, or Thai establishments.

The reason? These countries have the leanest, healthiest people, and much of that is due to the way they eat. And because the Chinese, for instance, have emigrated to so many countries around the world, it's usually possible to find a Chinese restaurant at least, whether in the United States, Canada, Australia, Europe, South America—or the Far East! But this doesn't mean you can't eat French, Italian, Mexican, Indian, or other foods. You just need to know what to order.

The trick, as ever, is to fill yourself up with the good stuff. That means having an appetizer and a main course, or just a main course, but not a dessert. It also means avoiding any breads, shrimp chips, or the like. In fact, it's best to ask the waiter to take it away, thus removing the temptation. Instead, ask them to bring some olives or a dish of hot pickles. Order water and say you won't be drinking anything else.

When you are choosing items from the menu, watch out for the hidden sugar and high-ⓖⓛ carbohydrates in sauces, pickles, and dips. For example, all Thai restaurants serve very tasty fish cakes and spring rolls. The fish cakes are better than the spring rolls because they have more protein. Both come with a sweet sauce, and you'll need to leave this on the side.

Where possible, choose food that hasn't been deep-fried. So go for boiled noodles rather than fried, or boiled rice rather than fried rice. Share a portion between two or even three people. Remember, you want about as much weight of the carbohydrate food as the protein-rich food, such as a steamed or poached fish.

Japanese restaurants are great, especially if you like fish. All offer wonderful fish dishes, from teriyaki salmon to sashimi. (Sushi isn't as good because it includes a lot of sweet white rice.) Sashimi can be very satisfying without filling you up with fast-releasing carbohydrates or saturated fat.

Always order some vegetable dishes, whether a salad or a side order of green beans or broccoli. Make sure you eat your greens and, if you haven't had enough, order some more.

By the time you get to the end of your main course, you should be full. This is the time to make your exit, asking for the bill and letting your perhaps dejected waiter know that the food was so good and filling that you don't want coffee or dessert!

Most of all, remember who is in charge of what goes in your mouth. Think of the menu as only a small selection of what's available, opening up the possibility of ordering off menu. For instance, if you like the sound of the fish, but not the cream sauce, ask for it without, or swap it for another method of cooking. Ask what's in various dishes and have a look around at what other people are eating.

Indian food uses a lot of vegetables, beans, and lentils, but there's also a lot of hidden sugar and fat in some of the sauces. You have to choose very carefully indeed in Indian restaurants, so I'd recommend going to them only as an occasional treat. The same applies to cheaper Italian restaurants that specialize in pizza and pasta. These dishes are based on high-**GL** carbohydrates and the pasta can come with fatty, cheesy, or creamy sauces, so they're best avoided. But authentic Italian and French restaurants will have plenty of excellent main dishes, such as grilled chicken, plus good salads and vegetables; be on the lookout for these.

Here are some typical items from Chinese, Thai, Japanese, Malaysian, and Indian restaurant menus to choose, or avoid.

CHOOSE

Sashimi	Steamed fish and other nonfried fish
Fish/chicken teriyaki	dishes
Tom yum soup	Tofu-based dishes

Thai fish/chicken/shrimp tikkas, curries (but avoid the creamier ones listed under "Avoid" below)

Fish/chicken satay (peanut-based sauce)

Indian bhunas or baltis—ask for less oil

Omelettes

Noodles with vegetables, such as chop suey (share a portion)

Vegetable dishes such as chana masala or dal (Indian) or stir-fried bean sprouts, bamboo shoots, water chestnuts, or mushrooms (Chinese)

AVOID

Fried fish/meat

Sweet-and-sour dishes

Creamy curries such as kormas and masalas

Rice (unless brown; then share a portion)

Potato dishes

Bread, such as naans and chapatis

Shrimp chips

The fallback in any restaurant is to choose something simple, without sauces with unknown ingredients. So you can't go wrong with grilled fish or chicken and vegetables or salad.

Restaurants are a good proving ground for your new relationship with food. Now that you understand so much more about why you feel the way you do and what food has to do with it, make good food your friend. Become the master of your own weight and health by becoming the master of your diet.

The best way to do this is to get your hands dirty preparing your own meals. Experiment. Make mistakes. Try new foods. Get involved with creating a way of eating that really works for you.

Choose to follow this diet because it makes sense and you want to change. I guarantee the results will be worth it. I want you to make this *your* diet, and simply use what's in this book as a springboard. That means finding the balance between eating out and eating in, breaking your addictions and having the odd treat. Be moderate in everything, including moderation.

20

Fatburning for Vegetarians

Being vegetarian is generally healthier than being a carnivore, but you have to know what you are doing. The key is making sure you get enough protein, vitamin B_{12}, and iron (see Chapter 21), and don't live off dairy and wheat, which are the most common allergy-provoking foods.

The Holford Diet's emphasis on vegetables and plant-based protein makes it very easy for vegetarians and vegans to follow. There are a number of delicious dishes listed in Chapter 28 that are suitable for anyone avoiding meat and fish, from Chestnut and Mushroom Pilaf and Quinoa Tabbouleh to Thai-Style Vegetable Broth and Pasta with Pumpkin Seed Pesto. The diet has also been designed to be as versatile as possible, so you can simply substitute tofu or legumes such as chickpeas or kidney beans for the meat or fish in most of the recipes.

To make this easier for you, in Part Four I have given recommendations for suitable replacements alongside recipes in the meat and fish sections, where appropriate. This is also a good opportunity to try some of the more unusual vegetarian- and vegan-friendly ingredients available. We've already had a look at some of these in Chapter 18, but let's delve a little deeper here and see how they can be used as dietary staples.

Soy stars

Plain, marinated, and smoked tofu (see page 180) are the protein stars of the vegetarian Holford Diet. You can now buy imaginative flavors of marinated tofu, such as sesame and ginger, or almond and hazelnut. Tempeh is made of fermented soybeans, and has a much nuttier taste and firmer texture than tofu. Rather like Marmite, it is not for everyone, but I love it. Silken tofu is a very soft type that is useful for blending to thicken sauces, dips or smoothies. There is a recipe in the vegetarian section of the main meals in Chapter 28 that makes use of smoked tofu, Japanese Noodles (page 272), and many in the meat sections that are easy to adapt.

A leg up with legumes

I've already discussed beans and lentils in Chapter 18, and as a vegetarian you're very likely highly familiar with legumes such as chickpeas and kidney beans. But we'll be cooking with many others, such as the delicious green-hued flageolet (Flageolet Bean Dip has a very delicate flavor and is a delicious and unusual alternative to hummus), while black-eyed peas add a great texture to salsas and in gazpacho soup. If you have previously dismissed lentils as mushy and bland, try French lentils cooked with a little vegetable stock. These green, shiny lentils hold their shape and texture when cooked, and are rightly considered a delicacy in France.

With the grain

You've seen how amazing quinoa is already. Containing all the essential amino acids for our protein requirements, it is a nutritionally perfect food as well as being very versatile, working as both carbohydrate and protein in a meal. You can use quinoa in all kinds of dishes, such as salads (Quinoa Tabbouleh), main dishes (Roasted Vegetables with Mediterranean Quinoa), and even desserts (Coconut Quinoa Pudding).

But good grains and seeds don't stop there. You can experiment with couscous, bulgur, and millet, which are excellent served with all sorts of casseroles. And the range of available yeast-free pumpernickel and other low-**GL** breads, as well as delicious flaked grains, increases yearly.

Not from the cow

If you are vegan, you can substitute soy milk or rice milk for dairy milk. Rice milk has a much higher **GL** and is therefore not so good. There are other milks now available in health food stores, from oat milk to quinoa milk. These have a lower **GL**.

21

Supplements

Good nutrition is achieved by eating the right foods, *and* by supplementing. There is no question that the levels of many nutrients required to help your body function at its best are above those easily achieved by diet alone. Such optimal levels of nutrients can also help you to reprogram your body to burn fat. If you want to know more about the vitamins and minerals that help you to burn fat, refer back to Chapter 10.

If you have never taken supplements before, you may find they have many beneficial side effects. In a survey at ION, 79 percent of people, after six months on a supplement program, reported improved energy, while 61 percent felt physically fitter and had fewer colds.

The basics

The starting point for any supplement program is a good, all-around multivitamin and mineral supplement plus 1,000 milligrams of vitamin C. Do check that the multivitamin/mineral that you've chosen meets the amounts shown on pages 128–29. You'll also probably need to supplement your diet with chromium (200 micrograms) separately—check the label on your multi.

So an ideal supplement program looks like this:

	Breakfast	*Lunch*	*Dinner*
High-strength multivitamin and mineral	1	1	
Vitamin C, 1,000mg	1		
Chromium, 200mcg	1		

A good-quality multivitamin will direct you to take two per day. This is simply because you can't fit adequate quantities of vitamins and minerals into a single tablet or capsule. To get the most value out of your multi, I recommend taking one with breakfast and the second with either lunch or dinner.

If you are struggling with your appetite or sugar cravings, I recommend you add hydroxycitric acid (HCA) and 5-HTP:

	Breakfast	Lunch	Dinner
HCA (450mg)		1	1
5-HTP (50mg)	1	1	1

HCA helps encourage fatburning and is good for everyone. Take it before meals.

5-HTP is especially good for those with sugar cravings and a tendency to mild depression. If you crave something sweet when your mood is low, try 5-HTP. It is best absorbed either on an empty stomach or with a piece of fruit. Try it with your midmorning and midafternoon snacks.

For details on suppliers and brands of supplements I recommend, see page 364 in Resources.

Fiber supplements

Generally speaking, fiber is not something you add to food. It's in food anyway, unless a food manufacturer has processed it out. The Holford Diet is a high-fiber diet. However, there is one special kind of fiber that can help you to lose weight by slowing down the release of carbohydrates. It is called glucomannan and comes from the Japanese konjac plant (see page 75 in Chapter 7 for more details).

Three grams of glucomannan a day has been proved to assist weight loss. Konjac extract, which is 60 percent glucomannan, comes in 500-milligram capsules. It's recommended that you take nine of these capsules a day. Take three, with a large glass of water, three times a day just before meals. Because glucomannan swells to a hundred times its volume by absorbing water, it is very important to drink a large glass of water whenever you take konjac extract or glucomannan. Suppliers are given on page 363.

The when and how of supplements

Vitamin and mineral supplements are best taken with food and, if they are involved in energy regulation, during the day. They should also be taken *every* day. While most people notice the effects of taking them after 30 days, it is best to stick to a supplement program for three months to see a real difference.

There are no dangers with taking any of these supplements on a long-term basis. However, once you've achieved your desired weight, you may wish to stop taking HCA, 5-HTP, and additional chromium. These are included specifically to help stabilize your blood sugar levels. Most decent multivitamin and mineral supplements will provide around 30 micrograms of chromium, which is enough when you're on the maintenance phase of the Holford Diet.

Exercise

While the main thrust of the Holford Diet is food, we've also seen how exercise helps you to keep your blood sugar level even and to burn fat. But it's important to do the right kind, and this is a combination of aerobic exercise and resistance or toning exercise.

To be a Fatburner, you need to exercise a minimum of 15 minutes a day, or 35 minutes three times a week. The exercise program you choose needs to include both aerobics, which burns fat directly, and toning exercises, which build fatburning muscle. If you are significantly underlean (see page 43), you may need to do more to build up enough lean muscle to keep you thin.

Earlier I suggested that you start to experiment with some of the exercises in this chapter right before you start the diet, to get used to including it in your week. Take that time to find an exercise routine that suits you. You may wish to join a gym, get a workout video, and find a friend to exercise with so you can keep each other motivated. Set yourself a specific time to exercise during the day. You may wish to double the time you exercise, and do it every other day, which will let you have more days off.

If you've never really exercised, or are very overweight or unfit, it's best to go to your local gym and get advice from a fitness instructor before you start. It's important, too, to let your doctor know what you're doing so that he or she can advise, if necessary.

Aerobic exercise

Aerobics has to be intense enough to raise your pulse rate into the training zone (see the chart below), but not so intense that you exceed your capacity to produce muscular energy using the oxygen you breathe. Sprinting, for example, is too intense—it demands more oxygen than is available, so the muscles switch to making energy anaerobically. This results in a buildup of toxic by-products.

Training heart rate zone (while exercising)

Age	65–80% of maximum heart rate	
	(beats in 1 minute)	(beats in 10 sec.)
20	130–160	22–27
22	129–158	22–26
24	127–157	21–26
26	126–155	21–26
28	125–154	21–26
30	124–152	21–25
32	122–150	20–25
34	121–149	20–25
36	120–147	20–25
38	118–146	20–24
40	117–144	20–24
45	114–140	19–23
50	111–136	19–23
55	107–132	18–22
60	104–128	17–21
65	101–124	17–21
70	98–120	16–20

The center column shows how many beats you should have in one minute; beginners should aim for the lower figure on the left-hand side (that is, 65% of the maximum heart rate for their age), then slowly increase to 80%. Do not exceed this higher level. The column on the far right gives you how many beats you should have in a 10-second pulse count. Beginners should stay at the lower end of their exercise range.

You may have never done aerobics, but don't view it as a hard slog before you've begun. It can be hugely fun. Think of swimming, a volleyball game with friends or colleagues, or a long ramble through stunning countryside.

Here are just some of your choices:

Walking	Aerobics
Rambling	Dance classes
Jogging	Cycling
Swimming	Team sports
Circuit training	Video workouts

But whichever you choose, you need to follow the same golden rules with each:

1. **Warm up first.** This is especially important if you are unfit and overweight. Warming up is necessary to prepare the body for an increased level of activity. The body needs time to transport the oxygen you breathe into your muscles. Gradually increasing a walk from a slow to a medium pace gives the body the time that is needed. Or starting with the breaststroke before you move on to the front crawl when swimming may be a good way to slowly increase the intensity.

If you start too quickly, then inevitably you will start to feel uncomfortable and will need to slow down in order to continue. This can be discouraging if you are new to exercise. Take 2–3 minutes to warm up. Think of it as a gradual increase rather than stop-start. It's like driving a car—you need to pull away in first gear and work your way up through the gears, slowly building up to a level you can maintain. If you tried to pull away in top gear when driving a car, it would struggle and stall. In the same way, you will feel very uncomfortable quickly if you do not warm up.

Remember: you warm up to work out, you don't work out to warm up.

2. **Exercise at a level that keeps you in your training zone for at least 15 minutes.** If you are swimming, for example, don't stop every couple of lengths. It is better to swim more slowly and keep going than to stop frequently and catch your breath. If you are attracted to team sports such as tennis, badminton, squash, or soccer, the trick is to keep moving. Short bursts of activity won't do you much good for developing aerobic fitness, which is what burns fat. In this respect squash, say, is better than soccer.

The purpose of training in your training zone is to develop your aerobic fitness. This will in turn increase your body's ability to use fat as a fuel. As you get fitter the body increases the cells where it produces energy. These cells (mitochondria) increase in size and number with activity that is continuous in nature and of a moderate intensity. They can turn you into an incredibly efficient fatburning machine. It is no surprise that distance runners and cyclists have the highest levels of these cells. Your goal is to build up to a level that allows you to keep exercising continuously for up to 35 minutes.

How will you know if you are exercising within your training zone? Well, it will be a faster pace than your normal walking speed but not so fast that you can't continue to talk to someone else at the same time.

If you are new to exercise, it's recommended that you start by increasing frequency and duration before increasing intensity. Think "More active, more often."

3. **Set yourself a realistic goal and gradually increase it.** Here's an example. If you like jogging around your local park, you might find that one circuit takes you 10 minutes. In your second week, can you get that time down to 9 minutes? Or you could increase the distance and/or how often you do it. In the beginning, make it easy to reach your goal. Then week by week, reach for higher goals. When you achieve them you'll know you're really fatburning—you'll be seeing, and feeling, the results.

Find some time in your schedule when you can do some exercise and make a date with yourself. As a benchmark, see how long you can exercise in your training zone. Let's say 5 minutes. Now that you know what you can manage, make sure you do 5 minutes of exercise more frequently. Your goal is to build up to 3–5 times a week. Alternatively, you may want to increase the time. Again, with 5 minutes as your starting point, try to add just 1 minute each time you exercise. Too often people try to add too much at the beginning, become uncomfortable, do not achieve their goal, and become discouraged.

Here's an example. If you plan to do more exercise, you may want to start with 10 minutes, three times a week. You could aim to add 1 minute each time you exercise, thereby gradually increasing the total duration. This would mean that in the first week you would complete three sessions: one of

10 minutes, one of 11 minutes, and one of 12 minutes. Within four weeks you will have doubled the time you initially exercised for, but the increase will have been so gradual that you'll hardly have noticed it.

	Monday	Wednesday	Friday	Week's total minutes
Week 1	10	11	12	33
Week 2	13	14	**15**	42
Week 3	16	17	18	51
Week 4	19	20	21	60

Within two weeks you will have reached the recommended 15-minute minimum and you can then focus on increasing the frequency.

Alternatively, you may want to increase the frequency first. This would require you to plan 15 minutes of exercise into your day. In the first week you might manage to fit in two 15-minute sessions. The following week you should aim to find time to add another session. This should continue gradually and soon you'll find that you are exercising for 15 minutes every day.

Once you have achieved this, you should try to find time elsewhere in your schedule so that you could carry out two 15-minute sessions in a single day. Perhaps you could look at alternatives to driving or taking public transportation to work: if you cycle, or get off your bus a few stops earlier, you could gain 15 minutes of exercise when traveling in and another 15 minutes when traveling home.

Your goals need to be achievable and manageable. You are better off planning and attaining small goals that gradually build your success rather than aiming too high initially. Remember that just becoming more active is an achievement. Finding time to be more active and planning exercise may be your initial goal.

4. **Vary the exercise so that you don't get bored.** Variety can add a dimension to your exercise routine. In the same way that you don't plan to eat the same meals every day, you can vary the types of exercise that you do. This will also allow you to work different muscles and develop your general fitness.

Try to find activities that you enjoy. If you don't enjoy one form of exercise, try something else. Finding the right environment can be very important.

Exercise won't always be fun. At times you may find it uncomfortable, time-consuming, or solitary. However, ask anyone who exercises on a regular basis and they will tell you that while they don't always enjoy the sessions, they do enjoy the results.

5. **Exercise with a friend, at a gym, or in classes for extra motivation.** When you start to plan your exercise program, consider several options.

Who do you want to exercise with? Some people prefer to exercise in groups or with other like-minded people. However, others prefer to exercise alone and use the time to think. You may want both. Time passes more quickly when you are with someone else.

Where do you want to exercise? The gym can be a really good place to get support. The fitness instructors want to help. They enjoy developing new exercise programs for people. You may prefer to take exercise classes. If you're not sure which would be most effective, ask for advice. Remember that you want something that is aerobic in nature rather than a "Legs, bums, and tums" class, which is better for toning.

Plan to reward yourself with something other than food for hitting certain targets. These rewards can be symbolic or practical—a new piece of training gear, a massage, or a new book, anything that will motivate you to achieve your goal.

6. **Drink plenty of water before, during, and after exercising.** The body is two thirds water and you lose significant amounts of it through sweating and breathing. Drink a glass of water for every half hour of exercise.

7. **Cool down when you finish and stretch the muscles you've been exercising.** If you have been exercising for 15 minutes, take 2–3 minutes to cool down before starting your stretches. The cool-down is the opposite of the warm-up. Again, think of your body as a car; you would not shift from fifth gear to first in one move. So make sure you slow down gradually.

Stretching will promote recovery as well as relaxing your muscles. It is often neglected; however, it is essential, to reduce the risk of injury, that you stretch the muscles you have worked. Depending on which muscles you've been working, stretch them out immediately after exercising. It is best to hold a stretch and count to 20, rather than stretching, releasing, and stretching again.

8. **Keep it up.** The real benefits of exercise are seen after weeks or months, not days. Make exercise a part of your daily routine.

It can be quite an achievement to plan and complete exercise on a daily basis. Remember that every exercise session that you complete takes you closer to your goal; every session missed keeps you further away. Try not to focus only on the physical changes to your body, as this does not recognize your accomplishment in being a regular exerciser (with all the planning and organization this entails).

Don't think of it as taking up exercise, but as giving up being inactive.

The psychological benefits of exercise are just as well established as the physical benefits. Not only will you enjoy a healthier, more efficient body, but you will also sleep more soundly, have more energy for other tasks, and think more clearly.

Toning exercises

By toning specific muscle groups you can lose inches as well as pounds. As we've seen, the more muscle you build, the greater your ability to burn fat: muscle uses up more calories. Some workouts include both aerobic and toning exercises. Alternatively, you could do a mainly aerobic exercise one day and a mainly toning exercise another.

The trick for toning exercises is to get some good advice. Your local gym is probably the best place for that. If you prefer to exercise as part of a group, ask your local gym for an exercise class. Classes focusing on toning exercises are very popular and you will often have a variety to choose from. Many celebrities swear by yoga—if you can't attend a class you could try one of the yoga videos for sale. There are different types of yoga and you need to find a style and level to suit you.

Ask your gym instructor to include compound exercises in your workout. These exercises use the large muscle groups and help keep the total number of exercises to a minimum.

Typical exercises used in circuit classes can be completed at home. Traditional push-ups and their modifications can be performed in the living room, as can many of the other body-weight movements. Here is an example of a set of exercises that could be performed one after another in a circuit fashion, to give you the toning effects you want. (For detailed descriptions of the exercises, please visit www.theholforddiet.com.)

Example circuit workout

Exercise	Circuit 1	Circuit 2	Circuit 3
Squats	10	12	15
Push-ups	10	12	15
Sit-ups	10	12	15
Upright rows	10	12	15
Back extensions	10	12	15
Triceps dips	10	12	15
Lunges	10	12	15
Side leg lifts	10	12	15
Lateral raises	10	12	15
Biceps curls	10	12	15

You do not have to start by doing all of the exercises at once or all three circuits the first time; you can build up to completing this over a period of time.

Psychocalisthenics®

One of my favorite exercise routines is Psychocalisthenics. You can learn it in five hours, by watching a video or, ideally, taking a class, and do it in about 15 minutes wherever you are.

Psychocalisthenics is a precise sequence of 23 exercises that leave you feeling fantastic. I've been doing it for 20 years and I've yet to find anything that keeps me trimmer and makes me feel better—not bad for 15 minutes a day! Each exercise is driven by the breath and, somehow, my body feels lighter, freer, and thoroughly oxygenated after this simple routine, which anyone can do.

Psychocalisthenics is the brainchild of Oscar Ichazo. Ichazo founded the Arica School in the 1960s as a school of knowledge for the understanding of the complete person. A practitioner of martial arts and yoga since 1939, he developed Psychocalisthenics to be a daily routine that can be done in less

For Exercise Enthusiasts

If you are already an exercise enthusiast and are clocking a significant amount of time each day doing exercise, you may find that the 40 ⓖⓛ rule for the food you eat does not fill you up. The same also applies if you are very tall, while the reverse applies if you are very short. The chart below helps adjust the total number of ⓖⓛ you eat, based on your height and your average level of exercise.

ⓖⓛ per Day

	Average exercise per day (mins.)						
	0	15	30	45	60	90	120
5 ft	35	35	40	45	45	50	55
5 ft 3	40	40	40	45	50	55	60
5 ft 6	40	40	40	45	50	55	60
5 ft 9	40	40	45	50	55	60	65
6 ft	45	45	50	55	60	65	70
6 ft 3	50	50	55	60	65	70	75
6 ft 6	55	55	60	65	70	75	80

than 20 minutes. At first glance it looks like a powerful kind of aerobic yoga. "In the same way that we have an everyday need for food and nourishment we have to promote the circulation of our vital energy as an everyday business," says Ichazo.

While most exercise routines simply treat the body as a physical machine that needs to be worked to stay fit, Psychocalisthenics is designed to generate both physical fitness and vital energy by bringing mind and body into balance. The key lies in the precise breathing pattern that accompanies each physical exercise. Energy generation happens when you have stable blood sugar, plus a good supply of oxygen. According to Jane Alexander of the *Daily Mail*, "Psychocalisthenics is exercise, pared to perfection. I wasn't sweating buckets as I would after an aerobics class. But I had exercised far more muscles. I was clear-headed and bright rather than wiped out."

The best way to learn Psychocalisthenics is to take a short course. For details see www.pcals.com. You can also teach yourself from a DVD, but it is best to learn it "live."

My ideal weekly fatburning exercise regime is to do Psychocalisthenics every other day, three or four times a week; walk, run, swim, or cycle three times a week; and take one Ashtanga yoga class a week that involves "resistance" training, building muscle more than stamina. Enjoy experimenting and finding your favorite routine—once you've done this, it'll be easier to stick to it.

Monitoring Your Results

Once you get going on the Holford Diet, you will feel and see the results. You may not be able to measure your new energy levels—but you can certainly monitor the pounds you're dropping and the inches you're losing. And here's how.

Weigh and measure yourself at the start of this diet and at the end of every week. Always weigh yourself in the morning, before breakfast, without clothes. Keep monitoring your progress week after week. If you have a bad week, notice what effect that is having on your progress, and get back on course. If you reach a "plateau," don't worry. This can happen. You can encourage weight loss by following the diet more precisely. Soon, you'll find what you need to do to lose weight and, once you've reached your ultimate goal, what you need to do to stay there.

There's a Fatburner progress report for each of the first four weeks in Appendix 4. Fill out the report for Week 1, setting your long-term goal weight and your weekly target weight (see page 147 for how to figure these out). You'll need an accurate pair of scales and a tape measure. Since scales do vary, it's best to weigh yourself on the same one each week. For the measurements, always take the widest part of, for example, your waist, your thighs, and your hips. For your thigh measurement, take the average of your left and right thighs.

Waist-hip ratio and total inch loss

I recommend that you also calculate your waist-hip ratio. This is your waist measurement divided by your hip measurement. The reason is that it's one of the most important measures in relation to your health. Abdominal weight gain is associated with insulin resistance—and hence, the risk of diabetes—much more than hip and thigh weight gain. Once you're above 0.95 for men or 0.85 for women, you do have an increased risk of obesity-related diseases. Broadly speaking, if your waist is greater than 46 inches (men) or 40 inches (women), you need to lose weight. (Obviously, this does depend a bit on your height.)

Your total inch loss is the sum of all the inches you have lost from your bust or chest, waist, hips, and thighs. (If you've lost an inch from each, your total loss is 4 inches.)

Progress, week by week

At the end of each week, ask yourself honestly how well you've stuck to the diet and exercise program. There's a space on the progress report to rate yourself out of 100 percent. This will help you to stay on course. If, at the end of the week, you feel your targets are too hard or too easy, you can adjust the rate of progress you're aiming for.

You'll also find a spare Fatburner progress report that you can copy for subsequent weeks. Keep all these weekly progress sheets and then, when you've reached your ideal weight, I'd greatly appreciate it if you'd fill out the Fatburner questionnaire on page 353. This is how I can get your feedback to keep making this diet even more effective.

With a little help from your friends . . .

Let your friends and your family know what you are doing. Show them this book. Maybe they'll want to join in, too! Going on the diet with a friend is great, because you can then give each other support. Encourage your family to support you by being tolerant with the new foods you'll be preparing, and not tempting you with forbidden foods. When you're invited out to dinner, let your hosts know about the diet. And when you throw your own dinner party, use the recipes in Part 4. There are plenty that are elegant enough for a formal meal, and they're all delicious.

You may also find it extremely helpful to carry out this diet with the help of a nutrition consultant, who can help you to get started and will work out a personalized vitamin program for you. He or she can also keep you on track and provide you with moral support and tips on how to deal with any problems you may have. (See the section on nutrition consultations on page 362 in Resources.)

Breaking the rules

Very few people stick to diets 100 percent, 100 percent of the time. No doubt there will be the odd occasion when you break the rules. This is not a disaster. In fact, it can be a good idea to give yourself two meals a month when you can eat what you like. This will help you to deal with special occasions and celebrations. So enjoy yourself.

Remember, though, that the more you break the rules, the slower your progress will be. And if you are really addicted, say to double espressos or binge drinking after work, be careful. You can't consume any addictive substance in excess and keep your weight down or your health up. They have a nasty habit of creeping back into your life and are best avoided if you really feel you can't control your consumption of them.

If you do indulge at a friend's wedding, or find yourself unable to resist pizza and gelato on your Italian vacation, the most important thing to do is to get back on track the next day. In one experiment, two groups of dieters were given an identical milk shake to drink. One group was told it was high in calories, the other that it was low. Each group was then given an unlimited amount of ice cream. Which group, do you think, ate more?

The answer is, the group that had been told the milk shake was high in calories. This shows a very common pitfall among dieters—the "If I've broken my diet, I might as well go whole hog" syndrome. Don't do it. If you blow it one day, get back on track the next.

The first 30 days

If you have more weight to lose and feel good on this diet, keep going for up to 90 days. An excellent target weight loss for an obese person is to decrease body fat percentage by 10 percent each month, or to lose 18 pounds in 90 days. The balance of protein, carbohydrate, and fat in the Holford Diet (25 percent protein, 50 percent carbohydrate, 25 percent fat) helps to reprogram your body to burn fat. This reprogramming is especially important for those of you with a degree of insulin resistance who show signs of sugar sensitivity (see the questionnaire on page 38), and sometimes it takes longer than 30 days.

If you've achieved your goal, you can ease up by eating 50 🄶🄻 a day. Chapter 25 is all about how to maintain your weight and health. But first, let's look at what to do if this diet simply isn't working for you.

What If It's Not Working?

Say you're on Week 4 of the diet, and you've really stuck with it. Congratulations! You've conquered your coffee addiction, you're feeling much more energetic, and you can definitely see the gloss back in your hair with all the omega-3s you're getting. You love the recipes and your new jogging regime. There's just one problem: you haven't shed a pound.

I can understand how frustrating this must feel. It's at this point that I have to say no single diet works for everyone, for the simple reason that there are many different causes of overweight or obesity.

But I also have to say that, in truth, I haven't yet had a case of a person failing to lose weight after they looked at all the possible reasons below, and discovered the one that's holding them back.

So let's look at some common problems.

You're not losing weight, but you are losing inches. This is okay for now. What it means is that you are making lean muscle, which is heavier, but has the capacity to burn more fat. Keep going. The weight loss will follow.

You are still insulin resistant. Have you quit alcohol, sugar, and/or caffeine? If not, and you're not losing weight, you'll have to bite the bullet and give them up.

You're not exercising. Exercise really does help kick-start your metabolism. If your weight isn't decreasing, then up your levels of activity.

You're not taking the supplements. Supplements do make a difference and, in addition to the basic multivitamin and vitamin C, the combination of chromium, HCA, and 5-HTP definitely gives you the edge in appetite control. They are well worth taking.

You have a hidden allergy. Don't underestimate this factor. Many people fail to lose weight until they have their food allergies checked. Your weight can really get stuck until you remove an offending food. Have a food-intolerance test (see page 366 in Resources) and avoid your food allergies.

You are estrogen dominant. Hormonal imbalances, especially of the thyroid, can keep you from losing weight. You need to get this checked by your doctor. You should also be tested for an underactive thyroid (see page 207).

Hormone imbalances and weight gain

It is not at all uncommon for weight gain to be precipitated by hormonal changes. In fact, according to the MyNutrition survey ION conducted on almost 30,000 people, those with hormonal issues were twice as likely as those without to have problems losing weight. For some women, the pounds pile on during pregnancy, only to stay on after giving birth. For others, going on or coming off the pill or hormone replacement therapy can trigger weight gain.

A common time for weight gain for many women is in the pre-menopausal years (usually from 40 onward) and, even more, at menopause, when menstruation ceases. Even more common than weight gain is a change in weight redistribution, which we'll look at now.

Apples and pears

Are you an apple or a pear? Excess weight on the hips and thighs, resulting in a pear-shaped body, is associated with excess estrogen, the feminizing hormone. Too much upper-body and waist gain is associated with excess androgens, the masculinizing hormones.

These hormonal differences are partly genetic and partly a consequence of how we live. Some people have more active adrenal glands, a factor encouraged by a stressful and competitive lifestyle. This leads to the release of more adrenal hormones, such as cortisol and adrenaline, as well as androgens, which all help to build protein and muscle.

Hence these "adrenal types" tend to be more muscular and have more weight in the top half of their bodies. For such people, it is very important not to live off adrenal stimulants (see Chapter 7) and to keep fat intake down. Too much fat, coupled with prolonged stress and a lack of exercise, leads to obesity. In fact, too much of the adrenal hormone cortisol can also lead to too much estrogen (produced in both the adrenal glands and fatty tissue, as well as the ovaries), which can lead to lower-body weight gain, too.

The two key female hormones are *estrogen* and *progesterone*. They're produced mainly in the ovaries and need to be in balance with one another. An increasingly common problem is that a woman produces too much estrogen in relation to progesterone. The problem usually stems from a progesterone deficiency, rather than actual excess estrogen.

Progesterone is produced by the ovaries only once an egg has been released, at ovulation. If a woman doesn't ovulate (which is increasingly com-

Hormones and their effects on weight distribution. Too much estrogen (or not enough progesterone) competes with the thyroid hormone thyroxine, resulting in a slow metabolism and weight gain, especially on the hips and thighs. Too much cortisol, the stress hormone, also affects thyroid function, slowing down the body's metabolism, which leads to weight gain, especially around the middle.

mon as a woman approaches menopause), then no progesterone is produced. After menopause, progesterone output falls to almost nothing, while estrogen levels sink very gradually. Estrogen is the feminizing hormone: it helps to lay down fat, especially on the hips and thighs, creating a more curvaceous shape. Many women gain weight in these places after the age of 35.

Full details on this subject are given in my book *Balancing Hormones Naturally,* coauthored with Kate Neil.

Men, too, can suffer from estrogen dominance. This is most likely to occur when their levels of the male hormone testosterone are low; testosterone counteracts the feminizing effects of estrogen. A diet high in meat, dairy, and pesticide-sprayed foods can make a contribution to developing estrogen dominance.

If you suspect that you have a hormonal imbalance and that this is contributing to your excess weight, the best thing to do is to see a nutritionist who can work with your doctor to have the necessary tests done and provide appropriate treatment if necessary.

Thyroid problems

The thyroid gland, found in the area at the base of the throat, controls your rate of metabolism by releasing a hormone called *thyroxine,* which stimulates cells to speed up energy production. Although they make up a relatively small percentage, some people with persistent weight problems do have underactive thyroids, which produce insufficient thyroxine. Excess estrogen can also interfere with thyroid function.

Some people have an underactive thyroid because their immune systems are attacking their thyroid tissue. This is known as *autoimmune thyroid disease.* You can have this checked by having an *antithyroid antibody test.* One in every 10 people who test positive has undiagnosed celiac disease (gluten sensitivity). It seems that you can become allergic to a food, and your immune system can then attack a part of you, thinking it's the food, perhaps because the food and you share similar proteins. So the next thing to do is get yourself tested for hidden food allergies.

If you've done everything I've mentioned in this chapter and it still isn't working, I recommend that you get professional advice from a qualified nutritional therapist. He or she can investigate your particular problem or perhaps give the necessary support and guidance you need. There are details on how to find one near you on page 362.

Controlling Emotional and Obsessive Eating

Eating is very nearly the first thing most of us do in life. Within minutes of being born, a baby receives sustenance from its mother. But suckling provides far more than food, as Harry Harlow's monkeys showed us.

In this famous experiment in the 1950s, infant monkeys were presented with the choice of two surrogate mothers—constructed dummies complete with teats. One provided nourishment, the other no milk but the tactile experience of fur. The baby monkeys chose the tactile sensation rather than food—comfort over nourishment.

Eating is emotive

For baby humans, the tactile sense and security of the breast are soon associated with food. Eating is an emotive business. And, later in life, eating can become associated with pleasing, rebelling, imitating, rewarding—even with punishment. For example, the girl who eats sparingly, like her mother, because she also wants to be thin; the boy who eats certain foods because they "make him big and strong" and develops aversions to other foods; the rebellion against "Eat it up or you won't get any dessert"; the reward of sweets if you do something good; the comfort of sweets when you're hurt. By adolescence, a multitude of psychological factors governs when, how, what, and how much we eat.

Does any of this ring a bell? Do you reach for chocolate when you're upset? Do you gain or lose weight when you are in love? Do you reward yourself with food? Do you always finish what's in front of you? Are you a fussier eater when you feel unhappy? Do you eat more when you are out with the guys?

"Five hundred people were asked what they fear most in the world and 190 answered that their greatest fear is 'getting fat,' " wrote Kim Chernin in *The Obsession*, a book about hunger. The fear of fat, and the love and hate of food, are a real social problem of epidemic proportions. With this fear, there has been a rapid rise in maladaptive eating behavior, compulsive eating, crash dieting, bulimia (weight control by vomiting), and anorexia nervosa.

Conflicting images

At least 95 percent of the sufferers are women, and there is little doubt that social pressures play a significant role. Torn between the advertising images of the sexually provocative "perfect" woman and perpetual sensory bombardment by tantalizing foods; between the image of the thin and sensuous woman, designed to attract her man, and the caring, providing "earth mother" image associated with fat, 21st-century women feel they must be all things to all people. And 21st-century men are also meant to bring home the bacon, yet look like Brad Pitt. But who has the time, the money, or the inclination to live at the gym, given today's work pressures?

There's a simple set of exercises that will help you get a handle on emotional eating so you have more choice about how to eat, rather than being a victim of your immediate desires or emotions. The exercises are divided into three steps called the three As:

Awareness
Acceptance
Action

STEP 1: AWARENESS

Awareness is the first: awareness of when, how, what you eat, and of your beliefs, facts, and fantasies about eating, being fat, and being thin. To get the most benefit from these exercises, answer each question accurately and write down your answer on a separate sheet of paper.

1. What do you weigh?
2. What is the heaviest you have ever been?

3. What is the lightest?
4. What is your ideal weight?
5. How long have you been overweight?
6. What personality characteristics do you associate with being fat?
7. What personality characteristics do you associate with being thin?
8. What do you fear most about being overweight? (Think about this in relation to health, sex, relationships, work, and so on.)
9. What do you like most about being overweight?
10. Imagine you're at a party and you are at your ideal weight. What feelings would you experience? How would this change the way you relate to the people around you?
11. Now imagine you become very overweight. How do you feel now, and how does this change the way you relate to others?
12. If you were at your ideal weight, how do you think your life would change? (Think of your feelings, relationships, sex, career, clothes, and sports.)

When

At this stage do not reason why, just observe your own behavior in relation to eating—the hows, whens, and whats. Now make a comprehensive list of all the circumstances that precipitate eating for you, other than hunger:

I eat when I'm bored.
I eat when I get home from work.
I eat when . . .
I eat when . . .

What

The next exercise will take a little longer.

Keep a food diary for one week, listing the circumstances in which you eat, your feelings before and feelings after each meal or snack, and, in detail, exactly what, and how much, you ate.

This can be done as shown in the chart on p. 211.

Be precise in your answers. They will help you become aware of the situations in which you eat, as well as showing you what you eat. You may find there are some foods or snacks you feel guilty about, that you would rather not commit to paper. You may make excuses to yourself—"I don't usually eat . . ." or "It would have been rude to refuse." Again, observe your own re-

Day 1 (time)	Food/drink	Circumstances	Feelings before	Feelings after
Monday 9 a.m.	Cup of coffee	Need to wake up	Tired	Bit more energy

actions as if you were watching your behavior and thoughts, without judgment, on a TV screen.

How

The next series of questions will help you examine how you eat. Answer these as precisely as possible.

1. What eating and mealtime rules did your parents teach you (such as "Always eat everything on your plate")?
2. Do you:
   a) eat your food very fast?
   b) eat your food at a normal rate?
   c) savor each mouthful and chew it well?
3. How fussy are you? What foods will you not eat and for what reasons?
4. When you shop for food, do you:
   a) go for the best quality even if it's a little expensive?
   b) go for the best value in terms of money?
5. Do you enjoy cooking and preparing food?
6. Do you usually work, read, or watch TV when you eat?
7. Do you have set mealtimes?
8. How much of what you eat is snacks and nibbles?
9. Do you usually eat beyond the point of feeling full?
10. Do you prefer to eat with other people or by yourself?

Now go back over all the questions and make any additions or changes until you are sure that you have a comprehensive picture of all aspects of your eating behavior. (If there are aspects of your eating behavior that are not covered by the questions, write these down, too.) Review your eating behavior by reading your answers back to yourself as if you were hearing an impartial commentary on someone else.

STEP 2: ACCEPTANCE

All eating behavior, however destructive or counterproductive, has a purpose. We may overeat to help us deal with anger or boredom, or as a rest after a hard day. Sometimes we overeat because we *want* to be fat. For some being fat is a mark of authority. Susie Orbach, in *Fat Is a Feminist Issue*, cites a number of clients for whom fat was a rebellion against the sexy, dependent, ineffective model imposed on women. By being fat one could be stating, "I'm a real person with ambitions and independence." Fat means many different things to many different people. For all, overeating has a purpose, is a means for compensation. The first step to acceptance is to understand this.

Only by seeing your eating behavior as it is—and understanding that, in the past and the present, this behavior has been an attempt to compensate, to find pleasure or security—is it possible to eat (and, on occasion, overeat) without guilt or remorse. However, to accept our habits is not to give in, to surrender to food. It's a step nearer to being in control of your eating behavior.

Acceptance is the opposite of resistance. To resist any desire or want means that desire will persist. Nothing is really solved. If you continually crave chocolate, you can resist for only so long. You may overeat "good" food with the hope that your craving for chocolate will go away. You may believe that eating chocolate is bad, that you're bad, and as you give in to this irresistible urge you may have feelings of guilt and self-disgust at your unhealthy tastes and lack of willpower. With these feelings can come more desire to eat, to compensate for these feelings. It is better to accept your initial desires and to understand them.

As an exercise in acceptance, go to your favorite food shops and buy all the foods you like most, whether "good" or "bad." Stock up your fridge and larder with all the foods you could possibly want. For one week, eat what you want, how you want it. If what you really want is the dessert, start with dessert.

STEP 3: ACTION

We are all programmed to survive. We have a built-in mechanism that makes us hungry when we are deprived of nutrition. Any baby will cry if it wants food. If the food doesn't satisfy the baby's nutritional needs, it will still feel hungry. We are no different.

For many of us, hunger is rarely the motive for eating. We have learned that eating suppresses feelings that certain foods are addictive, that it is sociable to eat and to encourage others to eat. We have learned how to eat against our instincts. Only when we unlearn these habits is it possible to discover or uncover our inbuilt desire to eat nutritious food in the right quantities.

From the questions on previous pages, you will have a list of when you eat and what you eat, as well as the feelings you associate with eating. These are some of the commonest "when"s from clients at my clinics:

- I eat when I'm bored.
- I eat when I'm happy.
- I eat when I'm frustrated/angry/upset.
- I eat when I'm sexually frustrated.
- I eat when I'm tired.
- I continually nibble after work from 6 P.M. onward.
- I eat when I'm under pressure at work.

According to the psychologist Oscar Ichazo, these are examples of using eating to compensate for feelings we cannot handle. For instance, boredom may result from our having more energy than we know how to deal with. Drinking or overeating is one way to dissipate that energy, leaving us psychologically in balance. It's as if we had a steam boiler full of energy, and when the pressure builds up we experience negative feelings like frustration or boredom. To compensate, we must let off steam by opening safety valves, one of which is gluttony, which includes overeating. Others include panic, phobia, overexertion, cruelty, and toximania (such as getting drunk).

Ichazo calls these "doors of compensation" because we develop the habit of losing energy through one "door" or another. (I've discussed these more fully in my book *Beat Stress and Fatigue*.) If, for example, gluttony or toximania is one of your favorite doors, then the goal is to find a better way to deal with the situation you are compensating for.

BREAKING THE HABITS

The object of the next exercise is to break each part of your overeating habits, initially for a period of one week. Only then are you in a position to decide whether curbing overeating is the most effective way to deal with the particular situation. With objective awareness and acceptance of our eating behavior and the following exercise, habitual eating becomes easier to stop.

Pick a "when," such as "I eat when I'm frustrated."

QUESTION 1. Is there any way you can deal with the situation directly? For example, how can you most effectively express the anger/frustration to achieve the results you want? Depression is often anger without enthusiasm!

QUESTION 2. Is there any way you can deal with the situation indirectly? For example, go for a run, call a friend, energetically do some housework, beat the hell out of a carpet, or rip the weeds out of your garden instead.

SET YOUR TARGET. Now set yourself this target for the next week:

"I eat as much as I want, when I want, and I do not eat when . . . [I'm frustrated]."

Write this down on a card and keep it in a prominent place. When you have completed your first target, reward yourself by doing something you really enjoy. You are now in a position to choose whether eating is the best way of dealing with this "when" situation. You are in control.

Now move on to your next "when." Ask yourself Questions 1 and 2 each time this situation arises. Set your target for the next week, write it down on a card, and keep it in a prominent place. Do this for each "when" until you've completed your list.

Remember: *you are not your eating behavior.* Your eating behavior consists of habits you have consciously or unconsciously learned as a result of experiences in the past. Some of these habits are still useful, and some of them are not. By stopping each eating habit for a week you put yourself in a position to choose how, when, and what you eat. You are in control.

These simple exercises will allow you get a handle on emotional and obsessive eating, helping you to follow my diet to its successful conclusion.

Maintenance

As I said at the start, the Holford Diet is all about optimum health, and weight loss is just one facet of this. This is a diet for life, and that's why 90 percent of the principles covered in this book are consistent with ongoing good health and weight maintenance. However, there are some aspects of the diet that you don't need to keep up forever.

Once you have lost most of the weight you wanted to lose, are feeling full of energy and vitality, and have lost any cravings for stimulants and sugary foods (check your score on the "Are you insulin resistant?" questionnaire on page 38), you don't need to keep eating quite so much protein every day. You can reduce the amount from 25 percent of your daily calories to between 15 and 20 percent. The chart below shows you what this means in practice.

Protein servings on the maintenance diet

Food	Weight/Vol.	Serving
Tofu	3 oz.	½ package
Textured vegetable protein	2½ oz.	2 tbsp.
Chicken (no skin)	1¼ oz.	¾ very small breast
Turkey (no skin)	1¼ oz.	¼ small breast
Quorn	3 oz.	½ cup
Salmon	1½ oz.	¾ small fillet
Tuna (water packed)	1¼ oz.	small can

Food (cont.)	Weight/Vol.	Serving
Sardines (water packed)	2 oz.	2 tinned fillets
Cod	1½ oz.	¾ small fillet
Clams	1½ oz.	¼ cup
Prawns	2 oz.	4 large prawns
Mackerel	2 oz.	¾ medium fillet
Oysters		11
Yogurt (natural, low-fat)	7 oz.	1 small tub
Cottage cheese	3 oz.	tub
Hummus	5 oz.	¾ small tub
Skim milk	1.4 cups	c. ⅔ pint
Soy milk	1.3 cups	c. ⅔ pint
Eggs (boiled)		1½
Quinoa	3¼ oz.	5 heaped tbsp
Baked beans	8 oz.	¼ can
Kidney beans	4½ oz.	1 tbsp (dry)
Black-eyed peas	4½ oz.	1 tbsp (dry)
Lentils	4½ oz.	1 tbsp (dry)

But, while you eat less protein-rich food, you'll eat more carbohydrate-rich food. Go by the chart on page 170, but this time aim to eat from half to two thirds of the protein portions given, and 1½ times to twice the carbohydrate portion. This means upping your daily Ⓖ score for what you *eat* from 40 to 55 points, which will include unchanged Ⓖ of 10 for two snacks, and 5 for drinks, sweets, and desserts. So each meal will have 15 Ⓖ.

As a result, you'll have to alter some of the recipes a bit to up the proportion of carbohydrate-rich foods. The chart below gives you some guidelines on common combinations.

Protein-rich food	Carbohydrate-rich food
¾ small breast/3 slices chicken	1 medium serving brown rice (⅔ cup)
¾ small fillet salmon	1 serving whole-wheat pasta (¾ cup)
12 oz. cottage cheese	6 small (new) boiled potatoes (5½ oz.)
1 tbsp. dried beans	6 oatcake crackers

Everyone is different, so you'll have to experiment with ratios of carbohydrate and protein till you find what suits you best. Your best guide is your body and your instincts. Eat what works for you.

Supplements for life

While it's a great idea to keep supplementing your diet with a good high-strength multivitamin and mineral, plus 1,000 milligrams of vitamin C, you don't need to keep taking additional chromium (provided there's 40 micrograms or more in your multi), HCA, or fiber supplements forever. So you can safely stop these, too, when you've achieved your final weight. Chromium is particularly helpful at keeping your blood sugar level stable, so if you ever find yourself craving stimulants or sweet things—perhaps when you're under a lot of stress—you may find it helpful to take additional chromium for a few weeks.

Stimulants—don't drift back

One of the most important, yet most difficult, times to stay on track is when you're stressed. This is when the old familiar stimulants (tea, coffee, chocolate, cigarettes, sugar) remind you of their existence. If you've really been addicted to one or more of these, don't let them creep back, even when you've achieved your final goal. The daily use of any stimulant is a bad sign. The odd cup of weak tea or coffee when you eat out or on vacation, or the odd chocolate dessert, is no big deal, though.

100 percent health

Losing weight and gaining all that energy is just the beginning. Why not go all the way, and start to incorporate into your diet and lifestyle all the advice

TOP TIP

Fatburner research

You can help with ongoing Fatburner research. If you've completed the diet for four or more weeks, let us know your results by filling out the simple questionnaire at the end of Appendix 4, on page 353. Answer as many questions as you can and send or fax the questionnaire to Fatburner Research, Healthy Directions, 7811 Montrose Road, Potomac, MD 20854-3369. Alternatively, you can fill in the information online at www.theholforddiet.com.

given in my books *The Optimum Nutrition Bible* and *Optimum Nutrition for the Mind?* Each encourages you to go deeper in both your understanding and your application of optimum nutrition, to help you achieve higher and higher levels of health in all aspects of mind and body. And you can produce even more delectable gourmet dishes with my *Optimum Nutrition Cookbook*, coauthored with Judy Ridgway.

References: Part Three

1. J. Warren, C. Henry, and V. Simonite, "Low Glycemic Index Breakfasts and Reduced Food Intake in Preadolescent Children," *Pediatrics,* vol. 112(5) (2003), p. 414.
2. D. Ludwig, "Dietary Glycemic Index and Regulation of Body Weight," *Lipids,* vol. 38(2) (2003), pp. 117–21.
3. K. Heaton et al., "Particle Size of Wheat, Maize and Oat Test Meals: Effects on Plasma Glucose and Insulin Responses and on the Rate of Starch Digestion in Vitro," *American Journal of Clinical Nutrition,* vol. 47 (1988), pp. 675–82.
4. E. Cheraskin, "The Breakfast/Lunch/Dinner Ritual," *Journal of Orthomolecular Medicine,* vol. 8(1) (1993), pp. 6–10.
5. J. T. Braaten et al., "High Beta-glucan Oat Bran and Oat Gum Reduce Postprandial Blood Glucose and Insulin in Subjects with and without Type 2 Diabetes," *Diabetic Medicine,* vol. 11(3) (1994), pp. 312–18.

Part Four

....

Food:
Menu Plans
and Recipes

27

Menus

You may have followed diets with insipid low-fat recipes, or, in the case of high-protein regimes, superrich and filling ones. The Holford Diet is all about freshness, flavor, zing—and satisfaction. And there's no end to the variety of meals you can make that fit within the Fatburner principles.

So now is the time to come to grips with all the new ingredients in your fridge and larder. I'll start with a menu plan for the first four weeks, which I recommend that you follow for at least the first week so you get a clear idea of the quantity and balance of foods on this diet. Once you're familiar with them and with the basic rules, you can use these recipes and your imagination to create a feast of fatburning gastronomic delights.

Should you wish to do it your own way and work out your menus yourself, that's fine, too. You can swap meals around from one day to another. However, do bear in mind that each day of the menus in this book is well balanced. The menus are also balanced for fat, giving you two measures of the essential fats (explained in Chapter 8) each day.

If you make up your own daily menus, make sure you are not getting too much or too little essential fat. Don't pick the highest-fat recipe and have that every day. Oily fish, for example, occurs in the menus no more than three times a week. So, as you work out each day's menu, ensure you have enough variation. Also, be sure to mix and match your snacks. Try a ripe pear with pumpkin seeds; a couple of oatcake crackers with a dollop of hummus; cottage cheese with berries; or a handful of delicious Spiced Chickpea Chews (page 292).

Bear in mind that desserts are a treat I recommend having just once a week, starting in Week 3.

If you're a vegan or vegetarian, you've got both recipes that you can go with right away and recipes in which you can substitute tofu, tempeh, or other protein sources for fish or chicken. Chapter 20 also has useful information and suggestions for the rich array of options this diet offers.

Please note the portion sizes you should consume for the following, as either snacks or components of a meal:

- Nuts/seeds—1¾ oz.
- Berries—½ cup
- Steamed vegetables (taken from the "unlimited" table on page 164)—half a full dinner plate, unless stated otherwise

WEEK ONE

Day 1

BREAKFAST: Oatmeal with berries or one chopped apple or pear and milk

LUNCH: Apple and Tuna Salad with three oatcake crackers

DINNER: Steam-Fried Vegetables with tofu with 2½ oz. brown basmati rice

SNACKS: Pear with pumpkin seeds/two oatcake crackers with hummus

DRINKS: Unlimited water, herbal teas, and coffee alternatives, plus one glass of diluted juice

Day 2

BREAKFAST: Fatburner Muesli

LUNCH: Fatburner Sandwich with Green Salad

DINNER: Chicken Tandoori with 2½ oz. brown basmati rice and steamed vegetables

SNACKS: Apple with sunflower seeds/cottage cheese with berries

DRINKS: Unlimited water, herbal teas, and coffee alternatives, plus one glass of diluted juice

Day 3

BREAKFAST: Fruit Yogurt/Yogurt Shake

LUNCH: Beany Vegetable Soup with two oatcake crackers

DINNER: Pasta with Pumpkin Seed Pesto

SNACKS: A pint of strawberries/one thin slice of rye bread with peanut butter

DRINKS: Unlimited water, herbal teas, and coffee alternatives, plus one glass of diluted juice

Day 4

BREAKFAST: Oatmeal with ½ cup berries or one chopped apple or pear and milk and yogurt

LUNCH: Quinoa Tabbouleh

DINNER: Tuna Steak with Black-eyed Pea Salsa and Arugula and Watercress Salad

SNACKS: An apple and five almonds/two oatcake crackers and peanut butter

DRINKS: Unlimited water, herbal teas, and coffee alternatives, plus one glass of diluted juice

Day 5

BREAKFAST: Fatburner Muesli

LUNCH: Fatburner Baked Potato with Coleslaw

DINNER: Chicken Chermoula with Oriental Green Beans

SNACKS: A small yogurt with blueberries/crudités (one carrot, two sticks of celery, and five broccoli florets) and hummus

DRINKS: Unlimited water, herbal teas, and coffee alternatives, plus one glass of diluted juice

Day 6

BREAKFAST: Fruit Yogurt/Yogurt Shake

LUNCH: Walnut and Three-Bean Salad with Green Salad

DINNER: Chestnut and Mushroom Pilaf with steamed spinach and broccoli

SNACKS: Pear with pumpkin seeds/two oatcake crackers with hummus

DRINKS: Unlimited water, herbal teas, and coffee alternatives, plus one glass of diluted juice

Day 7

BREAKFAST: Scrambled Egg with one thin slice of rye toast

LUNCH: Stuffed Peppers with Green Salad

DINNER: Thai Baked Cod with 2½ oz. brown basmati rice and Crunchy Thai Salad

SNACKS: Apple with sunflower seeds/cottage cheese with berries
DRINKS: Unlimited water, herbal teas, and coffee alternatives, plus one
            glass of diluted juice

WEEK TWO

By now you'll be getting a taste for the Fatburner recipes. Note the ones you
like, and remember that you can exchange lunches or dinner from one day
with another day. However, keep your choices varied, since some meals are
less balanced than others. By Weeks 3 and 4 you can add in one dessert per
week, and continue to introduce new and delicious recipes. Rather than suggest specific fruits or nuts and seeds for snacks in the following menus, I have
left it open for you to choose the particular fruits, nuts, and seeds that you
prefer. As always, keep your choices varied. For ideas, refer to Week One.

Day 1

BREAKFAST: Oatmeal
LUNCH: Fatburner Sandwich with Green Salad
DINNER: Ratatouille Sausage Bake with three steamed baby new
            potatoes and a quarter of a plateful of broccoli
SNACKS: Two pieces of fruit with nuts/seeds
DRINKS: Unlimited water, herbal teas, and coffee alternatives, plus one
            glass of diluted juice

Day 2

BREAKFAST: Fatburner Muesli
LUNCH: Thai-Style Vegetable Broth, Crunchy Thai Salad
DINNER: Trout with French Lentils and Roasted Tomatoes on the Vine
SNACKS: Two pieces of fruit with nuts/seeds
DRINKS: Unlimited water, herbal teas, and coffee alternatives, plus one
            glass of diluted juice

Day 3

BREAKFAST: Fruit Yogurt/Yogurt Shake
LUNCH: Smoked Salmon Pâté on two thin slices of toasted rye bread
DINNER: Thai Green Curry with a quarter plateful of steamed snow
            peas.
SNACKS: Two pieces of fruit with nuts/seeds

DRINKS: Unlimited water, herbal teas, and coffee alternatives, plus one glass of diluted juice

Day 4

BREAKFAST: Oatmeal

LUNCH: Flageolet Bean Dip with crudités (one carrot, two sticks of celery, and five broccoli florets) and three oatcake crackers

DINNER: Roasted Vegetables with Mediterranean Quinoa

SNACKS: Two pieces of fruit with nuts/seeds

DRINKS: Unlimited water, herbal teas, and coffee alternatives, plus one glass of diluted juice

Day 5

BREAKFAST: Fatburner Muesli

LUNCH: Fatburner Baked Potato with Green Salad

DINNER: Dal (Lentil Curry) with 2½ oz. brown basmati rice and steamed broccoli

SNACKS: Two pieces of fruit with nuts/seeds

DRINKS: Unlimited water, herbal teas, and coffee alternatives, plus one glass of diluted juice

Day 6

BREAKFAST: Fruit Yogurt/Yogurt Shake

LUNCH: Chestnut and Butter Bean Soup with two oatcake crackers

DINNER: Spiced Turkey Meatballs with 3 oz. of whole-grain spaghetti and one zucchini (sliced lengthways and grilled)

SNACKS: Two pieces of fruit with nuts/seeds

DRINKS: Unlimited water, herbal teas, and coffee alternatives, plus one glass of diluted juice

Day 7

BREAKFAST: Boiled Egg with one thin slice of rye toast

LUNCH: Gazpacho, Baba Ghanoush and one thin slice of rye bread

DINNER: Chicken Dumplings with Chili Dipping Sauce, with 3 oz. soba (buckwheat) noodles and steam-fried bok choy

SNACKS: Two pieces of fruit with nuts/seeds

DRINKS: Unlimited water, herbal teas, and coffee alternatives, plus one glass of diluted juice

WEEK THREE

Day 1

BREAKFAST: Oatmeal

LUNCH: Green Bean, Olive, and Roasted Pepper Salad in one whole-meal pita bread

DINNER: Cranberry Bean Bolognese with two steamed zucchini

SNACKS: Two pieces of fruit with nuts/seeds

DRINKS: Unlimited water, herbal teas, and coffee alternatives, plus one glass of diluted juice

Day 2

BREAKFAST: Fatburner Muesli

LUNCH: Hummus with crudités (one carrot, two sticks of celery, and five broccoli florets) and four oatcake crackers

DINNER: Fajitas with Mediterranean Tomato and Zucchini Salad

SNACKS: Two pieces of fruit with nuts/seeds

DRINKS: Unlimited water, herbal teas, and coffee alternatives, plus one glass of diluted juice

Day 3

BREAKFAST: Fruit Yogurt/Yogurt Shake

LUNCH: Beany Vegetable Soup with two oatcakes or one toasted pita bread

DINNER: Garlic and Lemon Roast Chicken with two small boiled new potatoes and steamed broccoli Chocolate Coconut Cookies

SNACKS: Two pieces of fruit with nuts/seeds

DRINKS: Unlimited water, herbal teas, and coffee alternatives, plus one glass of diluted juice

Day 4

BREAKFAST: Oatmeal

LUNCH: Blueberry and Cottage Cheese Salad with three oatcake crackers

DINNER: Chickpea Curry with 2½ oz. brown basmati rice or 1¾ oz. couscous and steamed Italian flat beans

SNACKS: Two pieces of fruit with nuts/seeds

DRINKS: Unlimited water, herbal teas, and coffee alternatives, plus one glass of diluted juice

Day 5

BREAKFAST: Fatburner Muesli
LUNCH: Fatburner Baked Potato with Mediterranean Tomato and Zucchini Salad
DINNER: Stuffed Peppers with Tomato and Red Onion Salad
SNACKS: Two pieces of fruit with nuts/seeds
DRINKS: Unlimited water, herbal teas, and coffee alternatives, plus one glass of diluted juice

Day 6

BREAKFAST: Fruit Yogurt/Yogurt Shake
LUNCH: Walnut and Three-Bean Salad with Coleslaw
DINNER: Sticky Mustard Salmon Fillets with 3½ oz. quinoa and steam-fried leeks and peppers
SNACKS: Two pieces of fruit with nuts/seeds
DRINKS: Unlimited water, herbal teas, and coffee alternatives, plus one glass of diluted juice

Day 7

BREAKFAST: Scrambled Egg with one thin slice of rye toast
LUNCH: Lentil and Lemon Soup with three oatcakes
DINNER: Indian Spiced Chicken with 2½ oz. brown basmati rice and steam-fried vegetables
SNACKS: Two pieces of fruit with nuts/seeds
DRINKS: Unlimited water, herbal teas, and coffee alternatives, plus one glass of diluted juice

WEEK FOUR

Day 1

BREAKFAST: Oatmeal
LUNCH: Fatburner Sandwich with Tomato and Red Onion Salad
DINNER: Grilled Goat Cheese on Portobello Mushrooms with mixed salad leaves (such as spinach, arugula, and watercress) and French or Tahini Dressing
SNACKS: Two pieces of fruit with nuts/seeds
DRINKS: Unlimited water, herbal teas, and coffee alternatives, plus one glass of diluted juice

Day 2

BREAKFAST: Fatburner Muesli
LUNCH: Spicy Pumpkin and Tofu Soup
DINNER: Chicken with Roasted Zucchini and Red Onion
SNACKS: Two pieces of fruit with nuts/seeds
DRINKS: Unlimited water, herbal teas, and coffee alternatives, plus one glass of diluted juice

Day 3

BREAKFAST: Fruit Yogurt/Yogurt Shake
LUNCH: Sardines on Toast with Celeriac Rémoulade
DINNER: Nick's Beef Burgers with Mexican Bean Dip and as much lettuce as you can squeeze into a toasted whole-meal pita bread
Individual Berry Cheesecake
SNACKS: Two pieces of fruit with nuts/seeds
DRINKS: Unlimited water, herbal teas, and coffee alternatives, plus one glass of diluted juice

Day 4

BREAKFAST: Oatmeal
LUNCH: Chestnut and Butter Bean Soup with a Green Salad on the side
DINNER: Tarragon and Lemon Roast Chicken Breast with 2½ oz. brown basmati rice and Mediterranean Tomato and Zucchini Salad (or steamed vegetables)
SNACKS: Two pieces of fruit with nuts/seeds
DRINKS: Unlimited water, herbal teas, and coffee alternatives, plus one glass of diluted juice

Day 5

BREAKFAST: Fatburner Muesli
LUNCH: Fatburner Baked Sweet Potato with Arugula and Watercress Salad
DINNER: Grilled Burgers with one whole-meal pita bread and mixed salad leaves (such as spinach, arugula, and watercress) with French or Tahini Dressing

SNACKS: Two pieces of fruit with nuts/seeds
DRINKS: Unlimited water, herbal teas, and coffee alternatives, plus one
            glass of diluted juice

Day 6

BREAKFAST: Fruit Yogurt/Yogurt Shake
LUNCH: Mexican Bean Dip and crudités (one carrot, two sticks of
            celery, and five broccoli florets)
DINNER: Trout with French Lentils and Roasted Tomatoes on the Vine
            with steamed zucchini
SNACKS: Two pieces of fruit with nuts/seeds
DRINKS: Unlimited water, herbal teas, and coffee alternatives, plus one
            glass of diluted juice

Day 7

BREAKFAST: Boiled Egg with one thin slice of rye toast
LUNCH: Quinoa Tabbouleh with Tomato and Red Onion Salad
DINNER: Chestnut and Mushroom Pilaf and mixed salad leaves (such
            as spinach, arugula, and watercress) with French or Tahini
            Dressing
SNACKS: Two pieces of fruit with nuts/seeds
DRINKS: Unlimited water, herbal teas, and coffee alternatives, plus one
            glass of diluted juice

28

Recipes

I n the end, all diets stand or fall by their recipes. Huge amounts of research, care, and thought may have gone into the principles behind them, but, if the food itself is tasteless or monotonous, the diet will fail.

The Holford Diet passes this test with flying colors. I promise you wonderful flavors, intriguing textures, fantastic freshness, and great variety. I've borrowed from the best in world cuisine to create dishes bursting with health and flavor. Hundreds of thousands of people have found these recipes seriously delicious, so, if you're ready, let's get going on them.

Almost all the recipes are sugar-free, using the natural sweetness present in food, or they use a proprietary product called xylitol, a natural plant sugar that has all the taste of sugar but a third of the calories, and does not disrupt your blood sugar, giving it a very low ⑤. Another added bonus is the fact that it protects your teeth from cavities. (See Resources for where to buy xylitol.)

The recipes are also high in fiber, so you don't need to add any. The foods used are naturally high in key vitamins and minerals. I recommend you buy the freshest ingredients, organic if possible, since these tend to contain more nutrients as well as being chemical-free.

As this diet is mainly based on fresh vegetables, fruits, beans, lentils, and whole grains, with some fish and chicken, you will find it very economical, too. You may, however, need to vary the fruits and vegetables depending on what's in season.

To follow the diet, all you need to do is select a breakfast, lunch and dinner for each day, based on the menus in the previous chapter. Not all the recipes have exactly the same balance of nutrients, so it's best to vary your choices.

Note that, unless otherwise stated, all lunches and main meals, except for things like sandwiches, give quantities for two people. If there's only one of you, halve the portion sizes or make enough for two meals and pop one in the fridge.

Bon appétit!

Breakfasts

Yes, it's true: breakfast *is* the most important meal of the day. It's all down, literally, to your body's sugar level, which is at its lowest ebb first thing in the morning. If you go to work very early, take your breakfast to work and have it during the first break you take. All recipes are for one person. (For the size of a serving of various kinds of fruits, see page 152.) Remember, breakfast can have a maximum 10 ⓖ.

ⓖ SCORES:

Recipe	Page number	ⓖ
Get Up & Go with berries	232	8.5
Fatburner Muesli	232	7
Oatmeal	233	8
Fruit Yogurt/Yogurt Shake	233	10
Scrambled Egg on rye toast	233	9
Boiled Egg with rye toast	234	10

GET UP & GO

Get Up & Go is a powdered breakfast drink, which is blended with skim milk or soy milk and banana or berries. Nutritionally speaking, it is the ultimate breakfast: each serving gives you more fiber than a bowl of oatmeal, more protein than an egg, more iron than a cooked breakfast, and more vitamins and minerals than a whole package of cornflakes. In fact, every serving of Get Up & Go gives you at least 100 percent of every vitamin and mineral and a lot more of some key nutrients. For example, you get 1,000 milligrams of vitamin C—the equivalent of more than 20 oranges.

Get Up & Go is made from the best-quality whole foods, ground into a powder. The carbohydrate comes principally from apple powder, the protein comes from quinoa, soy, and rice flour, the essential fats from ground flax-seed, ground sesame, sunflower, and pumpkin seeds, the fiber from oat bran, beetroot fiber, and citrus pectin, and additional flavor from almond meal.

It contains no sucrose, no additives, no animal products, no yeast, wheat, or milk, and it tastes delicious. Each serving, with half a pint of skim milk or soy milk and some fruit, provides fewer than 300 calories and, when mixed up, only 8.5 ⓖⓛ, making it ideal as part of the Holford Diet. It is nutritionally superior to any other breakfast choice and is totally suitable for adults and children alike. It is fine to have this for breakfast every day, if you choose.

Make it up with berries such as strawberries, raspberries, or blueberries, or a soft pear. If you use a banana have a small, less ripe banana or use half a large banana. It is widely available in health food stores.

● Get Up & Go

1 serving Get Up & Go powder
1 cup skim milk or low-fat soy milk
1 small banana, or ½ large banana, or 1 pear or 2 heaping tablespoons
  berries

Blend milk, fruit, and Get Up & Go powder.

● Fatburner Muesli

You can make this delicious muesli yourself. Experiment with fruit combinations. It tastes best when the oats/rye are soaked overnight in enough water to cover ingredients.

½ cup uncooked oats
½ cup oat bran
1 tablespoon ground seeds (see page 153 for the seed mix recipe)
as many berries as you want (strawberries, raspberries, blueberries)
2 tablespoons plain, natural yogurt

● Oatmeal

On a cold winter day nothing can be more warming than oatmeal. Oats have special properties, making them known to promote a healthy heart and arteries, and they are full of fiber and complex carbohydrates.

> 1 cup water
> 1 cup skim or soy milk
> 1 cup uncooked oatmeal
> 1 teaspoon honey
> 2 teaspoons ground flax and pumpkin seeds

1. Put the water and half the milk in a saucepan and sprinkle in the oats.
2. Bring to a boil and simmer for 3–5 minutes, stirring all the time.
3. Serve with milk, seeds and a little honey.

● Fruit Yogurt/Yogurt Shake

Low-fat, live, natural yogurt is a first-class food, unlike its commercial counterpart, in which most bacteria have been destroyed for a longer shelf life. Live yogurt is packed with friendly bacteria that have a spring-cleaning effect on your digestive system, as well as being a good source of protein.

> 10 ounces very-low-fat live yogurt
> 1 teaspoon honey
> 1 serving fruit—banana, apple, pear, berries, kiwi
> 2 teaspoons ground flax and pumpkin seeds

1. Combine all the ingredients. Use any fruit in season.
2. If you prefer, make a shake by processing the mix in a blender.

● Scrambled Egg

While eggs are rather high in fat, as part of a balanced diet they are a good source of protein and add variety. Limit to five a week, and seven a week in the maintenance phase.

(continued on next page)

1 large free-range egg
dash of skim or soy milk
1 tablespoon parsley
small pat of butter

1. Beat eggs with milk and parsley.
2. Melt butter in a small saucepan.
3. Pour in egg mixture. Cook slowly, stirring constantly.
4. Serve with one thin slice of rye toast.

● Boiled Egg

This simple breakfast makes a wholesome start to the day.

1 large free-range egg

1. Boil the egg to taste (3–4 minutes for soft-boiled).
2. Serve with very lightly buttered whole-grain rye toast.

Salads, soups, dips, and light meals

As you saw in the menus, you can include salads on the side with many of the main dishes. They add vitamins, crunch, and flavor to mealtimes and are all fast and easy to prepare.

A number of the soups in this section can take the place of main dishes. There's a wide and delicious selection. To save time, you may want to make enough for two or three days and store some in the fridge, or make in even larger batches and freeze some. If you're in a hurry, you could choose a serving of one of the better-quality soups now available commercially, such as Baxter's, Amy's Organics, or Wolfgang Puck. Remember to include a serving of protein if you choose a vegetable soup, and to avoid the creamy ones.

Most of these recipes would make great packed lunches for work, too (just invest in a thermos for the soups), and I have included some dips and dressings to liven up salads and vegetable accompaniments. Quantities given are for two servings unless otherwise stated.

Remember, salads and soups will make up a variable number of ⒼⓁ within your ultimate meal allowance of 10 ⒼⓁ.

GL SCORES:

SALADS

● French Dressing

This standard French dressing can be jazzed up by adding fresh and dried herbs. Also, experiment with other oils such as cold-pressed sesame oil or flax oil, which contains essential fatty acids. Use as little dressing as possible on salads.

> *3 tablespoons olive oil*
> *2 tablespoons Essential Balance Oil (from Omega Nutrition, whose address you'll find in Resources) or olive oil*
> *2 tablespoons cider or balsamic vinegar*
> *1 teaspoon French mustard*
> *1 clove garlic, crushed*

Put all the ingredients in a screw-top jar and shake vigorously. Any extra dressing can be stored in the fridge.

● Tahini Dressing

Tahini is made of crushed sesame seeds and their oil—it makes a dressing thicker and creamier.

> EITHER
> *2 tablespoons homemade French Dressing (see above)*
> *1 tablespoon tahini*

> OR
> *½ teaspoon honey*
> *1 teaspoon mustard*
> *2 tablespoons Essential Balance Oil (from Omega Nutrition—see Resources) or olive oil*
> *1 tablespoon tahini*
> *juice of ½ lemon*

Put all the ingredients in a screw-top jar and shake vigorously. Any extra dressing can be stored in the fridge.

● Arugula and Watercress Salad

Watercress is rich in iron and vitamin A and is delicious in salad.

> *2 good handfuls of arugula*
> *good handful of watercress, torn*
> *1 miniature Romaine lettuce, torn into pieces*
> *1 tablespoon watercress*

Combine all the ingredients and toss with 1 tablespoon French or Tahini Dressing.

● Green Salad

This simple green salad is a good accompaniment to any meal. It's subtly different because of the aniseed flavor from the fennel, and has plenty of crunch.

> *⅓ Romaine or other lettuce, torn into bite-sized pieces*
> *¼ bulb fennel, finely sliced, or 2 tablespoons fresh peas, uncooked or*
> *   just blanched (if you don't like fennel)*
> *¼ cucumber, finely sliced*
> *1 stalk celery, finely sliced*

Combine all the ingredients and toss with dressing.

● Mediterranean Tomato and Zucchini Salad

Raw zucchini has a subtle flavor that makes an interesting change from cucumber.

> *3 tomatoes, thinly sliced*
> *1 small zucchini, very thinly sliced in rounds (using a mandoline grater*
> *   is easiest)*
> *6 large, fresh basil leaves, roughly torn*
> *2 teaspoons olive oil*
> *2 teaspoons balsamic vinegar*
> *2 teaspoons pine nuts (lightly toasted in a dry pan if time)*
> *black pepper*

Toss all ingredients together and season.

● Crunchy Thai Salad

This is a variation on one of the most popular street food dishes in Thailand, where it is freshly made to order with a pestle and mortar. It originally comes from the northeast of the country. Now you can save the airfare and make it in your own kitchen!

> ¼ medium white cabbage, finely shredded
> 4 ounces snow peas, parboiled (for 2 minutes) and shredded sugar snap
>   peas, sliced
> ½ medium tomato, finely chopped
> 1 small, mild red chili, seeded and very finely chopped
> juice of 1 lime
> ½ teaspoon mirin (Japanese rice wine, available from supermarkets)
> 2 tablespoons tamari or soy sauce
> 1½ teaspoons sesame oil
> ½-inch chunk gingerroot, finely chopped
> 2 tablespoons sesame seeds (toast in a dry pan until they turn brown,
>   shaking from time to time)

Combine all ingredients in a large bowl and toss well. If you are not keen on hot food, leave out the chili, although if you are careful to remove the inner pith and seeds you will find it provides flavor without excessive heat.

● Tomato and Red Onion Salad

A classic salad with a strong taste, full of flavor and goodness.

> 1 beefsteak tomato, diced
> ½ red onion, finely sliced into rings
> 2 teaspoons extra-virgin olive oil
> juice of ½ lemon
> 2 teaspoons balsamic vinegar
> black pepper
> small handful fresh basil leaves, torn

Toss all ingredients together.

● **Coleslaw**

Cabbage is packed with vitamins and minerals. So are carrots, high in vitamin A, and onions, high in sulfur-rich amino acids, which help to remove
toxins from the body. This coleslaw is nothing like the limp supermarket
variety: it really packs in the power and crunch.

> *3 cups red or white cabbage, finely shredded*
> *¾ cup carrots, grated*
> *½ small onion, finely chopped*
> *1 tablespoon low-fat mayonnaise*
> *1 tablespoon very-low-fat live yogurt*

Mix all ingredients well in a large bowl.

● **Celeriac Rémoulade**

If you haven't eaten celeriac before, you'll find it's a revelation. This is a great
addition to a Fatburner picnic and the perfect alternative to store-bought
coleslaw.

> *½ bulb of celeriac, peeled and thinly grated*
> *½ teaspoon creamy mustard*
> *2 teaspoons chopped fresh parsley*
> *2 tablespoons live natural yogurt*
> *sea salt*

Stir all the ingredients until the celeriac is well coated and serve.

● **Oriental Green Beans**

Tender green beans go well with this dressing. This recipe works wonderfully
with tofu steam-fries.

> *2½ cups young green beans, cut in half crosswise*
> *1 clove garlic, crushed*
> *1 tablespoon tamari*

(continued on next page)

1 teaspoon sesame oil

*1 teaspoon sesame seeds, dry-roasted in a pan until golden (shake them
    occasionally)*

1. Steam the beans gently for around 3 minutes, or until tender.

2. Place the dressing ingredients in a bowl and stir together, then toss over
the beans and serve warm.

● Walnut and Three-Bean Salad

No foods are better than beans for satisfying your appetite and giving stamina. It helps if they're served in a delicious, crunchy salad such as this one.

*14 ounces canned mixed beans (such as chickpeas, navy, and flageolet
    beans)*

handful of walnuts, roughly chopped

½ apple, cubed

2 teaspoons fresh flat-leaf parsley or chives, chopped

1 tablespoon olive oil

1 tablespoon walnut oil (or olive oil)

juice of ½ lemon

1 stalk celery, finely chopped

black pepper

Combine all ingredients and serve with mixed salad leaves (such as
spinach, arugula, and watercress).

● Apple and Tuna Salad

Tuna is a fairly good source of essential fatty acids—which keep our hormones and brain in shape—as well as other vital nutrients and protein.
Combining it with apple is a bit unusual but highly successful in the flavor
stakes.

6 ounces water-packed tuna, drained

1 apple, chopped

1 stalk celery, sliced

1 miniature Romaine lettuce, ripped into bite-sized pieces

1 tablespoon low-fat mayonnaise
3 ounces natural live yogurt
2 teaspoons lemon juice
sea salt
black pepper

Drain the tuna and mix well with the apple, celery, lettuce, yogurt, mayonnaise, lemon juice, and seasoning.

● Green Bean, Olive, and Roasted Pepper Salad

A Spanish-style salad that goes well stuffed in a pita pocket. Or optionally add some black-eyed peas (5 ⓖ per half cup).

7 ounces French beans, tops and tails removed
2 medium eggs
1 small red onion, finely chopped
2 roasted red peppers, finely chopped
handful of black olives, pitted and halved
1 tablespoon olive oil
1 teaspoon red wine vinegar
black pepper

1. Hard-boil the eggs (8 minutes), then cool rapidly under cold water until they are cold. Shell and slice.
2. Steam the beans until al dente, then refresh under cold running water in order to keep the deep green color. Dry well on kitchen towel and put in a bowl.
3. Whisk the vinegar into the oil and season, then toss over the beans.
4. Place the beans in a serving dish, stir in the onion, red pepper, and olives, then gently scatter the egg over the top.

● Quinoa Tabbouleh

Using quinoa instead of bulgur wheat in this Middle Eastern dish provides first-class protein. You could double the quantities and keep some in the fridge to take to work.

(continued on next page)

5 ounces quinoa, uncooked

1¼ cups vegetable stock or bouillon made up into liquid (2 parts liquid to 1 part quinoa)

¼ medium-sized cucumber, sliced lengthwise into quarters, then finely sliced horizontally (making tiny triangles)

2 good handfuls of cherry tomatoes, chopped to the same size as the cucumber

4 scallions, finely sliced

good handful of fresh mint, finely chopped

good handful of fresh flat-leaf parsley, finely chopped

1–2 tablespoons olive oil

1 tablespoon lemon juice

2 teaspoons balsamic vinegar, or to taste

sea salt

black pepper

1. Bring the quinoa to a boil in a saucepan with the bouillon, then cover, reduce the heat, and simmer for approximately 10–15 minutes until the liquid is absorbed and the grains are fluffy. Place the quinoa in a bowl and leave to cool.

2. When at room temperature, mix in the chopped vegetables and herbs with a fork, then add the oil, juice, and vinegar and season. Taste to check the flavor and adjust accordingly.

3. Place in the fridge for at least an hour to allow the flavors to develop.

● Blueberry and Cottage Cheese Salad

Blueberries are one of the best sources of bioflavonoids, which are powerful antioxidants. Here they contrast beautifully in color and taste with apple and kiwifruit.

1 apple, thinly sliced

1 kiwifruit, peeled and thinly sliced

2 teaspoons lemon juice

8 ounces cottage cheese

2 handfuls of blueberries

4 fresh mint leaves, finely chopped

1. Arrange the apple and kiwifruit on individual dishes.

2. Sprinkle with lemon juice and top with cottage cheese, blueberries, and mint.

● Rice, Tuna, and Petits Pois Salad

This is unbelievably tasty—much more interesting than standard tuna salad. Peas are delicious raw, and of course retain more vitamins this way.

> 4 ounces brown basmati rice, cooked
> 4 ounces water-packed tuna, drained
> 1 teaspoon sesame oil
> 2 teaspoons tamari or soy sauce
> 2 teaspoons lemon juice
> 1 tablespoon fresh, uncooked petits pois (or blanched, according to taste)
> 1 carrot, julienned (finely sliced lengthwise)
> 1 scallion, finely sliced
> black pepper

1. Cook rice and allow it to cool.

2. Combine with all other ingredients, tossing thoroughly to mix all the flavors.

● Cottage Cheese, Radish, and Watermelon Salad

A refreshing summertime salad. Don't remove the watermelon seeds, because they are packed full of nutrients and are barely noticeable anyway.

> 8 ounces cottage cheese
> ¼ watermelon, sliced into thin triangles
> ⅓ cucumber, thinly sliced
> 6 radishes, trimmed and thinly sliced lengthwise
> 2 teaspoons lemon juice
> 4 fresh mint leaves, finely chopped
> black pepper

1. Lay the cucumber, watermelon, and radish slices out on a large platter and spoon the cottage cheese over the top.

2. Drizzle with the lemon juice and season with black pepper and mint.

SOUPS

● Beany Vegetable Soup

This one-pot winter warmer is crammed full of fiber and is just the thing to take in a thermos to work.

Serves 6

1 pound mixed root vegetables (such as carrot, rutabaga, and parsnip),
    peeled and chopped into bite-sized chunks
3 stalks celery, finely chopped
3 leeks, sliced
2 onions, chopped
2 14-ounce cans mixed legumes (or your choice of beans, such as
    kidney, chickpea, cranberry, butter, or flageolet)
3 cups vegetable stock
fresh flat-leaf parsley, roughly chopped
sea salt
black pepper

1. Put the onion, celery, leeks, root vegetables, stock, and seasoning in a large saucepan and stir.

2. Cover and bring to a boil, then reduce the heat and let the soup simmer for 20 minutes.

3. Stir in the mixed legumes, then cover and simmer for 5–10 minutes until the vegetables and beans are both tender.

4. Add the parsley, then season to taste before serving.

● Spicy Pumpkin and Tofu Soup*

A wonderfully warming soup that is a completely balanced meal, with hidden protein power from the tofu.

Serves 4

1 tablespoon olive oil
1 large onion, finely chopped
2 cloves garlic, crushed

* Courtesy of Cauldron Foods.

2 large butternut squash, seeded, peeled, and diced
1½ teaspoons cumin
1 teaspoon dried coriander
½ teaspoon ground nutmeg
¼ teaspoon chili powder
1 teaspoon fresh thyme, chopped
3 vegetable stock cubes dissolved in 3½ cups hot water
1 8-ounce container tofu, drained
sea salt and pepper to taste
parsley and chives, freshly chopped

1. Heat the olive oil in a large saucepan. Add the chopped onion and garlic and gently cook over low heat until the onion has softened.

2. Add the diced squash, cumin, coriander, nutmeg, chili, thyme, and stock. Bring to a boil, turn down the heat, and simmer for 15 minutes.

3. Blend the tofu in a food processor and set aside.

4. Once the soup has simmered for 15 minutes, allow to cool slightly, then blend until smooth and return to the pan.

5. Whisk in the tofu using a balloon whisk, a tablespoon at a time, and gently reheat. Season to taste, then add the fresh herbs and serve.

● Gazpacho

For a taste of Andalusia, serve this raw cold soup at al fresco meals such as barbecues, or keep for a perfect instant snack. It keeps well in the fridge for up to a week. Add black-eyed peas to make it a main meal—and an ice cube or two on really sultry days.

Serves 6

3 peppers (red, yellow, and orange are the sweetest)
1 cucumber
1 red onion
3 stalks celery
1 14-ounce can chopped tomatoes
1½ cups tomato juice
2 cloves garlic, crushed

(continued on next page)

½ jar Peppadew sweet baby peppers, drained and chopped
    (from supermarkets and delis)
black pepper
sea salt

1. Chop the fresh vegetables and put half in the food processor with the tomatoes, tomato juice, and garlic and process till smooth.
2. Add the remaining vegetables and the Peppadew peppers and season.

● Chestnut and Butter Bean Soup

Chestnuts have the lowest fat content of all nuts and a pleasantly sweet flavor that goes well with the smooth texture of the butter beans.

Serves 4

7 ounces cooked and peeled chestnuts (get the vacuum-packed or
    canned ones to save time)
1 14-ounce can butter beans, drained and rinsed
1 onion, chopped
1 carrot, peeled and chopped
couple of sprigs of thyme
4 cups vegetable bouillon or stock
black pepper

1. Place all the ingredients in a large saucepan, cover, and simmer very gently for 35 minutes.
2. Purée the soup until smooth and add black pepper.

● Lentil and Lemon Soup

The spices and lemony sharpness make this lentil soup anything but boring. A satisfying winter warmer.

Serves 4

1 tablespoon olive oil
1½ cups onions, chopped
4 cloves garlic, coarsely chopped
1½ cups red lentils, rinsed

4 cups chicken or vegetable stock
1 teaspoon ground cumin
1 teaspoon ground coriander
juice of ½ lemon
sea salt and black pepper

1. Heat the oil in a saucepan and add the onion and garlic, cooking them gently for 10 minutes until soft. Stir frequently to prevent sticking.

2. Add the lentils and cook for a further 2 minutes. Add the stock and bring to a boil before reducing the heat to a simmer for 30–45 minutes, until the lentils are almost soft.

3. In a nonstick frying pan, roast the herbs over high heat for 1–2 minutes until they release their aroma, then add to the soup. Bring soup back to a boil and add the lemon juice, then let it simmer for 5 minutes before seasoning lightly.

● Thai-Style Vegetable Broth

This soup is packed with flavor and phytonutrients, and, even better, tastes fabulous. Experiment with different vegetables such as bean sprouts.

Serves 4

4 thin slices ginger, cut into matchsticks
2 cloves garlic, cut into matchsticks
2 cups vegetable bouillon
1 head bok choy, finely shredded
2 shiitake mushrooms, sliced
1 carrot, cut in half lengthwise, then thinly sliced at a horizontal angle
    into half-moons
5 scallions, sliced thinly at an angle
2 ounces firm tofu, cut into ½-inch cubes
1 tablespoon tamari or soy sauce

1. Place the ginger and garlic in a saucepan with the stock. Bring to a boil, cover, and simmer for 3 minutes.

2. Bring the pan back to a boil and add the prepared vegetables and tofu. Season with the tamari, then reduce the heat and simmer for 2–3 minutes.

DIPS

● Mexican Bean Dip

This spicy red-bean dip is a tasty accompaniment to raw vegetables, but goes best of all with Nick's Beef Burgers (see page 277) with lettuce in a pita bread.

> ¼ onion, finely chopped
> 2 cloves garlic, crushed
> ¼ teaspoon chili powder
> 1 teaspoon lemon juice
> 5 ounces kidney beans, cooked and drained
> ½ cup cottage cheese
> ½ tablespoon olive oil
> 1 tablespoon yogurt
> sea salt
> black pepper

1. Sauté the onion and garlic gently in the oil for about 2 minutes, then add the chili powder and cook for a further 3 minutes. Cool.
2. Blend all the ingredients for a fairly smooth, creamy dip.

● Hummus

Chickpeas, also known as garbanzos, have a unique taste, which combines well with tahini, a paste of ground sesame seeds. You may prefer to buy ready-made hummus, which is widely available in supermarkets.

> 1 14-ounce can chickpeas, drained
> 2 cloves garlic, crushed
> 2 tablespoons olive oil
> juice of ½ lemon
> sea salt
> 2 teaspoons tahini
> cayenne pepper

1. Place all the ingredients, including a pinch of cayenne, in a food processor and blend until smooth and creamy, adding a bit of water if necessary. Check the flavor and adjust according to preference.
2. Garnish with a little cayenne pepper.

● Flageolet Bean Dip

This is an unusual, decorative, and tasty alternative to hummus that is delicious on oatcakes, whole-grain pita, or with crudités.

Serves 4 (keeps well in the fridge)

1 14-ounce can *flageolet beans, rinsed and drained*
5 scallions
1 clove garlic, crushed
handful of flat-leaf parsley, finely chopped
1–2 tablespoons lemon juice (according to taste)
1 tablespoon olive oil
around 1 tablespoon water (if the dip is too thick)
sea salt
black pepper

Place the beans, scallions, garlic, parsley, lemon juice, and oil into a blender, and blend until smooth. Add the water if necessary, then add the seasoning slowly, according to taste.

● Baba Ghanoush

I love this Lebanese eggplant dip on oatcake crackers or pumpernickel bread. Again, it's a great addition to a party, or can form part of an appetizer platter for an informal dinner, with Hummus and Quinoa Tabbouleh. Just add green and tomato salads.

2 cloves garlic, crushed
1 tablespoon olive oil
½ eggplant, cubed
juice of ½ lemon
½ cup sesame seeds
2 cups fresh cilantro
½ cup live natural yogurt (a healthier alternative to the common
*   supermarket yogurt)*
sea salt and freshly ground black pepper

(continued on next page)

1. Lightly sauté the garlic in the oil for a couple of minutes, then add the eggplant. Add a tablespoon or so of water to the pan, cover, and steam-fry the mixture for 8 minutes or so, until soft.

2. Put into a food processor and add the rest of the ingredients, then process till relatively smooth.

LIGHT MEALS

● Pumpkin Seed Pesto

This keeps in the fridge for two or three days and can be stirred into soup or pasta, or added to bean salads. It makes a pleasant change from the basil-and-pine-nut variety.

Serves 4

> *½ cup raw pumpkin seeds*
> *¾ cup flat-leaf parsley leaves*
> *2 cups basil leaves*
> *2 garlic cloves, crushed*
> *2 teaspoons lemon juice*
> *½ cup pumpkin seed oil (roasted if you can find it) or the same*
> *quantity of pumpkin seed butter instead of the separate seeds and*
> *oil (made by Omega Nutrition; see Resources)*
> *½ cup grated Parmesan*

1. Place the pumpkin seeds in a small blender or food processor with the herbs, garlic, salt, lemon juice, and Parmesan. Process until the mixture is blended but retains some texture.

2. Add the pumpkin seed oil or butter and mix until the pesto has an even consistency.

● Mashed Sweet Potato

A delicious and lower-Ⓖ version of mashed potatoes. Serve with meat, fish, or tofu and vegetables.

> *1 sweet potato (unpeeled)*
> *black pepper*

1. Slice the sweet potato into thin circles, then steam for about 12 minutes until soft.

2. Season with pepper and mash with a fork.

● Smoked Salmon Pâté

This could be a wonderful dinner-party starter. The cannellini beans provide great long-term energy and are a healthier alternative to the cream in most fish pâtés.

> *7 ounces smoked salmon*
> *7 ounces canned cannellini beans, drained*
> *juice of ½ lemon*
> *a drizzle of water or olive oil (to loosen the mixture if it's too thick)*
> *1 tablespoon chopped fresh parsley*
> *1 tablespoon chopped fresh dill*
> *black pepper*

Blend all the ingredients in a food processor until the mixture is really smooth, adding a little oil or water to loosen the mixture if preferred. Then chill and serve.

● Smoked Trout Pâté

Another lower-fat pâté, this time using cream cheese instead of cream.

> *2 smoked trout fillets, skinned, boned and flaked*
> *8 ounces low-fat cream cheese*
> *juice of ½ lemon*
> *black pepper*
> *1 teaspoon horseradish sauce (optional)*

Blend all the ingredients in a food processor or mash well with a fork. Serve with hot pita bread triangles (5 **GL** per half slice) and salad, or with rye bread (5 **GL** per slice).

● Curry-Roasted Celeriac

An unusual accompaniment to meat or fish.

> ½ bulb of celeriac, peeled and chopped into 1-inch chunks
> ¼ tablespoon mild or medium-strength curry powder
> 2 cloves garlic, unpeeled
> 2 tablespoons olive oil
> black pepper

1. Mix together the oil and curry powder. Toss the celeriac and garlic in the mixture and season with black pepper.
2. Roast in a roasting pan at 350 °F for 40–50 minutes, shaking the pan halfway through to recoat the pieces.

● Sardines on Toast

Sardines are endowed with lots of omega-3 fats and make a fast, delicious meal served this way. Just add a big green salad.

> 3 slices rye bread
> 2 tablespoons olive oil
> 2 tomatoes, sliced
> 6 ounces sardines in water, drained
> black pepper

1. Toast bread and drizzle with olive oil.
2. Place tomato slices and sardines on toast and season with black pepper.

● Hot-Smoked Fish with Avocado

The avocado provides healthy monounsaturated fat, while the fish gives plenty of omega-3 oils—just don't eat this more than once a week, to keep within your fat limit.

> 2 fillets hot-smoked salmon or trout
> 2-inch stalk cucumber, cut into bite-sized pieces

½ ripe medium-sized avocado
juice of ½ lemon
1–2 teaspoons chopped dill or chives
1–2 teaspoons chopped flat-leaf parsley
black pepper

1. Skin the fish and remove any bones, then flake into chunks. Place in a salad bowl with the cucumber.

2. Halve the avocado and cut one side into bite-sized pieces. (Leave the pit in the leftover half and drizzle with lemon juice to prevent discoloration, then cover and place in the fridge for future use.) Add the avocado to the bowl along with the lemon and herbs.

3. Season with black pepper and gently mix together.

● Fish in an Oriental-Style Broth

This dish is full of fresh, clean flavors and would be perfect for a special dinner.

½ cup vegetable bouillon
2 tablespoons mirin (Japanese rice wine, available from supermarkets)
2 tablespoons tamari
1 small chunk ginger, sliced
2 cloves garlic, crushed
2 slices lemon
2 fish fillets (haddock, flounder, or cod)
2 ounces broccoli, broken into very small florets
4 scallions, thinly sliced
2 ounces bok choy, finely shredded
2 ounces carrot, julienned (cut into matchstick-size pieces)
½ teaspoon sesame oil

1. Place the stock, mirin, tamari, ginger, garlic, and lemon in a wok and bring to a boil.

2. Measure the thickness of the fish fillets at their thickest points, then reduce the heat in the wok and slide the fish in. Poach for 10 minutes for every inch of thickness, or until the flesh turns opaque and flakes easily.

(continued on next page)

3. Lift the fish out of the broth and remove the skin, then divide the flesh between 2 soup bowls. Cover and keep warm.

4. Bring the broth back to a boil and add the vegetables in the following order, at 30-second intervals, cooking for a total of 2–3 minutes or until they are tender but still al dente: broccoli, carrots, bok choy, then scallions. Remove the vegetables and add to the bowls.

5. Boil the broth for a further 30 seconds, then remove the ginger and lemon slices and stir in the oil. Ladle over the fish and vegetables and serve immediately.

● Garlicky Butternut Squash and Eggplant

A wonderfully satisfying dish that goes well with anything from chicken to a simple Arugula and Watercress Salad with a good drizzle of Pumpkin Seed Pesto for protein.

> ½ butternut squash, peeled and diced into 1-inch pieces
> ½ medium eggplant, diced into pieces the same size as the squash
> 6 cloves garlic, unpeeled
> 1 teaspoon cumin
> 1 tablespoon olive oil
> sea salt
> black pepper

1. Put the squash, eggplant, and garlic into a bowl with the oil, cumin, and seasoning, mixing until all the vegetables are covered.

2. Place the mix in a roasting pan and put into a 350°F preheated oven for 40–45 minutes, or until the vegetables soften and start to brown.

3. Do eat the roasted garlic if you like the taste, squeezing out the softened flesh with a fork; otherwise simply discard and enjoy the flavor that will have permeated the rest of the vegetables.

● Smoked Salmon and Asparagus Omelet

A sophisticated light supper—or even breakfast in bed!

> 6 spears asparagus
> 4 eggs

sea salt
black pepper
2 teaspoons olive oil
2 ounces smoked salmon slices
2 slices lemon
2 sprigs flat-leaf parsley

1. Steam the asparagus until just cooked, then refresh by plunging the spears into cold water. Drain and set aside.

2. Beat the eggs with the seasoning.

3. Heat a medium-sized frying pan and add the oil, allowing it to heat up and coat the whole pan. Pour the egg into the pan and gently move around using a wooden spoon, allowing all of the egg to be exposed to the heat until the underside cooks through and colors slightly. Reduce the heat, loosen the eggs with a spatula, and flip over to cook the other side for a minute or so until just firm, then cut in half and tip each half onto a separate plate.

4. Lay the salmon on one half of each slice and place 3 asparagus spears on top, then fold the other half over to create a triangle. Top with a slice of lemon and sprig of flat-leaf parsley and serve immediately.

Main meals

From poached salmon to fajitas, there are enough delicious options here to keep you going through a year's worth of lunches, dinners, and dinner parties. Vegetarian options are included for many, and meat eaters' options are also included for some of the vegetarian dishes. Generally speaking, the recipes are designed for easy adaptation, as far as protein is concerned. If the menu suggests a meal you prefer not to have, simply choose an alternative.

Recipes given are for two people unless otherwise stated. Some of these dishes can be prepared in advance and frozen.

Ⓖ SCORES:

Recipe	Page number	Ⓖ
Steam-fried Vegetables with . . .	257	6–8
Fatburner Sandwiches	258	11–12
Fatburner Baked Potato or Sweet Potato	258	10–12
Tuna Steak with Black-Eyed Pea Salsa	259	8
Sticky Mustard Salmon Fillets	260	1

FAST AND EASY

● Steam-Fried Vegetables with . . .

This is a gentler alternative to stir-frying. Start off with a little oil in a wok and stir-fry the vegetables for a couple of minutes. Then add a couple of table-spoons of liquid (such as soy sauce or tamari, lemon juice, vegetable bouillon, or water) and place the lid on the wok to allow the food to steam inside. Check it after a couple of minutes—you can add more liquid if it has evaporated.

Versatility is the name of the game here. You can make this steam-fry with sauces ranging from Chinese to Mexican; throw in cauliflower and sugar snaps one night, carrots and mushrooms the next; use tempeh on Monday and chicken on Sunday—in short, anything goes. This is the perfect fallback recipe, using whatever's in the fridge and pantry for a truly tasty, convenient meal.

Vegetables
Scallions and garlic; then choose from carrots, broccoli, zucchini, cauliflower, sugar snap peas, Italian flat beans, water chestnuts, mushrooms, bean sprouts, peppers, bamboo shoots, and so on, ensuring there's enough to fill half your plate.

Seasonings
Thai: fresh cilantro, green curry paste, and a dash of coconut milk
Chinese: tamari or soy sauce, ginger and garlic
Japanese: ginger, tamari or soy sauce, teriyaki or yakitori sauce (try Kikkoman, available in supermarkets)
Mexican: fajita or enchilada dry seasoning or tomato salsa
Mediterranean: canned chopped tomatoes in juice with chopped basil and flat-leaf parsley, and a few chopped black olives if you wish
Indian: tomatoes with cilantro, cumin, and chili powder to taste

Protein-rich foods
11 ounces tofu, or tempeh, cubed
or 4 ounces boneless chicken, cubed
or 5 ounces filleted fish, cubed

1. Steam-fry onion and garlic in the chosen seasoning. Add protein-rich food and steam-fry until cooked.

(continued on next page)

2. Add your choice of vegetables, steam-fry briefly, then add a tablespoon of water and cover. Steam until vegetables are cooked but still crunchy.

● Fatburner Sandwiches

When it's lunchtime and you're starving, sometimes only a sandwich will do. To make this low-⑰ version, top two slices of rye bread or fill a whole-grain pita pocket with any one of the following combinations.

4 ounces cottage cheese, with cucumber slices and chopped chives
or *5 ounces hummus and lettuce*
or *1 small roast chicken breast (bones and skin removed) and 1 sliced tomato*
or *1 small smoked trout or salmon fillet with a smear of low-fat cream cheese or Pumpkin Seed Pesto (see page 250) and watercress*
or *2 ounces canned water-packed salmon or tuna, with cucumber and watercress*
or *egg "salad" (made with 2 hard-boiled eggs, a tablespoon of cottage cheese, a chopped scallion, and sea salt and black pepper)*

● Fatburner Baked Potato or Sweet Potato

Many diets give the humble spud short shrift, but a baked potato can be a great base for a satisfying lunch. It's also available at many sandwich shops in case you've forgotten to bring anything to work with you. All you need to remember is to choose a small potato so you don't overdo the carbs. Do eat the skins since they're full of fiber. When making your own, cook them for as short a time as possible (around 50–60 minutes, at 425–450°F), till done but still firm inside. Have them with any of the fillings below and a large salad or Coleslaw (see page 239). A sweet potato makes a delicious change.

2 ounces water-packed tuna blended with a teaspoon of cottage cheese or natural yogurt
4 ounces low-fat cottage cheese with chives and scallions
5 ounces hummus with a sliced tomato
7 ounces baked beans
1 mug Dal (see page 266)

1 small roast chicken breast (no skin, cubed) tossed in 1 tablespoon
    yogurt dressing (blended with paprika, black pepper, and fresh
    chives, basil, or parsley)

2 teaspoons Pumpkin Seed Pesto (see page 250) with 2 ounces cottage
    cheese and chopped chives

FISH

● Tuna Steak with Black-Eyed Pea Salsa

A robust summer dish. Vegetarians could substitute a thick slice of smoked
tofu for the fish.

FOR THE SALSA
2 tomatoes, seeded and chopped into bean-sized pieces
1 14-ounce can black-eyed peas, rinsed and drained
1 red pepper, chopped finely
1 mild, fresh red chili, seeded and finely chopped
2 cloves garlic, crushed
juice of 2 limes
2 teaspoons olive oil
2 teaspoons sesame oil
2 tablespoons fresh coriander or flat-leaf parsley, roughly chopped
black pepper

2 tuna steaks
1 tablespoon olive oil for frying

1. Mix together the salsa ingredients. Set to one side while you cook the
tuna steaks.

2. Heat a frying pan and spray or lightly drizzle with olive oil. When hot,
add the fish and press firmly into the pan to sear on both sides, before reducing the heat and cooking for a further 1–3 minutes (until the flesh flakes
easily).

3. Serve with the salsa on the side.

● **Sticky Mustard Salmon Fillets**

Salmon not only provides plenty of protein but is also a source of essential fats. Try to go for wild salmon, as it's a healthier option than farmed fish. Again, vegetarians could marinate tofu slices instead of salmon.

> *juice and zest of ½ orange*
> *1 teaspoon honey*
> *1 teaspoon whole-grain mustard*
> *2 skinless, boneless salmon fillets*

1. Preheat the oven to 350°F.
2. Whisk the orange juice and zest into the mustard and honey and marinate the salmon in the mixture for 30 minutes or longer, in the fridge.
3. Bake for 20–25 minutes at 350°F and serve with steam-fried spinach and red or yellow peppers and boiled baby new potatoes (5 ⒼⓁ per small serving) or brown basmati rice (5 ⒼⓁ per half serving).

● **Trout with French Lentils and Roasted Tomatoes on the Vine**

A simple but sophisticated dish that is perfectly balanced. Elegant enough to serve at a dinner party.

> *½ cup dried French lentils, washed*
> *1 teaspoon bouillon powder*
> *1 teaspoon mixed dried herbs (such as herbes de Provence)*
> *2 trout fillets, fully prepared*
> *cherry tomatoes on the vine (half a bunch, or 5–6 tomatoes per person)*
> *2 slices lemon*
> *handful of fresh flat-leaf parsley*
> *black pepper*

1. Cover the lentils with cold water and bring to a boil, then simmer for 20 minutes or so until the water is more or less absorbed, adding the bouillon powder and mixed herbs when the lentils are soft to the bite. (Do not worry if the lentils seem hard—French lentils retain their shape and have a satisfyingly chewy texture even when cooked.)
2. Place the fish in a nonstick roasting pan and lay the tomatoes around

them, then bake at 375°F for 12–15 minutes or until the fish is opaque and flaky.

3. Lay the fish on a dollop of lentils, with a slice of lemon and chopped parsley on each fillet and the tomatoes on the side. Sprinkle with black pepper.

● Grilled Herring

Norwegians are on to something: herrings are one of the best fish for omega-3 essential fats as well as protein and vitamins. The flavor is strong, so it needs little enhancement.

> *1 whole prepared herring (approximately 5 ounces)*
> *½ lemon*
> *black pepper*

Squeeze lemon juice and grind black pepper over the herring and place it under a medium broiler for 15–20 minutes, turning halfway through cooking.

● Spicy Mackerel with Couscous

The hint of North Africa in this spicy sauce is a wonderful complement to the rich taste of mackerel. It's partnered with couscous, an excellent source of carbohydrate that is very easy to prepare.

> *2 very small smoked mackerel fillets (skinned if preferred),*
> *or ½ medium fillet each (10 ounces total)*
> *1½ cups boiling water*
> *½ cup couscous*
> *1 teaspoon vegetable bouillon*
> *1 tablespoon olive oil*
> *1 small onion, finely chopped*
> *1 clove garlic, crushed*
> *¼ teaspoon chili powder*
> *1 teaspoon ground cumin*
> *1 red pepper, chopped*

(continued on next page)

1 zucchini, sliced
1 tablespoon tomato paste
1 teaspoon lemon juice

1. Pour the boiling water over the couscous, stir in the bouillon, cover, and let stand for 15 minutes, to allow it to absorb the water. Then fluff up and separate the grains with a fork.

2. Meanwhile, put the oil in a sauté pan and steam-fry the onion, garlic, chili powder, and cumin for 2 minutes.

3. Add the red pepper and zucchini and sauté for a further 2 minutes.

4. Add the tomato paste and lemon juice and steam-fry with the lid on until the vegetables are tender but still crisp.

5. Arrange each fillet on a mound of couscous and top with sauce.

● Thai Baked Cod

This dish is permeated with classic Thai flavors, which are clean and sharp, yet subtle. You can use any whitefish instead of cod if you prefer. It's even better if the fish is left to marinate in the sauce for a few hours before cooking. It goes very well with the Crunchy Thai Salad (see page 238) and soba (buckwheat) noodles (7 ⓒ per small serving).

juice and grated zest of 1 lime
½-inch piece gingerroot, grated
1 stalk lemongrass, sliced finely
2 cloves garlic, crushed
1 teaspoon tamari or soy sauce
1 mild, fresh, red chili, seeded and finely chopped
2 medium cod fillets

1. Mix together the lime juice, lime zest, ginger, lemongrass, garlic, tamari, and chili. *Beware:* when you chop the chili, wash your hands immediately after, since the oil is an irritant.

2. Place the cod fillets in a baking dish.

3. Pour the lime mixture over the fish, turning it so it is well coated. Leave to marinate in the fridge if possible.

4. Cover with lid or foil and bake in a 350°F preheated oven for around 20 minutes (or until cooked—this will depend on the thickness of the fish).

● Cod Roasted with Lemon and Garlic

A delicious, no-fuss fish dish that is perfect for a light summer supper.

> ½ tablespoon olive oil
> ½ tablespoon chopped fresh parsley
> 2 garlic cloves, crushed
> sea salt
> black pepper
> 2 cod fillets (or haddock or flounder)
> 1 lemon, sliced thinly

1. Mix together the oil, parsley, garlic, and seasoning and rub over fish, setting aside to marinate for 10 minutes.

2. Place the fish on a baking sheet and arrange the lemon slices on top. Bake in a preheated oven at 350°F for 15–20 minutes or until just done (and the flesh flakes easily).

3. Serve with Tomato and Red Onion Salad (see page 238).

● Poached Salmon

Salmon responds well to extremely simple treatments, as in this recipe. Fast food with a difference!

> 2 ounces salmon fillets
> 2 lemon wedges
> black pepper

1. Place salmon fillets in a shallow pan with just enough water to cover and poach them gently for around 15 minutes, depending on the thickness of the fillets.

2. Season and serve garnished with lemon wedges.

VEGETARIAN

● Cranberry Bean Bolognese

This is a mouthwatering vegetarian alternative to the classic spaghetti with tomato sauce. It can be prepared in batches and frozen for convenience.

(continued on next page)

10 ounces canned cranberry beans, drained and rinsed
1 onion, chopped
2 cloves garlic, crushed
4 ounces button mushrooms, sliced
1 tablespoon olive oil
1 teaspoon mixed dried herbs
1 teaspoon vegetable bouillon powder
1 tablespoon tomato paste
½ cup crushed or diced canned tomatoes
sea salt
black pepper

1. Sauté the onion and garlic in oil and herbs for 2 minutes, then add the mushrooms and cook till soft.

2. Add the vegetable bouillon powder, tomato paste, canned tomatoes, and beans, then season and simmer for a few minutes.

3. Serve on whole-grain spaghetti or other whole-grain pasta.

● **Pasta with Pumpkin Seed Pesto**

Sometimes at the end of a long day it is all you can do to boil water for some pasta. Luckily, this dish is pretty much instant, if you keep some Pumpkin Seed Pesto in the fridge. Serve with a Tomato and Red Onion Salad.

2 servings Pumpkin Seed Pesto (see page 250)
handful of fresh basil leaves
2 teaspoons pumpkin seeds (toasted in a pan if time)
freshly ground black pepper
6 ounces whole-wheat or buckwheat pasta

1. Cook the pasta according to package instructions, then drain well and return to the pan.

2. Stir in the pesto and put on plates.

3. Top with basil, pumpkin seeds, and black pepper.

● Roasted Vegetables with Mediterranean Quinoa

Quinoa is amazingly versatile and very special, because it is packed full of protein. It's a great foil for these Mediterranean flavors.

FOR THE ROASTED VEGETABLES
1 handful of cherry tomatoes
1 medium zucchini, cubed
1 red onion, sliced into wedges
1 red pepper, sliced
1 handful of button mushrooms
4 teaspoons olive oil
sea salt

FOR THE QUINOA
8 ounces quinoa
2 cups water
1 teaspoon vegetable bouillon or powder
4 black olives (Kalamata are delicious), pitted and roughly chopped
1 tablespoon fresh basil leaves, finely chopped
black pepper

1. Place all vegetables (except the cherry tomatoes) on a baking sheet, lightly drizzle with the olive oil, and lightly sprinkle with sea salt.

2. Bake in a preheated oven (350°F) for 40–50 minutes. Remove from the oven twice during cooking and shake pan to turn and recoat the vegetables. Add the tomatoes the second time you shake the vegetables, as they cook much more quickly.

3. Meanwhile, rinse the quinoa very well under cold running water.

4. Put it in a saucepan with the bouillon powder and the water, bring to a boil, cover, and simmer for 13 minutes or until the water has boiled away and the grains are light and fluffy.

5. Allow the quinoa to cool, and then mix in the basil and olives with a fork.

6. Serve a mound of the quinoa topped with vegetables. Add freshly ground black pepper.

● Dal (Lentil Curry)

This dish is a variation on a recipe given to me by a lady from Goa and is one of my favorites. It always goes down well with meat eaters as well as vegetarians. This is incredibly delicious and leftovers can be kept in the fridge and eaten with a baked potato for lunch the following day, or frozen.

Serves 4

11 ounces orange lentils
2 cups water
1 medium onion, chopped
4 cloves garlic, crushed
1 14-ounce can tomatoes
1 heaping teaspoon curry powder
4 teaspoons vegetable bouillon powder or 2 bouillon cubes

1. Rinse the lentils well in cold running water until the water runs clear.

2. Place the lentils in a saucepan with the water, onion, garlic, and bouillon powder.

3. Bring to a boil and simmer for 10 minutes.

4. Add tomatoes and curry powder and stir well. Cover and leave to simmer for a further 20 minutes, stirring occasionally to make sure the mixture does not stick to the bottom. If it starts to get too thick, add a little water, or, if it seems too watery, leave uncovered. The lentils should form a porridge-like paste.

● Chickpea Curry

Nutty-tasting and firm in texture, chickpeas appear in the cuisines of Spain, Mexico, southern Europe, the Middle East, and India. You can buy them dry, soak overnight, and cook them yourself (follow the package instructions), although this can take a while depending on the age of the chickpeas. I've used canned chickpeas for ease in this recipe, however.

1 14-ounce can chickpeas, drained and rinsed
1 large white onion, chopped
1 stalk celery, chopped finely

    1 medium carrot, chopped
    2 teaspoons olive oil
    2 tablespoons tomato paste
    2 cups vegetable stock
    2 cloves garlic, crushed
    1 teaspoon cumin
    ½ teaspoon turmeric
    ½ teaspoon mild or medium curry powder (according to taste)
    1 teaspoon ground ginger
    ½ teaspoon sea salt

1. Gently heat the oil in a large frying pan and sauté the garlic for a minute.

2. Add the onion and dry spices and cook for a further 2 minutes.

3. Toss in the vegetables and steam-fry in 2 tablespoons of the stock for a couple of minutes.

4. Add the chickpeas, the tomato paste, and the rest of the stock and let the curry simmer uncovered until the vegetables are tender and the sauce has thickened slightly (around 30 minutes).

● **Grilled Goat Cheese on Portobello Mushrooms**

A full-flavored dinner that will please anyone from vegetarian to hardened meat eater. Serve with a green salad, perhaps with a light dressing of walnut oil and balsamic vinegar or lemon juice.

    6 portobello mushrooms, cleaned with a dry brush or kitchen towel
    4 round slices of goat cheese (each about ¼ inch thick)
    1 tablespoon sun-dried tomato paste
    6 large basil leaves, torn
    1 tablespoon walnuts, roughly chopped
    2 teaspoons olive oil
    black pepper

1. Spread the sun-dried tomato paste on the undersides of the mushrooms, then sauté them in olive oil until the mushrooms start to go brown, taking care when you turn them over not to dislodge too much of the tomato paste.

(continued on next page)

2. Place mushrooms bottom side up on a broiler pan and top each with a slice of goat cheese. Broil gently till the cheese starts to bubble and turn golden on top.

3. Remove from the heat and place on a bed of salad greens (predressed if using dressing), then scatter the walnuts and basil on top and serve immediately.

● Sesame Steamed Vegetables with Quinoa

Steaming vegetables brings out their individual delicate flavors, but the dressing in this recipe adds real pizzazz, turning them into a light, delicious feast.

FOR THE QUINOA
1¼ cups quinoa
2 cups water
1 teaspoon vegetable bouillon powder or ½ bouillon cube

FOR THE DRESSING
2 teaspoons sesame oil
2 teaspoons tamari
1 tablespoon sesame seeds, toasted in a dry pan until golden
squeeze of lemon juice

FOR THE VEGETABLES
4 broccoli florets, chopped
handful of baby corn
2 handfuls of snow peas
2 scallions, chopped

1. Rinse the quinoa very well under cold running water. Put it in a saucepan with the water and bouillon, bring to a boil, cover, and simmer for 13 minutes or until the water is absorbed. Then fluff up the grains using a fork.

2. Mix the dressing ingredients in a cup.

3. Place the broccoli in a vegetable steamer and steam for around 4½ minutes before adding the snow peas and baby corn for a further 2 minutes or so, until the vegetables are just lightly cooked.

4. Serve the vegetables on a mound of quinoa and pour the dressing over the top, then sprinkle with the scallions.

• Chestnut and Mushroom Pilaf

The flavors in this dish go together beautifully. To add a bit of color, serve with steamed savoy cabbage or leeks.

> 6 ounces peeled, cooked chestnuts (vacuum-packed or canned)
> 1 tablespoon olive oil
> 2¼ cup brown basmati rice
> 1 small onion, chopped
> 2 cloves garlic, crushed
> ½ cup vegetable bouillon
> 1½ cups shiitake or button mushrooms, sliced
> 1-inch piece of gingerroot, peeled and finely chopped
> 2 teaspoons tamari or soy sauce
> ½ cup frozen peas

1. Gently heat the oil in a heavy frying pan and sauté the rice in it until it's pale brown (this will take around 3–4 minutes). Add garlic and ginger, stirring for 30 seconds, then add the onion, cooking for a further 3 minutes. Lastly, add mushrooms and cook for 3 minutes.

2. Stir in the bouillon and chestnuts, then cover and simmer until liquid is absorbed and rice is just tender (takes around 35 minutes).

3. Stir in the frozen peas at the end and allow to cook gently for a couple of minutes; they will turn bright green.

• Stuffed Peppers

You don't have to stop at peppers: eggplant and larger zucchini are excellent stuffed, too. Adding pine nuts makes a more interesting stuffing than the usual cheese and rice. Serve with salad.

> 2 large red peppers
> 1 tablespoon olive oil
> 1 medium onion, finely chopped
> 2 cloves garlic, crushed
> 1 tablespoon pine nuts
> 1 teaspoon vegetable bouillon powder

(continued on next page)

2–3 tablespoons water
½ cup brown basmati rice, cooked
6 ounces mushrooms, sliced
handful of fresh basil leaves, chopped
black pepper
1 teaspoon olive oil to grease baking sheet

1. Cut tops off peppers, remove seeds and pith, and slice off the bulbous part inside the pepper that sits below the stalk and contains most of the seeds. Reserve lid.

2. Put oil in a sauté pan and sauté the onion and garlic in it for 2 minutes. Add the mushrooms and bouillon and cook for a further 2–3 minutes.

3. In a large bowl, combine cooked mixture with the rice, pine nuts, and basil and season with black pepper.

4. Stuff peppers with the mixture and place tops back on.

5. Place on a lightly oiled baking sheet and bake in a preheated oven (400°F) for 35 minutes.

● **Grilled Burgers** *

Here is a homemade vegetarian alternative to the hamburger. Alternatively, many supermarkets now stock good ready-made vegetarian burgers and sausages, but you need to choose the ones without hydrogenated fat or additives.

8 ounces tofu, mashed
4 tablespoons tamari or soy sauce
1 medium carrot, grated
1 garlic clove, crushed
1 small scallion, chopped
2 slices rye bread, toasted and crumbed
1 tablespoon tomato paste
1 medium free-range egg
black pepper
1 tablespoon fresh cilantro, chopped
1 tablespoon olive oil

* Courtesy of Cauldron Foods.

1. Mix the tofu and soy sauce in a bowl, leave for 20 minutes, then squeeze out and discard any excess moisture.

2. In a bowl, mix the prepared tofu with all the rest of the ingredients except the oil and form into 4 burgers. Chill for 20 minutes.

3. Lightly brush the burgers with oil and cook under a medium broiler for 15 minutes, turning frequently.

4. Serve between slices of rye bread with sliced tomato and lettuce.

● Sweet Potato and Red Onion Tortilla

An interesting variation on traditional potatoes, with a lower ⓖ score. Cut this tasty Spanish-style tortilla into wedges and serve with a side salad or steamed broccoli.

> *1 large sweet potato, peeled and sliced horizontally into thin circles*
> *1 tablespoon olive oil*
> *2 large red onions, chopped*
> *2 cloves garlic, crushed*
> *4 medium eggs*
> *sea salt*
> *black pepper*

1. Steam the sweet potato for 10 minutes or so or until tender.

2. Heat half the oil in a pan and cook the onion and garlic over a very low heat for 12–15 minutes, covered, and stir occasionally until soft. Then remove from the heat to cool.

3. Beat the eggs and stir in the sweet potato and half the cooked onion. Season with sea salt and black pepper.

4. Heat the remaining oil in a shallow, medium nonstick frying pan until hot, then add the reserved onion. Pour in the egg mixture and cook over very low heat for 6 minutes or until the bottom is golden and the mixture looks set.

5. If the top is set at this point, simply take a spatula and loosen the edges of the egg tortilla so that you can slide it onto a plate and serve. However, if the top is still runny when the base has set, slide the tortilla onto a plate, and then tip it back into the pan upside down, to cook the top quickly before serving.

● Japanese Noodles

Soba (buckwheat) noodles complement this Japanese sauce and steam-fry perfectly.

FOR THE SAUCE
4 tablespoons dashi (Japanese stock made from bonito flakes, available from Oriental supermarkets)
1 tablespoon tamari or soy sauce
1 teaspoon mirin (Japanese rice wine, available from Oriental supermarkets)
1 teaspoon grated gingerroot
4 finely sliced shiitake mushrooms
1 teaspoon cornstarch mixed with 2 teaspoons water to form a smooth paste (optional)

FOR THE TOFU MIXTURE
11 ounces smoked tofu, cut into bite-sized pieces
finely sliced vegetables, choosing from carrots, bean sprouts, sugar snap peas, snow peas, broccoli pieces, or green pepper
4 ounces soba noodles

1. Combine the sauce ingredients and simmer in a saucepan. If preferred, add the cornstarch to thicken the sauce slightly.

2. Lightly broil the tofu until it begins to brown, turning to color both sides.

3. Add the broiled tofu, along with the vegetables, to the sauce and simmer for a few minutes until the vegetables have softened slightly.

4. Cook the soba noodles according to the package directions (they take almost no time), and toss the steam-fry through the noodles.

● Chili

This wonderful dish—just the thing for a crisp autumn evening—has fooled many a hearty meat eater. You can prepare this in double quantities and freeze it. It works well with brown basmati rice, on a small baked potato, or in a toasted tortilla wrap.

1 small onion, sliced
2 cloves garlic, crushed
½ green pepper, sliced

1 tablespoon olive oil

½ teaspoon chili powder

1 teaspoon paprika

1 teaspoon ground cumin

1 teaspoon ground coriander

2 ounces dried textured vegetable protein (TVP) (presoaked)
    or 6 ounces Quorn mince

7 ounces canned tomatoes, chopped

1 tablespoon tomato paste

4 ounces canned kidney beans, drained

1. Steam-fry onion, garlic, and pepper in oil with chili powder, paprika, cumin, and coriander.

2. Add presoaked TVP or Quorn mince and stir for 2 minutes.

3. Add tomatoes, tomato paste, and kidney beans. Mix well and leave to simmer for at least half an hour, stirring occasionally to prevent it from sticking or burning. If the mixture becomes too thick, add a little water.

MEAT

● Chicken Tandoori

It's the end of the week and you fancy some spicy food. What better than this fabulous Chicken Tandoori recipe? (For vegetarians, tofu would work just as well.) Even better, the herbs and spices in this dish lend it anti-inflammatory properties. Serve with brown basmati rice and steamed vegetables.

2 chicken breasts, boned, skinned, and chopped into bite-sized chunks

3 ounces natural yogurt

handful of sliced almonds

½ tablespoon lemon juice

2 garlic cloves, crushed

½ teaspoon grated fresh gingerroot

½ teaspoon ground cumin

½ teaspoon ground coriander

¼ teaspoon ground turmeric

pinch of cayenne pepper

black pepper

(continued on next page)

1. Place the chicken pieces in a shallow casserole.

2. Mix together the rest of the ingredients and spread over the chicken, then cover the dish and place it in the fridge to marinate for at least an hour.

3. Bake the chicken in the marinade at 400°F for 35–40 minutes until the meat is cooked thoroughly. Do not turn.

● Chicken Chermoula

Chermoula is a North African spice and herb mix that makes a wonderful marinade for chicken or tofu.

> ½ tablespoon olive oil
> 1½ tablespoon lemon juice
> 2 cloves garlic, crushed
> 1 tablespoon fresh parsley, chopped
> ½ tablespoon fresh cilantro, chopped
> ½ teaspoon ground coriander
> ½ teaspoon cayenne pepper
> ½ teaspoon ground cumin
> ½ teaspoon paprika
> black pepper
> 2 skinned, boned chicken breasts

1. Mix all ingredients except the chicken together in a bowl to make the marinade.

2. Cut several slashes in each chicken breast and rub the marinade into the meat. Cover the chicken and place in the fridge for 2 hours.

3. Take out and broil at medium heat for around 10–15 minutes or until the meat is cooked and the juices run clear, turning the chicken over halfway through.

4. Slice the breasts and spread on top of couscous or Quinoa Tabbouleh (page 241), or serve with Coleslaw (3 ⓖⓛ) (page 239) and Mashed Sweet Potatoes (7 ⓖⓛ) (see page 250).

● Garlic and Lemon Roast Chicken

Organic, free-range chicken is the best available. Once you've roasted the chicken, remove the skin before eating. Leftover meat can be used to make sandwiches or salads the next day.

½ lemon
1 teaspoon olive oil
4 cloves garlic: 2 crushed, 2 whole and unpeeled
1 medium chicken
sea salt
freshly ground black pepper

1. Mix together the juice of the lemon, oil, and crushed garlic and rub all over the chicken, then sprinkle with freshly ground black pepper and sea salt. Place the squeezed lemon and whole garlic cloves inside the chicken's cavity.

2. Put the chicken on a rack in a roasting pan (to allow the fat to drain) and bake in a preheated oven at 350°F for 20 minutes per pound, plus an extra 20 minutes. Baste with pan drippings two or three times during cooking.

● Chicken with Roasted Zucchini and Red Onion

Roasting vegetables with chicken is a great idea, as the vegetables absorb the flavor of the chicken. This version uses a Mediterranean-inspired mix of zucchini, new potatoes, and red onion.

2 zucchini, cut into chunks
2 red onions, cut into wedges
6 small baby new potatoes
1½ tablespoons olive oil
1–2 tablespoons balsamic vinegar, depending upon preference
4 sprigs fresh thyme
2 cloves garlic, unpeeled
pinch of sea salt
2 skinless, boneless chicken breasts
black pepper

1. Put the vegetables into a small roasting pan, pour over 1 tablespoon of the oil and half of the vinegar and add a pinch of salt and the thyme. Toss together and place the chicken breasts on top, pressing them into the mixture so that they nestle between the vegetables.

2. Drizzle the remaining vinegar and oil over the chicken and season.

(continued on next page)

3. Roast for 40–45 minutes at 350 °F, shaking the vegetables around to re-coat with oil and vinegar halfway through and turning the chicken, making sure that it doesn't dry out on top.

● Spiced Turkey Patties

A leaner alternative to beef burgers with a spicy kick, these patties go over well with teenagers and are perfect for barbecues. (If you do grill them, avoid charring the meat, because this promotes the development of harmful free radicals.)

Serves 4

2 large cloves garlic, crushed
1 large green chili, seeded and finely chopped
large pinch ground cumin
1 tablespoon olive oil
14 ounces lean ground turkey
sea salt
black pepper

1. Gently sauté the garlic, chili, and cumin in the oil for a couple of minutes and leave to cool.

2. Add to the turkey, season with a little sea salt and pepper, and mix thoroughly through the meat. Shape the mixture into 4 patties.

3. Broil or grill for 10 minutes or until cooked thoroughly, turning halfway through.

4. Serve with baked beans and grilled mushrooms and tomatoes, or whole-grain spaghetti (if using spaghetti, place lightly grilled or broiled zucchini pieces on top before topping with the patties: slice the zucchini lengthwise and drizzle with a little oil and sea salt—and lightly broil, turning halfway through).

● Ratatouille Sausage Bake

A no-fuss, warming dish, superb as a midweek supper. This seems like a lot of vegetables but they cook down quite a lot and any leftovers are delicious on a baked potato. Vegetarians could simply omit the sausages and add half a can of kidney beans with a pinch of chili powder per person to the ratatouille, and serve with baby new potatoes.

*4 lean, good-quality sausages (venison are the leanest; otherwise opt for
    lean pork, beef, or chicken)*
4 red, green, yellow, and/or orange peppers
2 red onions, sliced
2 zucchini, sliced
1 14-ounce can diced tomatoes
2 tablespoons tomato paste
2 cloves garlic, crushed
2 teaspoons dried mixed Italian herbs
black pepper

1. Place peppers, onions, and zucchini in a shallow casserole or roasting pan and mix in the tomatoes, tomato paste, garlic, and herbs, combining well so that the tomato sauce has coated everything.
2. Place the sausages on top of the vegetable base.
3. Bake in a preheated oven for around an hour at 350°F.
4. Grind black pepper on top when ready to serve.

● Nick's Beef Burgers

Created by a cavalry officer friend, this burger recipe will satisfy an army and is seriously delicious served with Mexican Bean Dip (4 ⓒⓛ; see page 248) and lettuce in a toasted pita bread (5 ⓒⓛ per half slice).

8 ounces extra-lean ground beef
1 tablespoon tamari or soy sauce
1 teaspoon Worcestershire sauce
1 tablespoon finely chopped fresh cilantro
¼ red onion, finely chopped
½ egg, beaten
½ teaspoon sea salt
½ teaspoon black pepper

1. Mix all other ingredients together, then add to the ground beef.
2. Knead the mixture thoroughly, then divide into 4 patties and flatten into a burger shape.
3. Place on a plate and cover before putting in the fridge to firm for approximately 10 minutes or until required.

(continued on next page)

4. Grill or broil under medium heat for approximately 7 minutes per side or to taste.

● Fajitas

Here's a low-fat take on this ever-popular Tex-Mex dish. Double or triple the recipe to make a fun family supper or a great informal meal for friends. Substitute a can of black-eyed peas if you do not eat meat.

FOR THE FAJITAS
2 onions, sliced
1 clove garlic, crushed
1 red and 1 yellow pepper, tops removed, seeded, and sliced lengthwise
olive oil
2 chicken breasts, boned, skinned, and cut into slices
⅔ tablespoon Old El Paso Fajita Seasoning
2 tortillas

FOR THE TOMATO SALSA
2 plum tomatoes, chopped
2 scallions, finely chopped
1 clove garlic, crushed
2 tablespoons fresh cilantro, finely chopped
1 tablespoon lime juice
1 tablespoon olive oil
pinch of sea salt
black pepper

1. Steam-fry the onion, garlic, and peppers in the oil.
2. Rub the seasoning into the chicken. If using black-eyed peas, broil them until cooked.
3. Mix the chicken or peas into the vegetables. (If you are using black-eyed peas, add the fajita seasoning to the steam-fry and cook for a further few minutes, then stir in the peas in and remove from the heat.)
4. To make the salsa, stir the ingredients together in a large bowl, then spoon onto each tortilla, add the chicken and vegetable or bean mixture, and roll up.

● Chicken Dumplings with Chili Dipping Sauce

These Oriental-flavored dumplings are steamed, making them much lower in fat than traditional fried meatballs. Turkey is equally tasty in this recipe.

> 2 skinless, boneless chicken breasts, cut into chunks
> 1 tablespoon tamari
> 1 red chili, seeded and finely chopped
> ¾-inch chunk fresh ginger, peeled and grated finely
> 4 scallions, roughly chopped
> 1 clove garlic, finely grated
> 1 tablespoon fresh cilantro, roughly chopped
> 2 tablespoons sweet chili dipping sauce

1. Place the chicken, tamari, chili, ginger, scallions, garlic, and cilantro in a food processor and blend until the mixture is coarsely chopped and combined.

2. Using your hands, shape the mix into 12 balls, then cover and chill for at least 20 minutes (and up to 8 hours).

3. When you are ready to cook the dumplings, place them in a steamer for 20 minutes, checking that the chicken is thoroughly cooked through, with no pink flesh showing inside.

4. Serve with Crunchy Thai Salad (4 **CL**; see page 238) and soba (buckwheat) noodles (7 **CL** per small serving).

● Thai Green Curry

The aromatic blend of spices and creamy coconut milk in this dish suits a number of protein-rich foods, so you can adapt this recipe whether you eat meat or not (simply add tofu chunks or shrimp as directed). Green curry paste, fish sauce, and kaffir lime leaves are now widely available in most supermarkets. If you can't find the last two, the curry will still be delicious.

> 1 small onion, chopped
> 2 cloves garlic, crushed
> 2 heaping teaspoons Thai green curry paste
> 1 teaspoon olive oil

(continued on next page)

> 1 small chicken breast, skinned, boned, and cubed
>   or 11 ounces firm tofu, cubed
>   or 6 ounces peeled shrimp
> 2 teaspoons fish sauce
> 1½ cups canned coconut milk
> 2 kaffir lime leaves
> 1 large zucchini, chopped
> handful of fresh basil leaves

1. Steam-fry onions, garlic, and curry paste in oil for 2 minutes.

2. Add chicken, tofu, or shrimp—whichever you choose—and steam-fry for a further 5 minutes.

3. Add fish sauce, coconut milk, and kaffir lime leaves. Stir well, cover, and leave to simmer for at least half an hour.

4. Approximately 5–10 minutes before serving, add zucchini and basil leaves and continue simmering.

● Indian Spiced Chicken

This dish should liberate you to experiment with different combinations of spices, although you can always just use a ready-made curry powder. Either way, it's irresistible.

> juice of 1 lemon
> 1 clove garlic, crushed
> ½ teaspoon turmeric powder
> ½ teaspoon ground cumin
> 1 teaspoon ground coriander
> dash of cayenne pepper
> 2 small chicken breasts, skinned

1. Blend the lemon juice, garlic, and spices.

2. Place rinsed chicken in a dish and toss it in the spice blend so it is well coated. Leave to marinate for at least 30 minutes, or ideally several hours.

3. Place under a medium broiler for 15 minutes (or until cooked—this will depend on the thickness of the chicken), turning once, halfway through cooking.

● Coronation Chicken Salad

A good leftovers meal. Full of crunch with a slightly sweet, spicy flavor. Perfect for packed lunches or picnics.

1 miniature Romaine lettuce, torn into bite-sized pieces
cold meat from ½ small roast chicken, skin removed
½ medium apple, cubed
1 stalk celery, chopped
1½ tablespoons low-fat mayonnaise
1½ tablespoons low-fat yogurt
2 teaspoons mango chutney
1 teaspoon tomato paste
1 teaspoon paprika

1. Create a bed of lettuce on a large plate.
2. Mix together the mayonnaise, yogurt, mango chutney, tomato paste, and paprika.
3. Combine the sauce with the chicken, apple, and celery.
4. Pile on top of the lettuce and serve in pita bread, or with any leftover boiled potatoes.

● Tarragon and Lemon Roast Chicken Breast

Tarragon and lemon lend extra flavor to roast chicken.

1 clove garlic, sliced
2 sprigs fresh tarragon
2 small chicken breasts (with skin)
2 teaspoons olive oil
1½ lemon

1. Place garlic slices and tarragon under chicken skin.
2. Place chicken breasts in a baking dish and drizzle with olive oil and lemon juice.
3. Place in an oven preheated to 375°F and bake for 15–20 minutes or until cooked through (this will depend on the thickness of the chicken). Before eating, remove and discard the skin.

● Spicy Pork Loin

A delicious way to serve pork, which should prevent it from drying out. Serve with steam-fried greens and Mashed Sweet Potatoes (7 ⓖ; see page 250).

> *12 ounces pork loin (fillet), fat trimmed*
> *1 tablespoon olive oil*
> *3 tablespoons tamari or soy sauce*
> *2 teaspoons tomato paste*
> *1-inch chunk gingerroot, peeled*
> *1 large mild, red chili, seeded*
> *1 garlic clove, peeled*
> *2 teaspoons honey or dark brown sugar*

1. In a blender, purée the tomato paste, garlic, tamari or soy sauce, chili, ginger, and honey or sugar until it forms a smooth paste.

2. Lightly boil the mixture in a pan for a couple of minutes, then cool.

3. Rub the marinade all over the pork, then cover and place in the fridge for around 20–30 minutes or until needed. Reserve marinade.

4. Bake the pork on a rack in a roasting pan for 30–35 minutes at 350 °F, basting in the marinade halfway through. Remove from the oven when cooked and let rest for 5 minutes under aluminum foil before serving.

● Venison Stroganoff

Venison is very tasty, is leaner than beef, and is not farmed intensively, making it less likely to be contaminated with chemical residues. Replace with extra mushrooms (allowing 2 handfuls per person) if you want a vegetarian version, and serve with quinoa instead of rice to make sure you get adequate protein.

> *1 tablespoon olive oil*
> *3 ounces cremini mushrooms, wiped clean and cut in half*
> *1 onion, sliced*
> *1 clove garlic, chopped*
> *sea salt*
> *black pepper*

7 ounces venison rump, trimmed of fat and sliced into ¾-inch strips
¼ cup water
¼ cup yogurt mixed with 1 rounded teaspoon cornstarch
½ rounded tablespoon chopped fresh tarragon
¼ teaspoon paprika

1. Heat half the oil in a frying pan and gently sauté the mushrooms, onion, and garlic for about 10 minutes. Season with salt and pepper and place in a bowl.

2. Increase the heat to high, add the rest of the oil, and put in the meat, quickly searing it and then stirring occasionally. When it is cooked, add to the reserved mushroom mixture, leaving any juices in the pan.

3. Add the water to the pan and heat gently for 5 minutes to reduce, stirring to mix in all the juices. Add the yogurt mixture and cook for another minute to allow the sauce to thicken.

4. Add the precooked ingredients, together with the tarragon and paprika.

5. Serve with Mashed Sweet Potatoes (7 ⓖⓛ; see page 250) or brown basmati rice (7 ⓖⓛ per small serving), sprinkled with paprika, and with steamed green beans on the side.

Desserts

This section is all about people who think life is sweet—and want to celebrate that, not succumb to seesawing blood sugar. You don't have to give up desserts on the Holford Diet. As you can see, cakes, pies, and puddings all have a part to play. Once your fatburning capabilities have hit their stride, have one of these a week if you like—or perhaps two, on the maintenance diet. Once your blood sugar is balanced, you can *really* enjoy desserts, because they're not ruling your life.

ⓖⓛ SCORES:

Recipe	Page number	ⓖⓛ
Individual Berry Cheesecake	284	5
Chocolate Coconut Cookies	285	5
Kiwi and Coconut Pudding	285	6
Cinnamon Steamed Pears with Summer Berry Purée	286	5

● Individual Berry Cheesecake

The base of this cheesecake uses chopped fruit and nuts for a much lower Ⓖ score. An easy-to-prepare dessert that can be made in advance.

FOR THE BASE
¾ ounce chopped walnuts and pecans (or other nuts)
4 dried apricots
½ teaspoon walnut oil

FOR THE CHEESE
8 ounces very-low-fat plain cream cheese
2 tablespoons lemon juice
zest of ½ lemon
3 teaspoons xylitol

FOR THE TOPPING
4 tablespoons berries (for example, raspberries, blueberries, or
* blackberries)*
1 tablespoon apple juice or water

1. Place nuts, apricots, and oil in a small blender and process until chopped into very small pieces and sticking together. Press into the bottom of 2 ramekins and chill.

2. In a bowl add the lemon juice to the xylitol and stir to allow the granules to dissolve.

3. Mix the dissolved xylitol and lemon juice and zest into the cream cheese until smooth and thoroughly combined, then spoon into the prepared ramekins, level off the top, and return to the fridge.

4. Place the berries in a small pan and gently stew them in apple juice or water until they soften and begin to burst. Remove from heat and cool before pouring onto cheesecakes.

5. Chill the cheesecakes once finished, until ready to serve.

● Chocolate Coconut Cookies

These miniature cookie bars are absolutely scrumptious served after a meal. A healthier version of a well-known chocolate bar!

Makes 12 (serves 4)

5 ounces dried coconut
3 egg whites
3 tablespoons xylitol
1 teaspoon lime or lemon juice
1 tablespoon cornstarch
3 small squares of good-quality dark chocolate, such as Ghirardelli

1. Combine the coconut, egg white, xylitol, cornstarch, and lime or lemon juice and mix well into a stiff paste.

2. Divide into 12 walnut-sized balls and shape into rectangles (like a piece of sushi rice) or flattish circles. Place on a lined baking sheet and bake at 350°F for 10 minutes, then reduce the heat to 300°F for a further 5 minutes. Remove from the oven.

3. Melt the chocolate in a double boiler or a microwave oven, then dip one half of each coconut bar into the chocolate and lay on a lightly greased or lined plate and chill in the fridge to set. Alternatively, drizzle the melted chocolate over the bars.

● Kiwi and Coconut Pudding

The easiest pudding ever, yet special enough for entertaining. This can be made in advance and kept in the fridge until needed.

2 ripe kiwifruit, peeled and cut into thin slices, crosswise
4 tablespoons Greek-style live yogurt
1 heaping tablespoon dried coconut

(continued on next page)

1. Divide the kiwi slices between two bowls or ramekins (glass dishes look best, because you can see the different layers of the finished pudding).

2. Stir coconut into yogurt.

3. Spoon the yogurt on top of both bowls.

● Cinnamon Steamed Pears with Summer Berry Purée

Steaming is much easier than poaching these pears, which are lovely served with puréed summer berries.

> 2 ripe pears
> ½ teaspoon cinnamon
> 1 teaspoon xylitol
> 2 heaping tablespoons summer berries

1. Slice the bottom off each pear, then remove the core using either a melon-ball scoop or a teaspoon.

2. Mix together the cinnamon and the xylitol, then sprinkle into the hollow core of each pear.

3. Lay the pears in a steamer and steam for about 8–10 minutes, turning halfway through, until they are soft when pierced with a knife. (Do not stand them up or all of the sweet juices from inside will escape.)

4. While the pears are steaming, purée the summer berries in a blender or stew slightly in a tablespoonful of water until they burst and release some juice.

5. Serve the pears still warm, with a dollop of the fruit purée.

● Almond Macaroons

These chewy little cookies will hit the spot if you have a carb craving, but, being made of egg and nuts, have a low ⓖⓛ.

Makes 12 miniature cookies (serves 3)

> 1 free-range egg white
> 2 ounces ground almonds
> 2 ounces xylitol
> ½ teaspoon ground ginger
> a few sliced almonds

1. Line a baking sheet with parchment.

2. Whisk the egg white until it forms stiff peaks.

3. Gently fold the ginger, ground almonds, and xylitol into the egg white with a metal spoon, taking care not to beat out all of the air.

4. Place teaspoonfuls of the mixture onto the baking sheet and lightly press a sliced almond onto the top of each macaroon.

5. Place in a preheated oven (350°F) and bake for 15–20 minutes, until firm to the touch.

6. When cooked and cooled, remove the macaroons from the baking sheet and peel or trim the paper from the edges of each macaroon. Store in an airtight container.

● **Apple Crumble**

Serve this to family and friends and I promise you no one will guess that you are on a diet. Experiment by adding different dried fruit and nuts, or pumpkin and sunflower seeds, to the crumble instead of walnuts.

FOR THE CRUMBLE
1 cup uncooked oats
½ cup chopped walnuts
2 tablespoons olive oil
2 tablespoons xylitol

FOR THE APPLE
2 Granny Smith apples, cored and diced
¾ teaspoon ground ginger or ½ teaspoon cinnamon
1 teaspoon xylitol
1 teaspoon lemon juice

1. Gently melt the 2 tablespoons of xylitol and oil together in a saucepan until the granules have dissolved, then add the dry crumble ingredients and mix well, stirring so that the oats just start to go crisp and become golden (around 3 minutes). Set to one side.

2. Place the apple, lemon juice, and teaspoon of xylitol in a new saucepan and gently stew until the apples soften and start to disintegrate, keeping them moving so that they do not stick.

3. Divide the apple between two ramekins and cover with the crumble topping. Serve while still warm.

● Almond Rice Pudding

This delicious, warming pudding is comfort food at its best, but the brown basmati rice, soy milk, nuts, and xylitol reduce the 🄶🄻 considerably. This is a very flexible recipe—simply add more or less milk and cook for more or less time to achieve the texture and consistency you prefer.

Serves 4

½ cup brown basmati rice
2½ cups soy milk (sweetened)
½ cup xylitol
¾ cup ground almonds
2 drops of vanilla extract
4 handfuls of sliced almonds, lightly toasted

1. Put half of the milk, the rice, vanilla extract, and xylitol into a saucepan and bring to a boil. Cover and leave to simmer for around 40 minutes (the rice will still be quite hard at this stage).

2. Add the rest of the milk and simmer without the lid on for another 30 minutes or so, until the mixture is soft and fairly gooey.

3. Stir in the ground almonds and cook for a further couple of minutes (add a bit more soy milk or some water if the mixture is too thick or is sticking to the bottom at this stage).

4. Spoon into 4 bowls and sprinkle almonds on each one before serving.

● Coconut Quinoa Pudding

A high-protein, low-🄶🄻 version of the comfort food classic rice pudding. This is not a glamorous-looking pudding, but it does taste delicious, especially served alongside a spoonful of Ginger Stewed Apricots (see next recipe).

½ cup quinoa, rinsed
½ cup low-fat milk or soy milk
1 tablespoon dried coconut
2 teaspoons xylitol

Place all the ingredients in a saucepan and bring to a boil, then reduce the heat, cover, and simmer until the quinoa is cooked (the grains will look light and fluffy and will be soft to the bite).

● Ginger Stewed Apricots

A spicy, warming dessert that goes beautifully with the Coconut Quinoa Pudding (see previous recipe) or simply a spoonful of crème fraîche.

4 ripe apricots, halved and pitted
1 tablespoon xylitol
¾ teaspoon ground ginger
1 tablespoon orange juice or water

Stew the apricot halves in a saucepan with the other ingredients until they are soft but still retain their shape.

● Fruit Kebabs

Just the thing for a late-summer barbecue, and a favorite with all ages.

1 apple
lemon juice
1 orange
4 black grapes
7 ounces natural yogurt
1 teaspoon honey

1. Cube the apples and coat with a little lemon juice to prevent them from going brown.
2. Peel the orange, removing all the pith, and cut into chunks.
3. Halve the grapes and remove the seeds.
4. Put the fruit onto skewers and broil under high heat or cook on a barbeque.
5. Blend the yogurt with honey and use as a dipping sauce.

● Raspberry Mousse

This fruit mousse tastes equally good made with strawberries or blackberries.

8 ounces raspberries (fresh or frozen and thawed)
4 ounces low-fat fromage frais

(continued on next page)

1–2 teaspoons honey
handful of fresh mint leaves

1. Blend raspberries, fromage frais, and honey.
2. Pour into individual serving dishes.
3. Garnish with a sprig of mint.

● Baked Apple with Spiced Blackberry Stuffing

A warming, fiber-rich dessert for autumn and winter. Alternatively, you could use blueberries.

2 teaspoons xylitol
¼ teaspoon cinnamon or ginger
1 heaping tablespoon blackberries
2 Granny Smith apples, cored to create a fairly large hole inside

1. Mix the cinnamon or ginger and xylitol into the berries.
2. Place the apples in an ovenproof dish and stuff with the berry mixture.
3. Bake in a preheated oven at 350°F for around 35–40 minutes, or until soft all the way through (test by inserting a skewer) but still standing (overcooking will cause the apples to collapse).

● Chocolate Ice Cream

This luscious ice cream shines if made with the highest-quality cocoa powder.

½ cup xylitol
1 cup whole milk
1 free-range egg, beaten
4½ heaping teaspoons dark chocolate cocoa powder
2 cups cream
1 teaspoon vanilla extract

1. Mix the xylitol, milk, and egg together in a bowl, then pour into a small pan and cook over medium-low heat, stirring constantly, until the mixture thickens—this takes about 10 minutes. Take care not to let it boil.

2. Remove from the heat and add the cocoa powder, stirring until the cocoa dissolves and is mixed in well.

3. Allow to cool for 15 minutes at room temperature before adding the cream and vanilla extract and placing in the freezer for at least 2½ hours. Remove 5 minutes before serving.

Drinks

The following drinks can be drunk without limit throughout the day:

- noncarbonated mineral water
- herbal teas
- dandelion coffee, Roma, Cafix, Teeccino

The following drinks are best limited to a small (6-ounce) glass a day:

- Izze
- other sugar-free juice blends (best diluted)

Also, you can have one of these a day (within your 5-ⓖⓛ allowance for drinks, sweets, and desserts):

- Fruit juices diluted 50 percent with water (see page 172 for quantities)

If you're prone to overindulging in alcohol, you'll need to stop drinking it for two weeks to a month at the start of the diet for maximum fatburning. Thereafter, limit your consumption of alcohol to a maximum of three units a week. A unit is:

- a small glass of wine
- a half-pint of beer
- a jigger of liquor

Snacks

As we saw in Chapter 15, you need never be bored at snack time. Have your snacks midmorning and midafternoon, away from main meals.

- You can have a piece of fruit, plus five almonds or two teaspoons of pumpkin seeds. Choose from apples, pears, plums, cherries, berries, peaches, grapefruit, and oranges. You can eat an entire pint or even more of strawberries (see the table on page 157), but avoid bananas; although they're fine with Get Up & Go for breakfast, they have too high a ⓖ to be eaten as an additional snack.
- Low-ⓖ bread with protein spreads and dips is a good savory option. Try one thin slice of rye, pumpernickel, sourdough, or other low-ⓖ bread with 4 ounces of cottage cheese, 4 ounces of hummus, or a tablespoon of sugar-free peanut butter. You could substitute a raw carrot or a selection of crudités for the bread.
- If you like, you can have a small, plain, low-fat natural yogurt (5 ounces), or 4 ounces of cottage cheese, with berries.

These should keep you going strong through the day.

Here's another delicious idea—if you bring these to work, you may have to hide them from your colleagues!

● Spiced Chickpea Chews

A low-fat, savory snack rich in combined protein and carbs.

Serves 3 (keep some in an airtight container for a handy snack)

1 can chickpeas, rinsed and drained
1 teaspoon olive oil
1 tablespoon lemon juice
1 teaspoon paprika or cayenne pepper
pinch of sea salt
black pepper

1. Toss the chickpeas in the oil and bake in a preheated oven (300°F) for 1 hour until crisp, shaking them around in the pan from time to time.

2. Take out, drizzle with lemon juice, and sprinkle the paprika or cayenne pepper and salt and pepper over the top.

3. Shake the chickpeas in the pan to coat thoroughly and then leave to cool.

Part Five

....

Hidden Benefits

29

Vitality Plus

Newton's Third Law of Thermodynamics, applied to what you eat, says that all the energy you consume as calories must go somewhere. You've been putting some of it into storage as fat.

But, as we've now amply seen, on the Holford Diet three things are going to happen. You'll start to burn off fat, you'll find yourself eating less without even trying, and your energy levels will shoot up.

When I first came into the field of nutrition, I was deeply impressed by the work of a (then) maverick named Dr. Roy Walford, professor of pathology at the UCLA School of Medicine in Los Angeles, who claimed he had discovered the secret of eternal youth. Dr. Walford (who sadly died of a rare genetic neurological disease called ALS), now respected as one of the truly pioneering gerontologists of our time, had proved how to increase the life span of any animal by up to 30 percent!

Walford fed laboratory animals food that had slightly fewer calories, but was of very high quality, with high levels of vitamins and minerals and a low glycemic load. These lucky animals clocked the equivalent of 130 human years! But what really impressed me was seeing them. His diet hadn't just added years to their life: it had clearly added life to their years. Compared with the "normal" animals, they looked healthy and lean and were very active and inquisitive.

I started following the human equivalent of his diet, which was very close to today's Holford Diet. And I've stayed lean and physically and mentally active, ever since. The research Dr. Walford started is now being tested on humans in a long-term study, and so far all the signs are good. His lucky volunteers have all the same positive characteristics that the animals displayed on his diet and are right on course for reaching 100 with the health of a 60-year-old. It's looking more and more as if you really can turn back the clock.

Energy, or the lack of it, is the bane of the 21st century. When ION conducted Britain's biggest-ever health survey in 2002, a staggering 76 percent of people said they felt tired much of the time. We also found that the more overweight a person was, the more likely he was to complain of fatigue. It's ironic that an overweight person should feel tired when his body is a storehouse packed full of energy-giving fat.

As I've shown, the trouble is that food is going straight to fat rather than straight to energy. When you change your body's metabolism to use the energy in your food more efficiently, you'll be off and running.

But don't take my word for it. I invited four magazines, *The Sunday Times Magazine, Time Out, She,* and *Woman's Realm,* to find volunteers and put my original Fatburner Diet to the test over a three-month period.

Woman's Realm tested it out on three people—Sabine, Ian, and Tina. Here's what they said:

> *Sabine complained of erratic weight and constant lack of energy. She's tried loads of diets that only ever gave temporary and limited success. It was her ambition to get down to 112 pounds and stay there, plus regain some of her get-up-and-go in the process!*
>
> *Sabine reached her target weight in just a few months. Her food weaknesses—midmorning nibbles on potato chips and chocolate—have completely gone. "Once I got used to eating lots of fruit, my craving for sugar and chocolate disappeared." Sabine now says her whole attitude toward food has changed. "I'm no longer obsessed with eating and automatically reach for healthy things when I shop and cook." Sabine says it's wonderful to feel so relaxed around food.*

Sabine lost 10 pounds in those three months—and gained energy, in leaps and bounds.

> *Ian's weight had hovered stubbornly around the 210-pound mark. He was also drinking and smoking heavily and wanted to reduce both significantly.*
>
> *Now only a few pounds off his target weight, Ian has managed to give up smoking and drastically reduce his alcohol consumption—a daunting*

task on top of his high-pressure job as a theater producer/actor. Ian started gradually, cutting out tea and coffee, then reducing his red-meat/ fried-food intake. Soon he was following the diet rigorously. Once he'd lost 14 pounds, Ian started to reduce his alcohol consumption—from two bottles of wine to two glasses per day—and eventually felt ready to stop the cigarettes, which he did overnight. Ian's comments: "I was very apprehensive at the beginning—I had a lot of vices to conquer. But once I got over my craving for caffeine it was easier to crack the weight problem."

Ian lost 19 pounds, and all his addictions.

Gina's problem was willpower. Having a huge appetite and a sweet tooth for chocolate and desserts, she admitted to eating throughout the day whether she was hungry or not!

First of all she reduced her tea and coffee intake and substituted fruit or healthy snacks for chocolate. Gradually, as she ate fewer foods high in saturated fat (like red meat), and more fruits and vegetables, her craving for sugar and sweet things lessened.

Gina lost 10 pounds and continues to lose 1 to 2 pounds a week.

She magazine selected ten volunteers. This is what they reported:

Increased alertness was a significant benefit. By the third day, everybody felt well—alert on rising, and three of us (including me) were bounding about full of the joys of spring. Two out of ten felt hungry, but the rest said that, as far as hunger was concerned, it was a comparatively easy diet to stick to. Mrs. Kilby noted by day four that her concentration had improved, and this was backed up by comments from other testers. Nobody had that weak and wobbly feeling associated with dieting. By the end of the week, everyone had stayed the course. Weight loss over the week varied from 3 pounds to 7 pounds, 4–5 pounds being the average.

The Sunday Times Magazine selected one volunteer. This is what she said:

After the first few days I began to feel wonderful—alert and fit and thoroughly detoxified with no more puffy eyes staring back from the bathroom mirror. There's no shortage of recipe ideas. I lost 10 pounds in a month and regained 2 pounds on vacation, but will whittle that off by eating sensibly.

This was *Time Out*'s comment:

> *Weight loss: 4 pounds to 7 pounds in four weeks. Verdict: Makes you look and feel good. Side effects: None.*

In the early days, when we put people on this diet, 86 percent reported a definite improvement in energy. The average "energy" score using our checklist was 7, and, three to six months later, the average score was 3. (Remember, the lower your score the better in this case.)

Now it's your turn to check your energy score. And in truth, you can expect even better results than the ones above from people on the prototype Fatburner Diet. That's because the Holford Diet incorporates new findings in obesity research, as well as even more feedback from thousands of volunteers over the years.

Energy levels are intimately linked to insulin resistance and blood sugar balance, as we've seen throughout this book. So, to figure out your energy score, go back to the insulin-resistance checklist on page 38.

If you answer yes to seven or more questions, you are struggling to keep your blood sugar level even, and you probably have serious energy slumps or feel exhausted much of the time.

If you answer yes to between seven and ten questions, you are beginning to show signs of a sugar sensitivity, which needs to be addressed. You may have several dips in energy a day.

If you answer yes to fewer than four questions, you are unlikely to have a blood sugar problem, and your energy level is on the upswing or consistently high.

Make a note of your score, then retest yourself in three months.

It's not all right to feel just "all right." I want you to feel full of energy, however old you are. Are you ready for it?

Warning:
This Diet Will Seriously
Undamage Your Health

As we've seen, extra energy is definitely on the agenda if you follow the Holford Diet. But I've hardly touched on the other side benefits—and they are something:

- better skin;
- younger looks;
- more even mood;
- sharper memory and concentration; and
- reduced risk for diabetes, heart disease, cancer, and arthritis.

This is a diet where you don't only lose weight. You look great and feel great—clear-headed, calm, glowing, and knowing that you are getting healthier as each week passes.

Eat yourself beautiful

Did you know your skin is new every 20 days? We are literally making new skin cells every day, and the healthier your diet, the healthier your skin. I know because, as I mentioned at the start of this book, I suffered for seven years with bad acne, and saw numerous specialists whose advice ranged from special cleansing routines to creams and antibiotics. Some of these substances made a mild difference, but none really worked. Then I discovered optimum nutrition and within one month the pimples were gone. Within three months, the scarring was visibly reduced. Why?

There are six secrets to having great skin, and all of them are fulfilled by following the Holford Diet.

INNER BALANCE

The first, and most important, is to keep your blood sugar level even. When your blood sugar level peaks too high, which is the fate of the insulin-resistant, the skin also receives excess sugar. Bacteria in the skin feed off sugar, and they are what cause acne. When the blood sugar level dips too low, the body produces adrenaline. This increases the production of sebum, an oily secretion in the skin, which in excess can block pores and cause an isolated pocket of infection to grow.

The reason excess sebum can block pores, as well as make the skin oily, is that the sebum gets oxidized, making it hard. The skin is always being bombarded with free radicals, rogue molecules that are sometimes called *oxidants*.

Major baddies as far as your skin and your health are concerned, oxidants originate from anything burned, especially fats. So they're in cigarette smoke (there are a trillion in each puff), fried food, burned meat, and exhaust fumes, as well as the air itself, since particles become damaged by the sun's burning rays. In truth, you are exposed to something like a bucketful of oxidants each year. These are damaging your skin every day and that is why people who live near the equator, or at high altitudes, and are therefore exposed to stronger sunlight, have much older looking skin.

There are only two things you can do to minimize oxidant skin damage: either limit your exposure to strong sunlight or rub on a sunscreen when you do, and take in more antioxidant nutrients through diet and supplements.

TOP TIP
You can feed the skin with antioxidants from the outside. The best two skin products I know of are Environ and Dermalogica. Both have antioxidant capsules that you pierce and rub on your skin. The results are amazing. (See page 365 for details.)

ESSENTIAL ANTIOXIDANTS

The Holford Diet is naturally full of antioxidants, partly by luck and partly by design. Some of the all-time best, low-🄖 fruits and vegetables also have the highest levels of antioxidants. To stay young and healthy you need to eat antioxidant-rich foods every day.

When I first came into the field of nutrition we used to measure the amount of antioxidant nutrients in food, including vitamin A, beta carotene, vitamin C, vitamin E, selenium, zinc, glutathione, and coenzyme Q10. We then started to discover more and more plant-based antioxidants. Examples of these phytonutrients are anthocyanidins in berries and allicin in garlic.

A method for measuring a food's total anti-aging antioxidant power was then invented, called the *ORAC score* of a food (ORAC stands for "oxygen radical absorption capacity"). The ORAC score of a food is the single best measure of a food's anti-aging potential. To give you some examples, I've listed some of the top common fruits and vegetables, starting with those with the highest ORAC scores.[1] I've also listed their 🄖 for a 100-gram serving.

Top anti-aging fruits

	ORAC PER 100 GRAMS	🄖 PER SERVING
Prunes	5,770	17
Raisins	2,830	46
Blueberries	**2,400**	1
Blackberries	**2,036**	1
Strawberries	**1,540**	1
Raspberries	**1,220**	1
Plums	**949**	5
Oranges	**750**	5
Grapes, red	739	7
Cherries	**670**	2
Kiwifruit	610	5
Grapefruit, pink	**495**	3
Cantaloupe	250	4
Bananas	210	10
Apples	207	5
Apricots	175	4
Peaches	170	4

While raisins and prunes have the highest ORAC rating, they also send your blood sugar soaring. Remember, the ⓰ limit for a snack on the Holford Diet is five points. I've put the best all-rounders in this list—berries, plums, oranges, cherries, and pink grapefruit—in bold, because these fruits will both help you lose weight and keep your skin healthy.

Be aware, however, that these are the scores for the whole fruit, not the juice. While an orange is the equivalent of 5 ⓰ points, and therefore a perfect snack for the diet, an 8-ounce glass of orange juice, which normally contains the juice and the sugar of between two and three oranges, has a ⓰ of 13 points. That's too much.

In the chart below I've picked out the best vegetables, both for their ORAC score and their ⓰, highlighted in bold.

Top anti-aging vegetables

	ORAC PER 100 GRAMS	⓰ PER SERVING
Kale	**1,770**	**1**
Garlic	**1,662**	**1**
Spinach	**1,260**	**1**
Broccolini	**1,183**	**2**
Pumpkin/squash	**1,150**	**3**
Brussels sprouts	**980**	**2**
Broccoli	**890**	**2**
Beets	840	5
Avocados	**782**	**1**
Beans, baked	503	7
Beans, kidney	460	7
Onions	450	2
Sweet corn	400	9
Peas, frozen	375	3
Potatoes	300	16
Sweet potatoes	295	17
Carrots	200	3
String beans	200	2
Tomatoes	195	3

As you can see in the chart above, the best antioxidant vegetables are also the best fatburning vegetables, with a low ⓰ score. I recommend you have a serving of one of these top scorers every day, with the exception of avocado—don't have more than three a week.

Of all the antioxidant nutrients, the two most important for the skin are vitamins A and C. Vitamin A is what protects your skin from sun damage. Vitamin C makes collagen, a substance that's a bit like "glue," holding your cells together. When you lack vitamin C, your skin loses its tone and wrinkles develop. On the Holford Diet I not only recommend that you eat foods naturally rich in these nutrients, but I also recommend that you supplement with a multivitamin containing at least 1,500 micrograms of vitamin A, plus 1,000 milligrams (or even 2,000 milligrams) of vitamin C, which is the optimal amount for both fatburning, anti-aging, and boosting your immune system.

FATS AND FLEXIBILITY

The third secret for healthy skin is to eat the right fats. Essential fats, found in seeds and fish, are vital for your skin and, without them, it can look dry and old. Skin cells contain these essential fats, which not only keep skin looking young and flexible but also are needed to reduce skin inflammation. Omega-3 fats are very powerful anti-inflammatory agents that can reduce redness and swelling in conditions such as eczema.

The Holford Diet recommends that you eat foods naturally high in essential fats, such as oily fish, seeds, and nuts. These essential fats not only help your skin, they also help you to burn fat. You may also choose to use them as supplements, as I do every day. I take a supplement that contains a combination of EPA and DHA, which are the most powerful omega-3 fats, and GLA, the most powerful omega-6 fat. (See also Chapter 8.)

LIQUID LOVELINESS

The final secret for healthy skin is to drink enough water—and that means eight glasses a day. The body is 66 percent water and you need to keep it topped up with water to function properly, from the cellular and chemical levels up. Here, essential fats are invaluable, helping to maintain perfect water balance in the body by keeping the right amount of it inside your cells.

Drinking enough water to stay hydrated is not only good for your health. It also helps to reduce your appetite, as we often mistake thirst for hunger.

THE CALORIE CONNECTION

Skin cells are not much different from other cells in your body and, for this reason, those four secrets for healthy skin—balance your blood sugar, eat an antioxidant-rich diet, get enough essential fats, and drink eight glasses of water a day—are also the top tips for staying young and slowing down the aging process. And there are two more.

In the last chapter I told you about the excellent research of Dr. Roy Walford, who proved that if you cut down on calories you live longer. Calorie restriction, however, is not the same as malnutrition. It is about giving the body exactly what it needs and no more.

That's exactly what the Holford Diet is all about. Many foods in today's diet provide "empty" calories. That is, they provide sugar or saturated fat, but none of the micronutrients needed to process them. These foods are out if you want to lose weight and extend your life span. Nutrient-dense foods such as fish, beans, nuts, and seeds provide as many nutrients as calories, plus, in the case of fresh fruit and vegetables, plenty of essential and calorie-free water.

Since the first animal experiments in 1935, studies on several species have shown that animals eating 30 to 40 percent fewer calories can extend their life span by a third to (in the case of fish) a half. However, it isn't just about limiting calories. These animals were given optimum nutrition as well as fewer calories, with good intakes of antioxidants.

There's every reason to assume the same principle applies to humans. Consider the Japanese islanders of Okinawa. They eat 17 to 40 percent fewer calories than other Japanese and have more centenarians than any other population. According to Dr. Walford, "You can extend longevity by restricting food even after full adulthood and middle age."

Having a high-quality diet with minimal calories also means minimal oxidative stress on the body. You are giving yourself exactly what you need and no more. But how much is that? Dr. Walford said that you can extend life span by cutting calories by 10 to 25 percent. He ate between 1,500 and 2,000 calories a day, compared with the average intake of 2,500 to 3,000 calories. And that is exactly what I recommend you do. The recipes in the Holford Diet, and the menus based on them, are designed to be less calorific, yet fill you up and satisfy your appetite in the healthiest way possible.

Life insurance companies know well the correlation between weight and longevity. Based on these statistics, weight charts give an ideal weight range for your height. You can see one of these in Appendix 1. Generally, the ideal weight for increased life expectancy is the low end of this range. Even more important, as we've seen in this book, is keeping your body fat percentage down, which can also be greatly helped by regular exercise. Appendix 1 also shows you how to calculate this percentage.

THE HOMOCYSTEINE FACTOR

Homocysteine is a toxic amino acid (a building block of protein) found in the blood. You may not have heard of it yet, but you certainly will.

Your homocysteine level is a stronger predictor of having a heart attack or stroke than your cholesterol level. This is quite literally the most important medical breakthrough of the twenty-first century and I can't do it justice here—which is why I've written a book, *The H Factor,* with Dr. James Braly, an expert on this subject. No fewer than 6,000 medical studies have linked high levels of this amino acid to about 100 medical conditions, including obesity.

A comprehensive research study at the University of Bergen in Norway, published in 2001 in the *American Journal of Clinical Nutrition,*[2] measured the homocysteine levels of 4,766 men and women ages 65 to 67 in 1992, and then recorded any deaths over the next five years. During this time, 162 men and 97 women died. The researchers then looked at the risk of death in relation to their homocysteine levels. This is what they found: "A strong relation was found between homocysteine and *all* causes of mortality." They discovered that the chances of a 65- to 67-year-old dying from any cause increased by almost 50 percent for every five-unit increase in homocysteine!

So how can you lower levels of this toxic amino acid? It all hinges on something called SAMe.

Put simply, if you have a high homocysteine level, it means you've got a blockage in your body's ability to turn protein into one of the most important anti-aging nutrients of all, s-adenosyl methionine. SAMe is what's called a *methyl donor.* Every single second of your life there are a billion chemical reactions in your body, in which one chemical is turned into another by adding on what's called a methyl group. The regulation of insulin, adrenaline, and serotonin, three body chemicals that are vital to weight control, all depend on methyl reactions.

If you've got fully functional methyl reactions, you will be very healthy, happy, and "connected." I call this having a high "methyl IQ," and this is indicated by a low homocysteine level in your blood. If you have a high homocysteine level, that means you have a poor methyl IQ and are likely to gain weight easily, have insulin resistance, and suffer from depression, and are at greater risk of developing diabetes, heart disease, strokes, and Alzheimer's later in life.

The average "H" score is 10 to 11 units. The ideal is 6. I often see patients with levels of 20 or more. With every five-unit drop in your H score, you almost halve your risk of dying prematurely. If, for example, your H score was 16, and you drop it to 6 or less and maintain it there, you can probably add around ten years to your life!

High-homocysteine and methylation problems, on the other hand, literally age your cells faster, drain vitality from you, and make you feel old far beyond your years. Homocysteine ages the body directly. If, for example, you expose the cells that line arteries throughout your body to homocysteine, the cells get older much more quickly.[3]

So finally we are discovering that the reason we age is twofold. Cells, and their replacement "instructions," get increasingly damaged by poor methylation and excessive oxidation, both of which are reflected by your homocysteine score.

This is great news because it's easily remedied. The right diet and supplements can rapidly reverse both poor methylation and excessive oxidation, bringing your homocysteine level into the superhealthy range below 6 units. This is important because it means you really can measure where you are regarding homocysteine, and adjust your diet and supplements accordingly. By the way, you can measure your own homocysteine level using a home test kit.

The key homocysteine-busting nutrients are vitamins B_2 and B_6, folic acid, vitamin B_{12}, zinc, and magnesium. The high-strength multivitamin I recommend taking, along with the Holford Diet, provides optimum amounts of these. In fact, the diet is the perfect way to lower your homocysteine level and improve your health.

Eat to beat the blues

Being overweight and feeling blue are connected in more ways than one. Being overweight can be depressing in its own right—you don't look as good as you could, you may be tired, it may be harder to walk up stairs or run for the bus. However, scientists are discovering a much closer connection between these two conditions after looking at what happens in the brains of those prone to depression and weight gain.

A consistent finding is that both overweight people and depressed people have low levels of serotonin in the brain. This is the brain's "happy" chemical, and it also controls your appetite. SSRI antidepressants help promote serotonin in the brain and not only relieve depression in up to 50 percent of people, but also reduce appetite.

However, the side effects of SSRIs are in themselves depressing, so much so that most SSRI drugs are now banned in children up to the age of 18 and are under review for adults. Although there are more than 25 reported side effects, the main concern is that something like one in ten adolescents was found to develop suicidal tendencies as a result of taking these drugs. Talk about out of the frying pan into the fire!

PROTEIN AND SEROTONIN

Serotonin is made directly from a nutrient that you and I eat every day. It's an amino acid called *tryptophan,* found in protein foods. If you take tryptophan out of a person's diet, two things will happen. First, they'll become depressed, and second, they'll crave carbohydrates.

When you eat protein foods such as chicken or fish you will raise blood levels of tryptophan. Tryptophan then turns into 5-hydroxytryptophan (5-HTP), small amounts of which are also present in beans, fish, and other protein foods, and then into serotonin. The body stores 5-HTP in the platelets in the blood before passing it to the brain.

Now, you might logically think that a high-protein diet, for example bacon and eggs for breakfast rather than a high-carbohydrate choice such as a croissant, toast, or cereal, would increase the brain's levels of serotonin best. It doesn't. Research by Professors Richard Wurtman and Judith Wurtman at the Massachusetts Institute of Technology (MIT) has consistently shown that meals containing carbohydrate, rather than protein, raise serotonin best.[4]

The reason for this apparent anomaly is that tryptophan in the blood-stream competes very badly with all the other amino acids in protein, so little gets across into the brain. However, when you eat a carbohydrate food such as an apple, this causes some insulin to be released into the blood-stream, which carries the tryptophan and 5-HTP into the brain, and causes serotonin levels to rise.

This may be why many depressed people crave sweet foods to give them a lift. So, if you find sugar makes you feel happier, you are probably low in serotonin. The trouble is, a vicious cycle lies this way: most carbohydrate snacks are high in refined sugar and fat, and make you fat, which is depressing.

Judith Wurtman, who directs the Program in Women's Health at the MIT Clinical Research Center, says that when you stop eating carbohydrates on a high-protein diet, your brain stops regulating serotonin, leading to low mood and food cravings.

"When serotonin is made and becomes active in your brain, its effect on your appetite is to make you feel full before your stomach is stuffed and stretched," she says. "Serotonin is crucial not only to control your appetite and stop you from overeating; it's essential to keep your moods regulated."

CARBOHYDRATE CRAVINGS

This explains the common craving of high-protein dieters (especially women) for carbohydrates. Women have much less serotonin in their brains than men, so a serotonin-depleting diet will make women feel irritable. Some people feel down in the afternoon or early evening and crave carbohydrate.

According to Wurtman's clinical studies, if the carbohydrate craver eats protein instead, he or she will become grumpy, irritable, or restless. Furthermore, filling up on fatty foods such as bacon or cheese makes you tired, lethargic, and apathetic. This is another reason why I don't favor the high-protein/low-carbohydrate diets.

One way to guarantee healthy serotonin levels is to supplement with 5-HTP. This not only improves your mood, but also will reduce your appetite, especially for sugary foods. And aside from all the problems with sugar we've seen—unstable blood sugar, exhaustion, and weight gain—it has even been implicated in aggressive behavior,[5,6,7,8,9,10] anxiety,[11,12] hyperactivity and attention deficit,[13] depression,[14] eating disorders,[15] fatigue,[16] learning difficulties,[17,18,19,20] and PMS. So it's a good idea to ditch the stuff, and the best way of doing that is by following the Holford Diet.

A sharper mind

The effect of nutrition on the brain is a matter of keen interest these days. We now know that memory and concentration, as well as mood, depend largely on what we put in our digestive systems. Keeping an even blood sugar level is key, as is an optimal intake of essential fats and antioxidants.

To illustrate just how vital these essential Fatburner nutrients are, consider these studies. One measured the amount of DHA, an omega-3 fat, in the umbilical cord of newborn babies and found those with higher levels were faster thinkers eight years later. Another gave infants extra DHA for the first four months and found that they thought faster six years later. These benefits of essential fats are seen at both ends of the age spectrum. A person's risk of developing Alzheimer's falls by 60 percent if he or she eats a diet high in omega-3 fats, especially DHA, according to recent research by Dr. Martha Morris at Chicago's Rush Institute for Healthy Aging. Vitamins E and C, both in diet and in supplements, have also been shown to cut the risk of age-related memory problems by more than 60 percent![21, 22, 23]

Then there's the homocysteine factor (see above). Dropping your homocysteine level by five points halves the risk for Alzheimer's, according to a study published in the *New England Journal of Medicine*.[24] You'll be getting all of these nutrients—B vitamins, antioxidants, vitamins E and C, plus essential fats—on the Holford Diet.

Staying cool

We had a look at the effect stress has on mind and body in Chapter 7. A mild dose of stress can actually stimulate memory and mental alertness, but long-term stress is definitely bad news: it puts too much of the hormone cortisol into circulation, and this literally damages the brain. Another factor that causes the release of too much of the stress hormone cortisol is blood sugar peaks and troughs. When your blood sugar level crashes, the body produces more cortisol. It thinks you are being starved and goes into panic mode.

Raised levels of cortisol have been linked to poorer memory and a shrinking of the brain's memory-sorting center. This is probably why either high stress or high sugar worsens memory and concentration. After only two weeks of the raised cortisol levels of stress, the dendrite "arms" of brain cells, which reach out to connect with other brain cells, start to shrivel up, according to research carried out at Stanford University in California by Robert Sapolsky, professor of neuroscience.

The good news is that such damage isn't permanent. Stop the stress and the dendrites grow back. And one way to reduce your stress levels is to reduce your intake of sugar and stimulants. The more dependent on stimulants you are, and the more your blood sugar levels fluctuate, the more you are likely to react stressfully to life's inevitable challenges.

With the right nutrition and the right attitude, age-related memory loss doesn't need to happen to you. You can build new brain cells at any age. Research clearly shows that healthy, well-educated elderly people can show no decline in mental function right up to death, and no increased rate of brain shrinkage even after 65. It's a "use it or lose it" situation.

fighting disease

If you have heart disease, diabetes, breast cancer, osteoporosis, or arthritis, or any of your close family members (mother, father, sister, or brother) has suffered from any of these conditions, especially early in life, the Holford Diet may literally be a lifesaver for you.

The principles upon which it is based—the product of the results of 20 years of research at ION, reviewing thousands of scientific studies, testing our ideas with more than 100,000 now-healthy volunteers—can reverse most major life-threatening illnesses. Let's examine a few.

Diabetes. Since the Holford Diet is specifically designed to stabilize blood sugar levels, I hardly need to say that it is the diet of choice for diabetics. Professional diabetes associations around the world are adopting ⓖⓛ counting as an essential part of managing diabetes. Hundreds of studies now prove that a low-ⓖⓛ diet helps to improve blood sugar balance and hence reduce the need for medication. These are well summarized in a recent review article in the *Journal of the American Medical Association* for those who want the science.[25]

In Chapter 21 you'll see that I recommend supplementing with the mineral chromium, at least for the first three months of the Holford Diet. Chromium not only helps reduce your appetite, but it also improves the symptoms of diabetes and reduces the need for medication.

Heart disease and strokes. Just about every vital statistic of the Holford Diet is good news for your heart and arteries. If your blood pressure or your cholesterol, homocysteine, or triglyceride level is high, you can expect them to come down.

Here's what happened to Mike:

In mid-April I had my blood checked and found my cholesterol to be 255. I do eat really healthily and felt that my condition was due to hereditary cholesterol rather than dietary factors. A friend had reduced hers through the supplements recommended in your book, so I thought it was worth a try.

Five weeks later I went for a second blood test to find my cholesterol had dropped to 190. My GP couldn't believe it! He would not wholeheartedly acknowledge the success, but he didn't knock it either, saying, "Whatever you're taking is working—come back in a year!"

Valerie, age 73, is another case in point. She had suffered from high blood pressure for over 30 years, as well as a touch of arthritis. Her doctor had given her two drugs, captopril and a baby aspirin, every day. They had helped a bit, but her blood pressure was still high, often as high as 160/80.

She decided to have a homocysteine test. Her homocysteine score was 42.9, putting her in the very-high-risk category, so she went on my diet and the supplement program recommended in my book *The H Factor*. After two months she was retested and her H score had dropped by 88 percent to a healthy 5.1. Her blood pressure has also dropped and stabilized at 132/80 and she no longer needs medication. Her arthritis has improved, causing her much less joint pain, and she feels altogether better.

Take a look at the chart below, which shows the kind of risk reduction you can expect by normalizing your levels of homocysteine, cholesterol, and triglycerides, and your blood pressure, as well as correcting any insulin resistance.

Medical statistics	Estimated potential risk reduction
High blood cholesterol (low HDL, high LDL)	60 percent
High blood fats (triglycerides)	30 percent
High blood pressure	30 percent
High blood homocysteine	60 percent
Insulin resistance	30 percent

Diet and lifestyle changes	
Reducing saturated fat, increasing omega-3 fats	30 percent
Reducing alcohol	30 percent
Quitting smoking, increasing antioxidants	50 percent
Increasing B vitamins	30 percent
Less sodium, more potassium, magnesium, and calcium	30 percent
Increasing exercise	30 percent
Decreasing weight	30 percent
Reducing stress (cortisol)	30 percent

Ten good trials have shown that eating low-ⓖ foods alone will lower your cholesterol, especially the "bad" LDL cholesterol, and triglycerides.[26] In a study involving 75,000 nurses, those with a high-glycemic-load diet doubled their risk of heart disease.[27] Then there are the beneficial effects of reducing oxidants and increasing antioxidants, reducing saturated fat and increasing essential fats, having more B vitamins, and getting more exercise. The National Heart Forum estimates that if you could normalize your cholesterol and blood pressure, do some exercise on a regular basis, quit smoking, and lose weight, that alone would reduce your risk by almost a third.[28] Couple this with the proven benefits of a low-ⓖ diet high in essential fats, plus supplementing with antioxidants and homocysteine-lowering B vitamins, and there's a good chance you could eradicate your risk completely.

Cancer. Most people are still not aware that the primary risk factor for cancer is diet. When the World Cancer Research Fund examined more than 5,000 studies on diet and cancer, they concluded that you could halve the risk of cancer by changing your diet.[29] Many people mistakenly think that cancer is largely genetic. It isn't, and the following study, which involved 45,000 pairs of twins, will show you why I can say this with confidence.

This study, published in the *New England Journal of Medicine,* looked at whether people with the same genes had the same risk of cancer. What they found was that cancer is more likely to be caused by diet and lifestyle choices than by genes. Identical twins, who are genetically the same, had no more than a 15 percent chance of developing the same cancer. This suggests that the cause of most cancers is about 85 percent environmental—that is, due to factors such as diet, lifestyle, and exposure to toxic chemicals. This study concluded that diet, smoking, and (lack of) exercise accounted for up to 82 percent of cancers studied.[30]

To some extent you can divide cancer into two kinds. First there are cancers of the lungs and digestive tract—esophagus, stomach, and colorectal cancer. These are strongly linked to diet, with alcohol, smoking, hot drinks, and meat the major culprits. Burnt meat is by far the worst offender—eating burned or browned meat every day significantly increases your risk.

The other kind are hormonal cancers, most notably breast and prostate cancer. Both of these, and especially breast cancer, are linked to "estrogen dominance" and to high-ⓖ diets. Estrogen is the hormone that encourages breast and uterine cell growth, and an excess of estrogen signals (or a lack of progesterone, which counters the effects of estrogen) can trigger breast cancer.

Ten years ago I went public with my views on HRT, saying that it was an unacceptable risk factor for breast cancer, a view that is finally being accepted by government bodies around the world. But many women's diets are also to blame. The reason is twofold.

First, as you start to lose blood sugar balance and become overweight and insulin resistant, the resulting excess fat produces estrogen. Yes, fat cells—not just the ovaries—produce estrogen. This leads to a lifetime of extra exposure to estrogen. That's risk number one.

Here's risk number two. Increased consumption of high-🄖 foods leads, as we've seen, to insulin resistance, present in the majority of overweight people and 25 percent of those not overweight. Insulin resistance in turn can lead to polycystic ovary syndrome (PCOS). With this condition, women have more and more cycles in which they don't ovulate. Only if a woman ovulates is progesterone produced, so estrogen, unopposed by progesterone, can then trigger breast cancer. (If you want to go deeper into this subject read my book *Say No to Cancer*.)

The Holford Diet is a perfect diet in all respects for preventing both digestive cancers and hormonal cancers. Once again, the low-🄖 foods, high in antioxidants, essential fats, and B vitamins, all help to keep your body in fighting trim. The emphasis on fresh, organic foods wherever possible is important here, too. In fact, in all its essentials this diet matches the recommendations of the World Cancer Research Fund for reducing cancer risk. Supplementing with a good high-strength multivitamin, plus 1 or 2 grams of vitamin C, further boosts your body's natural immunity.

I have seen this approach not only keep thousands of women free from breast cancer, but even reverse the cancer in women who have it. That's what happened to Betty, who first consulted me in 1986. Here's what she says:

I feel moved to tell you I consulted you in 1986 with a recurrence of breast cancer. Now, 13 years later, I am pleased to tell you I have just celebrated my seventy-fifth birthday and am fit and well, taking no medication and attending no clinics. I am sure this is in large part due to the advice I received from you.

Arthritis. If you've got aching joints, welcome to the club. Nine out of ten people have arthritis by the time they're 60. I want to make sure you're one of the one in ten who don't. It's a vicious circle because once you develop aching joints you don't want to exercise, and then weight gain is just around the corner.

However, you will be pleased to hear that the principles of the Holford Diet work extremely well for repairing arthritic joints. That is because the five main causes of inflammation and damage to joints are all reversible. These are:

- glycation, which means damage caused by sugar;
- inflammation caused by a lack of essential fats;
- too much oxidation, not enough antioxidants;
- allergy; and
- lack of joint-building minerals and nutrients such as glucosamine.

Glycation is inflammation caused by glucose imbalance and insulin resistance. Glucose can damage joints in the same way it damages arteries. That's why there is a strong link between diabetes and arthritis. While ordinarily the adrenal hormone cortisol—the body's best anti-inflammatory agent—can handle such problems, out-of-control blood sugar results in adrenal exhaustion. So it's far better to restore blood sugar balance to avoid the damage in the first place. Reducing your use of stimulants such as caffeine and nicotine also helps.

The next cause of inflammation is a lack of what are called prostaglandins, the hormonelike substances made from essential fats, especially omega-3 fats. A diet high in meat and dairy products, which are high in saturated fats, promotes pain and inflammation, while a diet high in fish and seeds, high in essential fats, reduces it. That's what the Holford Diet achieves.

Then there are free radicals, or oxidants. In much the same way that oxidants from exhaust fumes or cigarettes damage your skin, oxidants in the bloodstream damage joints. That's why a diet high in antioxidants, backed up by supplements, helps to reduce inflammation.

The final common cause of arthritis is having unidentified food allergies. John is a case in point. He could barely walk 100 yards without pain and had to go up the stairs on his hands and knees, despite being on a lot of medication. He took YorkTest's IgG allergy test and discovered he was allergic to certain foods. Once he eliminated these from his diet, he began to feel less pain. He gradually reduced his medication and now needs none. He no longer experiences pain and has regained his mobility.

Once inflammation is under control, joints can and do repair themselves.

This, of course, requires a good supply of bone-building minerals such as calcium, magnesium, and zinc, all abundant in the whole foods I recommend you eat on the Holford Diet. Seeds are an especially good source of these nutrients, as well as an excellent source of essential fats. When you put all this together with appropriate supplements, you have an incredibly powerful anti-arthritis strategy.

Take Ed. I met him after he had retired from a highly successful business career. He had the money, he had the time, but he could barely walk without pain, let alone pursue his passion for golf. I advised him on how to change his diet and what supplements to take. It took him three months to become pain-free. Here's what he said:

> *I used to have constant pain in my knees and joints, could not play golf or walk more than ten minutes without resting my legs. Since following your advice my discomfort has decreased 95–100 percent. It is a different life when you can travel and play golf every day. I never would have believed my pain could be reduced by such a large degree, and not return, no matter how much activity in a day or week.*

If you'd like to find out more specifically about arthritis, I recommend you read my book *Say No to Arthritis*.

I know you just want to lose weight—and you will. But I hope I have convinced you that the diet you are about to start will change your life for the better. Not only will you feel the benefits in the next few weeks, but you will live the benefits for years to come. The Holford Diet is a diet for living your life to the fullest.

- If you choose to eat low-Ⓖ foods that are also high in antioxidants you will improve your skin. These include berries, plums, grapefruit, and oranges, as well as kale, spinach, broccolini, broccoli, beets, Brussels sprouts, and avocados.
- You need some carbohydrate to make serotonin in the brain, which keeps you happy and reduces your appetite.
- By controlling your blood sugar and providing brain-friendly nutrients, the Holford Diet helps sharpen your memory and concentration.
- You can slow down the aging process and extend your life span by following the Holford Diet because you'll be eating less quantity (calories) and more quality (optimum nutrition).

- The Holford Diet also helps to lower many vital statistics that mean greater risk for disease, including your cholesterol, triglycerides, homocysteine, and blood pressure.
- The Holford Diet helps to prevent heart disease, cancer, diabetes, Alzheimer's, and arthritis and is consistent with the cutting-edge science of disease prevention through nutrition.

References: Part Five

1. *Agricultural Research,* November 1996, pp. 4–8 (see ORAC Chart and the Watsons' approach to optimal health and longevity at http://optimal-health.cia.com.au/OracLevels.htm); Ronald Prior et al., Jean Mayer USDA Human Nutrition Research Center on Aging at Tufts, Boston, Mass, in *Journal of Agriculture and Food Chemistry,* vol. 46 (1998), pp. 2686–93, and *American Society for Horticultural Science* (1999); *Journal of Agriculture and Food Chemistry,* vol. 49(11) (2001), pp. 5165–70.

2. S. E. Vollset et al., "Plasma Total Homocysteine and Cardiovascular and Noncardiovascular Mortality: The Hordaland Homocysteine Study," *American Journal of Clinical Nutrition,* vol. 74(1) (2001), pp. 130–6.

3. D. Xu, R. Neville, and T. Finkel, "Homocysteine Accelerates Endothelial Cell Senescence," *Federation of European Biochemical Societies Letters,* vol. 470 (2000), pp. 20–4.

4. R. Wurtman and J. Wurtman, "Carbohydrates and Depression," *Scientific American,* vol. 260(1) (1989), pp. 68–75.

5. D. Benton et al., "Mild Hypoglycaemia and Questionnaire Measures of Aggression," *Biological Psychology,* vol. 14(1–2) (1982), pp. 129–35.

6. A. Roy et al., "Monoamimes, Glucose Metabolism, Aggression Toward Self and Others," *International Journal of Neuroscience,* vol. 41(3–4) (1988), pp. 261–4.

7. A. G. Schauss, *Diet, Crime and Delinquency,* Parker House (1980).

8. M. Virkkunen, "Reactive Hypoglycaemic Tendency Among Arsonists," *Acta Psychiatrica Scandinavica,* vol. 69(5) (1984), pp. 445–52.

9. M. Virkkunen and S. Narvanen, "Tryptophan and Serotonin Levels During the Glucose Tolerance Test Among Habitually Violent and Impulsive Offenders," *Neuropsychobiology,* vol. 17(1–2) (1987), pp. 19–23.

10. J. Yaryura-Tobias and F. Neziroglu, "Violent Behaviour, Brain Dysrythmia and Glucose Dysfunction: A New Syndrome," *Journal of Orthomolecular Psychiatry,* vol. 4 (1975), pp. 182–5.

11. M. Bruce and M. Lader, "Caffeine Abstention and the Management of Anxiety Disorders," *Psychological Medicine,* vol. 19 (1989), pp. 211–14.

12. W. Wendel and W. Beebe, "Glycolytic Activity in Schizophrenia," in D. Hawkins and L. Pauling (eds.), *Journal of Orthomolecular Psychiatry* (1973).

13. R. Prinz and D. Riddle, "Associations Between Nutrition and Behaviour in 5 Year Old Children," *Nutrition Reviews,* vol. 43 (1986), suppl.

14. L. Christensen, "Psychological Distress and Diet—Effects of Sucrose and Caffeine," *Journal of Applied Nutrition,* vol. 40(1), 1988, pp. 44–50.

15. D. Fullerton et al., "Sugar, Opionoids and Binge Eating," *Brain Research Bulletin,* vol. 14(6) (1985), pp. 273–80.

16. I. Christensen, "Psychological Distress and Diet—Effects of Sucrose and Caffeine," *Journal of Applied Nutrition,* vol. 40 (1988), pp. 44–50.

17. M. Colgan and L. Colgan, "Do Nutrient Supplements and Dietary Changes Affect Learning and Emotional Reactions of Children with Learning Difficulties? A Controlled Series of 16 Cases," *Nutrition and Health,* vol. 3 (1984), pp. 69–77.

18. J. Goldman et al., "Behavioural Effects of Sucrose on Preschool Children," *Journal of Abnormal Child Psychology,* vol. 14(4) (1986), pp. 565–77.

19. M. Lester et al., "Refined Carbohydrate Intake, Hair Cadmium Levels and Cognitive Functioning in Children," *Nutrition and Behaviour,* vol. 1 (1982), pp. 3–13.

20. S. Schoenthaler et al., "The Impact of Low Food Additive and Sucrose Diet on Academic Performance in 803 New York City Public Schools," *International Journal of Biosocial Research,* vol. 8(2) (1986), pp. 185–95.

21. M. Morris et al., "Vitamin E and Vitamin C Supplement Use and Risk Incident Alzheimer Disease," *Alzheimer's Disease and Associated Disorders,* vol. 12 (1998), pp. 121–6.

22. M. Morris et al., "Dietary Intake of Antioxidant Nutrients and the Risk of Incident AD," *Journal of the American Medical Association,* vol. 287(24) (2002), pp. 3230–7; see also pp. 3223–61.

23. M. Sano et al., "A Controlled Trial of Selegiline, Alpha Tocopherol or Both as Treatment of AD," *New England Journal of Medicine,* vol. 336 (1997), pp. 1216–22.

24. S. Seshadri et al., "Plasma Homocysteine as a Risk Factor for Dementia and AD," *New England Journal of Medicine,* vol. 346(7) (2002), pp. 476–83.

25. D. S. Ludwig, "The Glycemic Index," *Journal of the American Medical Association,* vol. 287(18) (2002), pp. 2414–23.

26. Ibid.

27. S. Liu et al., "A Prospective Study of Dietary Glycemic Load, Carbohydrate Intake, and Risk of Coronary Heart Disease in US Women," *American Journal of Clinical Nutrition,* vol. 71(6) (2000), pp. 1455–61.

28. "Nutritional Aspects of Cardiovascular Disease," Department of Health [U.K.] (1994).

29. World Cancer Research Fund, "Food, Nutrition and the Prevention of Cancer. A Global Perspective" (1997).

30. P. Lichenstein et al., "Environmental and Heritable Factors in the Causation of Cancer," *New England Journal of Medicine,* vol. 343(2) (2000), pp. 78–85.

Appendices

Appendix 1

Ideal Weight, Body Mass Index, and Body Fat Percentage

Weight in relation to height

The following table gives you your ideal weight range depending on your height and sex.

Your Ideal weight for height

Men age 25 and over		Women age 25 and over	
Height (feet)	Weight (pounds)	Height (feet)	Weight (pounds)
5' 1"	112–129	4' 8"	92–107
5' 2"	115–133	4' 9"	94–110
5' 3"	118–136	4' 10"	96–113
5' 4"	121–139	4' 11"	99–116
5' 5"	124–143	5' 0"	102–119
5' 6"	128–147	5' 1"	105–122
5' 7"	132–152	5' 2"	108–126
5' 8"	136–156	5' 3"	111–130
5' 9"	140–160	5' 4"	114–135
5' 10"	144–165	5' 5"	118–139
5' 11"	148–170	5' 6"	122–143
6' 0"	152–175	5' 7"	126–147
6' 1"	156–180	5' 8"	130–151
6' 2"	160–185	5' 9"	134–155
6' 3"	164–190	5' 10"	138–159

Body mass index

Even better than knowing your ideal weight for your height is to calculate your body mass index, or BMI, a measure of fat based on your height and your weight. Your BMI is a reliable indicator of total body fat. The score is valid for both men and women, but does have some limits:

- It may overestimate body fat in athletes and others who have a muscular build.
- It may underestimate body fat in older people and those who have lost muscle mass.

Your BMI can be used to work out whether you are overweight or obese. Here are the scores:

Underweight = 18.5 or less
Normal weight = 18.5–24.9
Overweight = 25–29.9
Obese = 30 or more

Body mass index table

BMI	Normal							Overweight				Obese										Extreme obesity															
	19	20	21	22	23	24	25	26	27	28	29	30	31	32	33	34	35	36	37	38	39	40	41	42	43	44	45	46	47	48	49	50	51	52	53	54
Height (inches)												Body weight (pounds)																								
58	91	96	100	105	110	115	119	124	129	134	138	143	148	153	158	162	167	172	177	181	186	191	196	201	205	210	215	220	224	229	234	239	244	248	253	258
59	94	99	104	109	114	119	124	128	133	138	143	148	153	158	163	168	173	178	183	188	193	198	203	208	212	217	222	227	232	237	242	247	252	257	262	267
60	97	102	107	112	118	123	128	133	138	143	148	153	158	163	168	174	179	184	189	194	199	204	209	215	220	225	230	235	240	245	250	255	261	266	271	276
61	100	106	111	116	122	127	132	137	143	148	153	158	164	169	174	180	185	190	195	201	206	211	217	222	227	232	238	243	248	254	259	264	269	275	280	285
62	104	109	115	120	126	131	136	142	147	153	158	164	169	175	180	186	191	196	202	207	213	218	224	229	235	240	246	251	256	262	267	273	278	284	289	295
63	107	113	118	124	130	135	141	146	152	158	163	169	175	180	186	191	197	203	208	214	220	225	231	237	242	248	254	259	265	270	278	282	287	293	299	304
64	110	116	122	128	134	140	145	151	157	163	169	174	180	186	192	197	204	209	215	221	227	232	238	244	250	256	262	267	273	279	285	291	296	302	308	314
65	114	120	126	132	138	144	150	156	162	168	174	180	186	192	198	204	210	216	222	228	234	240	246	252	258	264	270	276	282	288	294	300	306	312	318	324
66	118	124	130	136	142	148	155	161	167	173	179	186	192	198	204	210	216	223	229	235	241	247	253	260	266	272	278	284	291	297	303	309	315	322	328	334
67	121	127	134	140	146	153	159	166	172	178	185	191	198	204	211	217	223	230	236	242	249	255	261	268	274	280	287	293	299	306	312	319	325	331	338	344
68	125	131	138	144	151	158	164	171	177	184	190	197	203	210	216	223	230	236	243	249	256	262	269	276	282	289	295	302	308	315	322	328	335	341	348	354
69	128	135	142	149	155	162	169	176	182	189	196	203	209	216	223	230	236	243	250	257	263	270	277	284	291	297	304	311	318	324	331	338	345	351	358	365
70	132	139	146	153	160	167	174	181	188	195	202	209	216	222	229	236	243	250	257	264	271	278	285	292	299	306	313	320	327	334	341	348	355	362	369	376
71	136	143	150	157	165	172	179	186	193	200	208	215	222	229	236	243	250	257	265	272	279	286	293	301	308	315	322	329	338	343	351	358	365	372	379	386
72	140	147	154	162	169	177	184	191	199	206	213	221	228	235	242	250	258	265	272	279	287	294	302	309	316	324	331	338	346	353	361	368	375	383	390	397
73	144	151	159	166	174	182	189	197	204	212	219	227	235	242	250	257	265	272	280	288	295	302	310	318	325	333	340	348	355	363	371	378	386	393	401	408
74	148	155	163	171	179	186	194	202	210	218	225	233	241	249	256	264	272	280	287	295	303	311	319	326	334	342	350	358	365	373	381	389	396	404	412	420
75	152	160	168	176	184	192	200	208	216	224	232	240	248	256	264	272	279	287	295	303	311	319	327	335	343	351	359	367	375	383	391	399	407	415	423	431
76	156	164	172	180	189	197	205	213	221	230	238	246	254	263	271	279	287	295	304	312	320	328	336	344	353	361	369	377	385	394	402	410	418	426	435	443

Source: Adapted from Clinical Guidelines on the Identification, Evaluation, and Treatment of Overweight and Obesity in Adults: The Evidence Report. National Institutes of Health.

Measuring percentage of body fat

A more important statistic than your BMI is your body fat percentage. Following is an equation to work out an approximation of this percentage. (Your local gym may offer a service for measuring your body fat percentage more accurately using calipers or testing equipment.) An ideal percentage of fat for a man is less than 15 percent; for a woman it's less than 22 percent. You can reduce your body fat percentage by around 10 percent a month on the Holford Diet.

STEP 1

Find your body weight (BW) on the chart on page 325 and write down the corresponding conversion factor. For every pound over the figures given, add 1.08 to the conversion factor.

So: if you weigh 175 pounds, your conversion factor is 189.36.

If you weigh 132 pounds, your conversion factor is 142.83 (140.67 + 2 × 1.08).

STEP 2

Find your waist girth on the chart and write down the corresponding conversion factor.

So: if you have a 35-inch waist, your conversion factor is 145.26.

STEP 3

Subtract the waist conversion factor from the body weight conversion factor.

So: 189.36 − 145.26 = 44.1.

STEP 4

To the result, add 98.42 for men or 76.76 for women. This gives you your lean body weight (LBW).

So: 44.10 + 98.42 = 142.52.

STEP 5

To calculate your fat weight (FW), subtract the LBW from the BW:

BW − LBW = FW.

So: 175 − 142.52 = 32.48.

STEP 6

To determine the actual percentage of your body fat, divide FW by BW and multiply by 100:

FW ÷ BW × 100 = % BF.

So: 32.48 ÷ 175 × 100 = 19%.

Body fat percentage calculation chart

Body weight	Conversion factor	Waist girth	Conversion factor
100	108.21	25	103.75
105	113.62	25.5	105.83
110	119.03	26	107.9
115	124.44	26.5	109.98
120	129.85	27	112.05
125	135.26	27.5	114.13
130	140.67	28	116.2
135	146.08	28.5	118.28
140	151.49	29	120.35
145	156.9	29.5	122.43
150	162.31	30	124.51
155	167.72	30.5	126.58
160	173.13	31	128.66
165	178.54	31.5	130.73
170	183.95	32	132.81
175	189.36	32.5	134.88
180	194.77	33	136.96
185	200.18	33.5	139.03

(continued on next page)

Body weight	Conversion factor	Waist girth	Conversion factor
190	205.59	34	141.11
195	211	34.5	143.18
200	216.41	35	145.26
205	221.82	35.5	147.33
210	227.23	36	149.41
215	232.64	36.5	151.48
220	238.05	37	153.56
225	243.46	37.5	155.63
230	248.87	38	157.71
235	254.28	38.5	159.78
240	259.69	39	161.86
245	265.1	39.5	163.93
250	270.51	40	166.01
255	275.92	40.5	167.08
260	281.33	41	170.16
265	286.74	41.5	172.23
270	292.15	42	174.31
275	297.56	42.5	176.38
280	302.97	43	178.46
285	308.38	43.5	180.53
290	313.79	44	182.61

Appendix 2

The Complete Glycemic Load of Foods

Glycemic index

The glycemic index is about the *quality* of the carbohydrate within a food, not the *quantity*. In other words, the glycemic index (GI) of a food remains the same whether you eat 10 grams or 100 grams. It is a comparison of how one type of carbohydrate (for example, that in bread) compares with another type of carbohydrate (for example, sugar). It's worked out by feeding volunteers however much of the food in question they would need to eat to consume 50 grams of "available" carbohydrate. (Some carbohydrate, such as fiber, is not available to the body for its energy needs.)

If, for example, a food contains half available carbohydrate, the volunteers would be fed 100 grams of the food to obtain 50 grams of the available carbohydrate. The extent to which this raises blood sugar levels (see figure on page 66), compared with the extent to which 50 grams of glucose does, determines the food's GI score. Glucose, by definition, scores 100 on the glycemic index. So, if a food creates half the increase in blood sugar compared with glucose, its GI score will be 50. This means that you could eat twice as much carbohydrate in the form found in this food to match the effect of glucose on your blood sugar level.

Glycemic load

The glycemic load of a food (**GL**) is basically the GI of a food divided by 100, multiplied by the amount of available carbohydrate in a particular serving. So, the **GL** actually tells you what that specific serving, cookie, or slice of bread will do to your blood sugar.

The **GL** of a food is worked out as follows:

GI score divided by 100 multiplied by the available carbohydrate (carbohydrates minus fiber) in grams.

So, in our example above this would be:

50 (GI score) ÷ 100 × 50 (50 grams of carbohydrate in a 100-gram serving) = 25

So a 100-gram serving of our example food has a **GL** of 25.

Take watermelon as another example. Its glycemic index (GI) is pretty high, about 72. According to the calculations by the people at the University of Sydney's Human Nutrition Unit, in a serving of 100 grams it has 6 grams of available carbohydrate per serving, so its glycemic load is pretty low, 72 ÷ 100 × 6 = 4.32 (rounded to 4).

So, as long as you know the glycemic index of a food, the size of the serving you wish to use, and the amount of available carbohydrate in the food, you can calculate the **GL** yourself. However, I have calculated the **GL** for a comprehensive range of foods, which can be found in the chart on pages 330–340.

Please note that the glycemic index for some foods has not been published. In these instances we have estimated the **GL** based on the GI for very similar foods. These foods are marked "E."

The most accurate way to gauge whether or not you should eat a food is the glycemic load of a food, which is a calculation based on both the quantity of carbohydrate in a food, and the quality of that carbohydrate.

A **GL** of 10 or less is good, **shown in bold**
A **GL** of 11–14 is OK, shown in normal text
A **GL** of 15 or more is bad, *shown in italics*

However, even this is only a guide, because the amount of a food you eat will obviously alter its effect on your blood sugar, and hence your weight.

So, while generally I say to liberally eat the **bold** foods with low ⑪, limit the normal-text foods, and avoid the *italic* foods, what is most important is to limit the total glycemic load of your diet.

If you want to lose weight and feel great, eat no more than 40 ⑪ a day. This means roughly 10 for breakfast, 10 for lunch, 10 for dinner and 5 each for your two snacks, midmorning and midafternoon. You can also drink 5 ⑪, so your total daily intake from food and drink is 45 ⑪. If you choose the good, low-⑪ foods you'll be able to eat more food. If you choose the bad, high-⑪ foods you'll be eating much less.

In the chart which follows mainly select from the bold foods, then use the right-hand column to work out how much to eat for 5 ⑪, which is the serving for a snack, or 10 ⑪, which is a serving for a main meal. If you are not sure what a "serving" means, look at the amount of grams for 5 ⑪ and check the grams on the package of the food in question. Foods containing no carbohydrate, composed entirely of protein or fat (meat, fish, eggs, cheese, mayonnaise) have, in effect, a ⑪ of 0, and are not included in this chart.

Remember that foods marked with an "E" have an estimated value, while other foods have measured values. As the ⑪ of more foods is calculated, this table will be expanded on www.theholforddiet.com.

GLYCEMIC load GL of common foods

Item	Serving size (in oz.)	GL per serving	10 GLs	5 GLs	5 GLs (in oz.)
BAKERY PRODUCTS					
Muffin, apple, made without sugar	2.1	9	1 muffin	½ muffin	1.2
Muffin, apple muffin, made with sugar	2.1	13	1 small muffin	½ small muffin	0.8
Muffin, apple, oat, raisin, made from mix	1.8	14	1 small muffin	½ small muffin	0.6
Muffin, bran	2.0	15	½ muffin	¼ muffin	0.6
Muffin, blueberry	2.0	17	½ muffin	¼ muffin	0.6
Muffin, carrot	2.0	20	½ muffin	¼ muffin	0.5
Banana cake, made without sugar	2.8	16	1 small slice	½ small slice	0.9
Croissant	2.0	17	½ croissant	¼ croissant	0.6
Doughnut, cake	1.6	17	½ doughnut	¼ doughnut	0.5
Sponge cake, plain	2.2	17	½ slice	¼ slice	0.7
BREADS					
Pumpernickel bread	1.1	6	2 slices	1 slice	0.9
Sourdough rye	1.1	6	2 slices	1 slice	0.9
Rice bread, high-amylose	1.1	7	2 small slices	1 small slice	0.7
Rice bread, low-amylose	1.1	8	2 thin slices	1 thin slice	0.7
Whole-grain rye bread	1.1	8	2 thin slices	1 thin slice	0.7
Wheat tortilla	1.8	8	1½ tortillas	Less than 1 tortilla	1.1
White bread, high-fiber	1.1	9	1 thick slice	1 thin slice	0.6

Whole-wheat bread	1.1	9	1 thick slice	1 thin slice	0.6
Gluten-free fiber-enriched bread	1.1	9	1 thick slice	½ thick slice	0.6
Gluten-free multigrain bread	1.1	10	1 slice	½ slice	0.5
Light rye	1.1	10	1 slice	½ slice	0.5
White bread	1.1	10	1 slice	½ slice	0.5
Pita bread, white	1.1	10	1 pita	½ pita	0.5
Wheat flour flatbread	1.1	10	1 slice	½ slice	0.5
Gluten-free white bread	1.1	11	1 slice	½ slice	0.5
Corn tortilla	1.8	12	1 tortilla	½ tortilla	0.7
Middle Eastern flatbread	1.1	15	⅔ slice	⅓ slice	0.4
Baguette, white, plain	1.1	15	1/20 baguette	1/40 baguette	0.4
Bagel, white	2.5	25	½ bagel	¼ bagel	0.5
BREAKFAST CEREALS					
Oatmeal made from rolled oats	1.1	2	as much as you like	1 very large bowl	2.6
Get Up & Go with strawberries and ½ pint of milk	30	5	1 cup	½ cup	5 fl. oz.
All-Bran	1.1	6	2 small servings	1 small serving	0.9
Muesli, gluten-free	1.1	7	2 small servings	1 small serving	0.7
Muesli, Natural	1.1	10	1 serving	½ serving	0.5
Raisin Bran™	1.1	12	1 small serving	⅓ serving	0.5
Weetabix™	1.1	13	2 biscuits	1 biscuit	0.4
Bran flakes	1.1	13	1 small serving	⅓ serving	0.4
Special K™	1.1	14	1 small serving	⅓ serving	0.4

Item	Serving size (in oz.)	GL per serving	10 GLs	5 GLs	5 GLs (in oz.)
Shredded wheat	1.1	15	1 very small serving	⅓ serving	0.4
Cheerios™	1.1	15	1 very small serving	⅓ serving	0.4
Frosted Flakes™	1.1	15	1 very small serving	⅓ serving	0.4
Grape-Nuts™	1.1	15	1 very small serving	⅓ serving	0.4
Rice Krispies™	1.1	21	½ serving	¼ serving	0.2
Corn Flakes™	1.1	21	½ serving	¼ serving	0.2
CANNED SOUPS					
Tomato soup	8.8	6	1 can	½ can	7.3
Minestrone	8.8	7	1 can	½ can	6.3
Lentil	8.8	9	⅔ can	⅓ can	4.9
Split pea	8.8	16	½ can	¼ can	2.7
Black bean	8.8	17	½ can	¼ can	2.6
CEREAL GRAINS					
Semolina	5.3	6	1 very large serving	1 small serving	4.4
Taco shells, cornmeal-based, baked (Old El Paso)	0.7	8	2 shells	1 shell	0.5
Quinoa	5.3	8	1½ cups	¾ cup	3.3
Cornmeal mush	5.3	9	a very large serving	small serving	2.9
Buckwheat	5.3	16	1 small serving	⅓ serving	1.6
Kamut	5.3	9	a very large serving	small serving	2.9
Pearl barley	5.3	11	1 serving	½ serving	2.4

Cracked wheat (bulgur)	5.3	12	1 serving	½ serving	2.2
Rice, brown basmati	5.3	13	1 small serving	½ serving	2.0
Rice, brown	5.3	18	1 small serving	⅓ serving	1.5
Rice, long grain, white, instant (Uncle Ben's)	5.3	19	½ serving	¼ serving	1.4
Rice, white basmati	5.3	22	½ serving	¼ serving	1.2
Rice, white	5.3	23	½ serving	¼ serving	1.2
Rice, long grain	5.3	23	½ serving	¼ serving	1.2
Couscous	5.3	23	½ serving	¼ serving	1.2
Millet	5.3	25	½ serving	¼ serving	1.1

CRACKERS/CRISPBREADS

Rough oatcake crackers	.4	2	5½ crackers	3 crackers	1
Rye crispbread	.9	11	2 crackers	1 cracker	0.4
Water cracker	.9	13	2 crackers	1 cracker	0.2
Puffed-rice cakes	.9	17	2 rice cakes	1 rice cake	0.2

DAIRY PRODUCTS AND ALTERNATIVES

Plain yogurt (no sugar)	7.0	3	3 small cups	1½ small cups	11.7
Nonfat yogurt (plain, no sugar)	7.0	3	3 small cups	1½ small cups	11.7
Milk, whole	8.8	3	3½ cups	1¾ cups	14.1 fl. oz.
Milk, skim	8.8	4	2½ cups	1¼ cups	10.9
Custard, home made from milk	3.5	7	1 small cup	½ small cup	2.4 fl. oz.
Ice cream, regular	1.8	8	2 scoops	1 scoop	1.0 fl. oz.
Soy yogurt	7.0	7	2 small cups	1 small cup	5.3

Item	Serving size (in oz.)	🍷 per serving	10 🍷s	5 🍷s	5 🍷s (in oz.)
Soy milk (no sugar)	8.8	7	2 small cups	1 small cup	6.0 fl. oz.
Soy milk (sweetened with apple juice concentrate)	8.8	8	2 small cups	1 small cup	5.3 fl. oz.
Soy milk, reduced-fat (1.5%)	8.8	8	2 small cups	1 small cup	5.3 fl. oz.
Soy milk (sweetened with sugar)	8.8	9	1½ small cups	¾ small cup	4.7 fl. oz.
Low-fat yogurt, fruit (with sugar)	7.0	10	1½ small cups	⅔ small cup	3.5
Rice milk	8.8	14	1 small cup	½ small cup	3.2
Milk, condensed, sweetened	*1.8*	*17*	*1 teaspoon*	*½ teaspoon*	*0.5*
FRUIT AND FRUIT PRODUCTS					
Blackberries	4.2	1	2 pints	1 pints	21
Blueberries	4.2	1	2 pints	1 pints	21
Raspberries	4.2	1	2 pints	1 pints	21
Strawberries	4.2	1	2 pints	1 pints	21
Cherries	4.2	3	14 oz. or 1 lb.	1 basket or ½ lb.	7
Grapefruit	4.2	3	1 large	1 small	7
Pear	4.2	4	2 large pears	1 large pear	5.3
Melon/Cantaloupe	4.2	4	1 small melon	½ small melon	5.3
Watermelon	4.2	4	2 big slices	1 big slice	5.3
Peaches (raw or canned in natural juice)	4.2	5	2 peaches	1 peach	4.2
Apricots	4.2	5	8 apricots	4 apricots	4.2
Oranges	4.2	5	2 large	1 large	4.2
Plum	4.2	5	8 plums	4 plums	4.2

Apples	4.2	6	2 small	1 small	3.5
Kiwifruit	4.2	6	2 kiwis	1 kiwi	3.5
Pineapple	4.2	7	2 thin slices	1 thin slice	3.0
Grapes	4.2	8	20 grapes	10 grapes	2.6
Mango	4.2	8	½ mango	¼ mango	2.6
Apricots, dried	2.1	9	6 apricots	3 apricots	1.2
Fruit cocktail, canned (Del Monte)	4.2	9	1 small can	½ small can	2.3
Papaya	4.2	10	½ small papaya	¼ small papaya	2.1
Prunes, pitted	2.1	10	6 prunes	3 prunes	1.1
Apple, dried	2.1	10	6 rings	3 rings	1.1
Banana raw	4.2	12	1 banana	½ banana	1.8
Apricots, canned in light syrup	4.2	12	⅔ small can	⅓ small can	1.8
Lychee, canned in syrup and drained	4.2	16	½ (7 oz.) can	¼ (7 oz.) can	1.3
Figs, dried	2.1	16	2 figs	1 fig	0.7
Raisins	2.1	28	20	10	0.4
Dates, dried	2.1	42	2 dates	1 date	0.2
JAMS/SPREADS					
Pumpkin seed butter	0.6	1	3 large jars	1½ large jars	26.8
Peanut butter (no sugar)	0.6	1	3 large jars	1½ large jars	26.8
Blueberry spread (no sugar)	1.1	4	4 tablespoons	2 tablespoons	0.7
Apricot spread, reduced sugar	1.1	7	2½ tablespoons	1¼ tablespoons	0.7
Orange marmalade	1.1	9	2½ tablespoons	1¼ tablespoons	0.6
Strawberry jam	1.1	10	2 tablespoons	1 tablespoon	0.5

Item	Serving size (in oz.)	● per serving	10 ●s	5 ●s	5 ●s (in oz.)
LEGUMES					
Hummus	1.1	1.5	8 oz.	4 oz.	4
Soy beans, canned	5.3	1	6 cups	3 cups	26.3
Peas, dried, boiled	5.3	2	3 cups	1½ cups	13.1
Pinto beans	5.3	4	2 cups	1 cup	6.5
Lentils	5.3	5	2 cups	1 cup	5.3
Butter beans	5.3	6	1½ cups	¾ cup	4.4
Split peas, yellow	5.3	6	1½ cups	¾ cup	4.4
Baked beans, canned	5.3	7	½ can	¼ can	3.7
Kidney beans, canned	5.3	7	¾ can	⅓ can	3.7
Chickpeas, dried, cooked	5.3	8	1½ cups	¾ cup	3.3
Navy beans, canned	5.3	12	½ can	¼ can	2.2
Black-eyed peas, boiled	5.3	13	1 cup	½ cup	2.0
PASTA AND NOODLES					
Ravioli, durum wheat, meat filled	3.2	7.5	2 small servings	1 small serving	2.1
Vermicelli, white	3.2	8	a large serving	½ large serving	2.0
Pasta whole-wheat	3.2	8	a large serving	½ large serving	2.0
Fettuccine, egg	3.2	9	1 serving	½ serving	1.8
Spaghetti	3.2	9	1 serving	½ serving	1.6
Spaghetti, durum wheat	3.2	10	1 serving	½ serving	1.5
Instant noodles	3.2	9	1 serving	½ serving	1.6

Macaroni, plain	3.2	11	1 very small serving	½ very small serving	1.4
Rice noodles	3.2	11	1 very small serving	½ very small serving	1.4
Udon noodles, plain	3.2	15	⅔ serving	⅓ serving	1.1
Gnocchi	3.2	16	1 very small serving	½ small serving	0.9
Brown rice pasta	3.2	17	1 very small serving	½ small serving	0.9
SNACK FOODS (SALTY)					
Olives, in brine	1.8	1	4 cups	2 cups	9.5
Peanuts	1.8	1	18 oz.	9 oz.	8.8
Cashews, salted	1.8	3	6 oz.	3 oz.	2.9
Popcorn, salted, no sugar	0.7	8	0.9 oz.	0.45 oz.	0.4
Potato chips, plain, salted	1.8	11	1.6 oz	0.8 oz.	0.8
Pretzels, oven-baked, traditional	1.1	16	8	4	0.3
Corn chips, plain, salted	1.8	17	13 chips	7 chips	0.5
SNACK FOODS (SWEET)					
Granola bar containing dried fruit	1.1	13	less than 1 bar	less than ½ bar	0.4
Chocolate, milk, plain	1.8	14	less than ½ bar	less than ¼ bar	0.6
Apricot fruit bar (dried apricot filling in whole wheat pastry)	1.8	17	1 bar	½ bar	0.5
Twix	2.1	17	1 stick	½ stick	0.6
Snickers	2.1	19	⅔ bar	⅓ bar	0.6
Jelly beans, assorted colors	1.1	22	4 jelly beans	2 jelly beans	0.2
Mars bar	2.1	26	½ bar	¼ bar	0.5

Item	Serving size (in oz.)	⬤ per serving	10 ⬤s	5 ⬤s	5 ⬤s (in oz.)
SUGARS					
Xylitol	0.7	2	6 tablespoons	3 tablespoons	1.8
Agave nectar	0.7	2	7 tablespoons	3 tablespoons	1.8
Fructose	0.7	4	3 tablespoons	5 teaspoon	0.9
Sucrose (table sugar)	0.7	14	3 teaspoons	1½ teaspoons	0.2
Honey	0.7	16	2 teaspoons	1 teaspoon	0.2
Maltose (malt)	0.7	22	2 teaspoons	1 teaspoon	0.2
VEGETABLES					
Tomato	2.5	2	5 medium	2½ medium	6.1
Broccoli	3.5	2	5 handfuls	2½ handfuls	8.8
Kale	2.6	1	10 handfuls	5 handfuls	13.1
Avocado	6.7	1	10	5	33.3
Onion	6.3	2	5 medium	2½ medium	15.8
Asparagus	4.4	2	5 handfuls	2½ handfuls	11.0
Green beans	2.6	1	10 handfuls	5 handfuls	13.1
Carrots	2.8	3	2 carrots	1 carrot	4.7
Green peas	2.8	3	5 tablespoons	2–3 tablespoons	4.7
Pumpkin	2.8	3	9 oz.	3 servings	4.7
Beets	2.8	5	4 small	2 small	2.8
Rutabaga	5.3	7	2 small servings	1 small serving	3.8
Plantain, green	4.2	8	1 small	½ small	2.6

	Serving size (in oz.)	GL per serving	10 GLs	5 GLs	5 GLs (in oz.)
Fava beans	2.8	9	**2 tablespoons**	**1 tablespoon**	**1.5**
Corn	2.8	9	1 serving	½ serving	1.5
Parsnips	2.8	12	1 small	½ small	1.2
Yam	5.3	13	1 small serving	½ small serving	2.0
Boiled potato	5.3	14	2 small	1 small	1.9
Microwaved potato	5.3	14	2 small	1 small	1.9
Mashed potatoes	5.3	15	2 tablespoons	1 tablespoon	1.8
New potatoes, unpeeled and boiled	5.3	16	4 very small	2 very small	1.6
Instant mashed potatoes	5.3	17	2 tablespoons	1 teaspoon	1.5
Sweet potato	5.3	17	1 small	½ small	1.5
Baked potato, with skin	5.3	18	1 large	½ large	1.5
Baked potato, without added fat	5.3	26	½ medium	¼ medium	1.0
French fries	5.3	22	8–10	4–5	1.2

Glycemic load (GL) of common drinks

Item	Serving size (in oz.)	GL per serving	10 GLs	5 GLs	5 GLs (in oz.)
Tomato juice, canned, no added sugar	8.4	4	1 pint	½ pint	10.6
Carrot juice, freshly made	8.4	10	⅔ cup	⅓ cup	4.2
Grapefruit juice, unsweetened	8.4	11	⅔ cup	⅓ cup	3.9
Apple juice, unsweetened	8.4	12	⅔ cup	⅓ cup	3.5
Orange juice, unsweetened	8.4	13	⅔ cup	⅓ cup	3.2

Item	Serving size (in oz.)	GL per serving	10 GLs	5 GLs	5 GLs (in oz.)
Pineapple juice, unsweetened	8.4	16	*1 cup*	*½ cup*	2.7
Cranberry juice drink (Ocean Spray)	8.4	16	*1 cup*	*¼ pint or ½ cup*	2.7
Coca-Cola	8.4	16	*½ cup*	*¼ cup*	2.7
Orange soft drink (Sunkist)	8.4	23	*⅔ cup*	*⅓ cup*	1.7

Most of the GI and GL values of foods listed here are derived from research published by K. Foster-Powell, S. H. Holt, and J. C. Brand-Miller, "International Table of Glycemic Index and Glycemic Load Values," *American Journal of Clinical Nutrition* 76 (1) (2002): 5–56.

NOTES

Serving Size

All pasta serving sizes are for cooked food. For the equivalent in dry weight, halve the figure. So, if you wish to cook spaghetti and the serving size is 4 ounces, that means you should put 2 ounces in the pot.

Portion Guide at a Glance

All servings provide 7 ⓖⓛs.

Food	Dry weight (oz.)	Looks like	Looks like when cooked
Rice	1.4	1½ tablespoons	2½ tablespoons
Pasta	1.4	2 handfuls	4 handfuls
Quinoa	2.4	3 tablespoons	4 rounded tablespoons
Couscous	0.9	1 tablespoon	½ cup

Personalize your GL allowance

While 45 ⓖⓛs per day is the average, what if you're tall or short, or very active? This table shows you how to tailor-make your ⓖⓛ allowance to suit your build and lifestyle:

Height	Average exercise per day (mins.)						
	0	15	30	45	60	90	120
5'	35	35	40	45	45	50	55
5' 3"	40	40	40	45	50	55	60
5' 6"	40	40	40	45	50	55	60
5' 9"	40	40	45	50	55	60	65
6'	45	45	50	55	60	65	70
6' 3"	50	50	55	60	65	70	75
6' 6"	55	55	60	65	70	75	80

Appendix 3

The Dangers of High-Protein Diets

There are big problems with high-protein diets, especially in the long term, that I'd like you to know about. While I agree that high-protein diets do help balance your blood sugar, and hence cause weight loss, the reason I'm not a fan of this approach is that I believe the risks and restrictions outweigh the benefits. The most famous high-protein diet is the Atkins Diet. Headlines the world over have warned of heart and cancer risk, kidney damage and bone mass loss—and quite rightly so. Let's examine these causes of concern.

Kidney problems. Protein produces breakdown products that are hard work for the kidneys. If your kidneys are healthy and your protein excess isn't too high, no problem. But how far can you push it? Researchers found that about 30 percent of women between the ages of 42 and 68 had a mild kidney problem. They also found that, in women who had normal kidney function, there was no link between high protein intake and a decline in renal function.

However, those who already had a mild kidney problem and ate a high-protein diet—particularly one high in meat protein—showed some deterioration. Interestingly, dairy and vegetable proteins were not associated with worsening kidney function. And the parameters here for "high protein" were much narrower than for what you'd normally eat on the Atkins Diet. Ironically, one of the first signs of poor kidney function is water retention (see

Chapter 9), which leads to weight gain. However, the consequences are much more serious as kidney function starts to decline, leading to the need for dialysis.

Bone problems. Protein is acidic, and excess amounts need to be neutralized. The Nurse's Health Study, conducted in the U.S. and analyzed by the Harvard School of Public Health, recently found that women who consumed 95 grams of protein a day, as compared with those who consumed less than 68 grams a day, had a 22 percent greater risk of forearm fractures.[1] In another study, eating more than 80 grams of protein a day, which is equivalent to bacon and eggs for breakfast and a steak for dinner, was found to increase your risk of osteoporosis.[2]

This happens because protein is made of amino acids. Too much acid is neutralized by the body's release of calcium, an alkaline mineral, from the bones—a finding that has been confirmed by "metabolic ward" studies in which people are kept in a controlled environment, fed precise diets, and measured for their calcium loss. Such studies have found that a negative calcium balance is created when 95 grams of protein is consumed while a person eats 500 milligrams of calcium. The calcium intake must be raised to 800 milligrams before calcium balance is achieved—that is to say, when the calcium entering the body is the same as the amount leaving.

Dr. Shalini Reddy from the University of Chicago conducted a six-week study on ten healthy adults eating a low-carb diet. Volunteers lost an average of 9 pounds over the course of the study—that's 1½ pounds a week.

That's the good news. The bad news is that the acid excretion in the urine, which is an indication of acid levels in the blood, rose by 90 percent in some volunteers. There was also a sharp rise in the amount of calcium excreted in the urine during the low-carbohydrate, high-protein diets, and even during the "maintenance" diets for these regimes, despite only a slight decrease in calcium intake. This means the people were losing calcium from the body. Also, urinary citrate, a compound that inhibits kidney stone formation, decreased, implying an increased risk of kidney stone formation.[3]

According to Dr. Reddy, "Consumption of a low-carbohydrate, high-protein diet for six weeks delivers a marked acid load to the kidney, increases the risk for stone formation, decreases estimated calcium balance, and may increase the risk for bone loss." These studies all suggest that such high-protein diets may increase the risk of bone loss over the long term. Of course, we are going to have to wait a while to find out, but I'd rather you weren't the guinea pig.

Breast and prostate cancer risk. After reviewing thousands of studies on diet and cancer, the World Cancer Research Fund states that there is an unequivocal link between high meat consumption and cancer incidence, especially for breast, colon, and prostate cancer.[4] For breast and prostate cancer the link is strongest in relation to high dairy and dairy meat (beef) consumption. People in countries where beef and dairy products are not eaten have a fraction of the risk. In China, for example, the chances of a woman's dying from breast cancer are 1 in 10,000, while her chance in the UK is 1 in 10. For prostate cancer the difference is even greater. In rural China the incidence is 0.5 in 100,000, yet it is estimated that, by 2015, 1 in 4 men in the UK. will have a diagnosis of prostate cancer at some point in his life! Why?

The most likely cause of prostate and breast cancer is that these hormone-sensitive cells go into overgrowth due to exposure to abnormal levels of hormones or hormonelike substances, which include many of the man-made pollutants, from pesticides to PCBs, and dioxins to DDT. These tell a cell to continue growing. The hormone estrogen does this too, which is why estrogen HRT increases the risk of developing breast cancer.

Milk is high in estrogen, but it's also high in other growth-stimulating chemicals, which, as we've seen, is hardly surprising, since milk is designed to make baby calves grow massively. It's called insulin-like growth factor. There are different types—IGF-1, IGF-2, and so on, although much of the focus is on IGF-1, which is very abundant in milk and beef. The amount in modern milk is double this, partly because cows have been selectively reared to produce milk during pregnancy. On top of that, in the United States cows are treated with BST (bovine somatotrophin), a growth hormone capable of further increasing milk yield by about 12 percent.

All this means a cow's daily milk production has gone up from 3 to 30 liters. Not surprisingly, this milk has two to five times the amount of IGF-1, while the beef from a BST-treated animal has about double the IGF. Casein, the protein in milk, then helps to carry the IGF into us.

But what does IGF-1 do, and why is it a strong candidate for increasing the risk of cancer? We make IGF, but very little in adulthood. It's produced mainly in childhood to stimulate growth. Normally, it is produced by the liver, especially during puberty. In girls it stimulates the growth of breast tissue, encouraging cells to divide and grow. In boys it stimulates growth of the prostate. There's nothing wrong with IGF-1, just as there's nothing wrong with estrogen. It's a perfectly normal hormone. It's just that we aren't designed to be eating sources of it in adulthood. And that makes me very worried when a nation of dieters starts living off meat and cheese.

When IGF levels in the blood increase by 8 percent, the risk for prostate cancer increases seven times. Levels of IGF are, on average, 9 percent higher in meat-eating omnivores and dairy-eating vegetarians than in vegans. Recent research from Shangai, China, has found that the higher a woman's IGF-1 levels, the higher her risk for breast cancer. This study found that women in the top 25 percent of IGF-1 scores had two to three times the risk of women in the bottom 25 percent of IGF-1 levels.[5]

A study from York University in the U.K. on the link between IGF and prostate cancer risk in men found a similar result. Men in the top 25 percent of IGF levels had three times the risk of prostate cancer.[6] These are just two of a dozen trials finding a strong link between circulating levels of IGF-1 and prostate cancer. There are many more linking IGF with breast cancer, with the combination of being insulin resistant and having high IGF and excessive levels of estrogen increasing the risk most greatly.[7,8,9] The way to reverse this risk is to correct insulin resistance by eating low ⒼⓁ carbohydrates, reduce your consumption of milk and beef, eat organic where possible, and stay away from HRT.

Underactive thyroid. What's more, high-protein diets can lead to an underactive thyroid. Just two weeks without carbohydrates suppresses the body's production of thyroxine, which controls your metabolic rate. It also promotes the stress hormone cortisol, which makes you even more insulin resistant (see pages 38–39). This, in turn, even further reduces thyroxine production, the major symptom of which is weight gain. Thyroxine is now the second most commonly prescribed drug in the United States. So don't be surprised if your metabolism slows down and you experience rebound weight gain after being on a high-protein, very-low-carb diet.

Other problems. Cancer is not the only disease associated with this type of high-protein, high-meat, and high-dairy diet. Other research strongly suggests that high consumption of meats and dairy products can lead, or at least contribute, to heart disease, type II diabetes, gallbladder disease, osteoporosis, kidney failure, kidney stones, multiple sclerosis, rheumatoid arthritis, constipation, diverticulosis, hemorrhoids, and hiatal hernia.[10] Recent research in mice has also shown substantial reduction in the ability to conceive in females placed on high-protein diets.[11]

Dr. Atkins argued, justifiably, that if you can correct blood sugar problems, you can reduce your risk for many of these diseases. And, while you *can* correct blood sugar problems with a high-fat/high-protein diet, unless caution is exercised you may put yourself at risk of all of the negative effects associated with such a diet. The fact is, you can control your blood sugar just as well, if not better, by eating the right kinds of carbohydrate, the right kinds of fat, plus sufficient—not excessive—protein and less saturated fat. That's what I'm recommending to you in the Holford Diet because I believe it's safer, tastier, easier, and more effective.

Ironically, if you follow the development of the Atkins Diet, you'll see that it is edging in this direction. The earliest version was really low on carbs, while the latest version ends up with 30 percent carbohydrates, 30 percent protein, and 40 percent fat. In my opinion, this still falls short of the ideal diet for painless weight loss, weight maintenance, and overall lifelong health.

The other argument sometimes given in favor of high-protein, high-fat diets is that they mimic the diets of our hunter-gatherer ancestors. I would dispute this—even in the most carnivorous phases of our evolution, our ancestors would never have eaten the amount of fat advised on a conventional high-protein, high-fat diet. Why? Because it wasn't in the meat. Today's animals are fattened up. Almost all meat you buy is marbled with fat, even if you buy the lean stuff. Real meat, as our ancestors ate, was real *lean* meat. However, our ancestors really thrived when they switched from the higher-protein "hunter-gatherer" diet to the lower-protein, higher-carbohydrate "peasant farmer" diet. That's when humanity multiplied and become dominant. Of course, these diets were also low-ⒼⓁ.

Appendix 4

Keeping Track and
Contributing to the Research

Follow the instructions in chapter 23 to monitor your progress week by week using the Fatburner progress report on the following pages. There's a progress report for each of the first four weeks, and a spare progress report for subsequent weeks.

The Fatburner progress reports

WEEK No. 1   Starting date: / /   Ending date: / /

THIS WEEK

Initial weight _____ Bust/chest _____ Waist _____ Hips _____ Thighs _____

Final weight _____ Bust/chest _____ Waist _____ Hips _____ Thighs _____
(at end of week)

Target weight _____ Bust/chest _____ Waist _____ Hips _____ Thighs _____

PROGRESS THIS WEEK

Weight lost _____ Total inch loss _____

How many aerobic sessions? _____ How many toning sessions? _____

How well did you follow the diet? _____ % The exercises? _____ %

PROGRESS TO DATE

Initial weight _____ Initial total inches _____
(at start of diet)   (bust+waist+hips+thighs)

Weight lost to date _____ Inches lost to date _____

WEEK No. 2   Starting date: /   /   Ending date: /   /

THIS WEEK

Initial weight _____ Bust/chest _____ Waist _____ Hips _____ Thighs _____

Final weight _____ Bust/chest _____ Waist _____ Hips _____ Thighs _____
(at end of week)

Target weight _____ Bust/chest _____ Waist _____ Hips _____ Thighs _____

PROGRESS THIS WEEK

Weight lost _____ Total inch loss _____

How many aerobic sessions? _____ How many toning sessions? _____

How well did you follow the diet? _____ % The exercises? _____ %

PROGRESS TO DATE

Initial weight _____ Initial total inches _____
(at start of diet)   (bust+waist+hips+thighs)

Weight lost to date _____ Inches lost to date _____

WEEK No. 3   Starting date: /   /   Ending date: /   /

THIS WEEK

Initial weight _____ Bust/chest _____ Waist _____ Hips _____ Thighs _____

Final weight _____ Bust/chest _____ Waist _____ Hips _____ Thighs _____
(at end of week)

Target weight _____ Bust/chest _____ Waist _____ Hips _____ Thighs _____

PROGRESS THIS WEEK

Weight lost _____   Total inch loss _____

How many aerobic sessions? _____   How many toning sessions? _____

How well did you follow the diet? _____ % The exercises? _____ %

PROGRESS TO DATE

Initial weight _____   Initial total inches _____
(at start of diet)   (bust+waist+hips+thighs)

Weight lost to date _____   Inches lost to date _____

WEEK No. 4   Starting date: /   /   Ending date: /   /

THIS WEEK

Initial weight _____ Bust/chest _____ Waist _____ Hips _____ Thighs _____

Final weight _____ Bust/chest _____ Waist _____ Hips _____ Thighs _____
(at end of week)

Target weight _____ Bust/chest _____ Waist _____ Hips _____ Thighs _____

PROGRESS THIS WEEK

Weight lost _____ Total inch loss _____

How many aerobic sessions? _____ How many toning sessions? _____

How well did you follow the diet? _____ % The exercises? _____ %

PROGRESS TO DATE

Initial weight _____ Initial total inches _____
(at start of diet)   (bust+waist+hips+thighs)

Weight lost to date _____ Inches lost to date _____

WEEK No. ☐   Starting date: / /   Ending date: / /

THIS WEEK

Initial weight _____ Bust/chest _____ Waist _____ Hips _____ Thighs _____

Final weight _____ Bust/chest _____ Waist _____ Hips _____ Thighs _____
(at end of week)

Target weight _____ Bust/chest _____ Waist _____ Hips _____ Thighs _____

PROGRESS THIS WEEK

Weight lost _____ Total inch loss _____

How many aerobic sessions? _____ How many toning sessions? _____

How well did you follow the diet? _____ % The exercises? _____ %

PROGRESS TO DATE

Initial weight _____ Initial total inches _____
(at start of diet)   (bust+waist+hips+thighs)

Weight lost to date _____ Inches lost to date _____

Fatburner research

You can help with ongoing Fatburner research. If you've completed the diet for four or more weeks, let us know your results by filling in this simple questionnaire, answering as many questions as you can, and sending or faxing it to Fatburner Research, Healthy Directions, 7811 Montrose Road, Potomac, MD 20854-3369. You can complete the feedback questionnaire online at www.theholforddiet.com.

FATBURNER RESEARCH QUESTIONNAIRE

Your full name: _____

Address: _____

_____

_____

Contact number: _____

What was your initial weight? _____ pounds

How many weeks have you been following/did you follow the Holford Diet ?
_____

What was your final weight? _____ pounds

Bust/chest _____ inches   Waist _____ Hips _____ Thighs _____

Body fat percentage _____ (if known)

How well did you follow the diet indications? _____ percent

How well did you follow the exercise indications? _____ percent

How easy was the diet to stick to? Easy/reasonable/hard/very hard (circle answer)

How were the recipes? Excellent/good/fair/not good (circle answer)

Did you mainly follow the rules or the recipes? _____ percent (half and half would be 50 percent)

How did you feel while on the diet? _____

_____

_____

Did you notice any other changes to your health? _____

_____

_____

What do you think made the biggest difference? _____

_____

_____

Any other comments? _____

_____

_____

_____

_____

_____

Appendix 5

Figuring Out Your
Training Heart Rate Zone

The best way to know that you are exercising at an intensity that will burn fat and boost your metabolism is to measure your pulse while exercising. If it is within your training heart rate zone for 15 minutes or more, then your exercising is having a fatburning effect.

To find your training heart rate zone, you need to subtract your age from 220, then calculate 65 percent of this amount for the lower end of your training zone and 80 percent for the upper end:

$$220 - \text{age} \_\_\_ \times .65 = \text{lower limit}$$
$$220 - \text{age} \_\_\_ \times .80 = \text{upper limit}$$

For example, for a 30-year-old:

$$220 - 30 = 190 \times .65 = \text{lower limit} = 124 \text{ beats per minute}$$
$$220 - 30 = 190 \times .80 = \text{upper limit} = 152 \text{ beats per minute}$$

To find your pulse rate, you will need a watch with a second hand. There are two points at which the pulse can be felt easily: the neck on either side of the Adam's apple (the carotid pulse), and the wrist (the radial pulse). To find your pulse, apply light pressure with your fingers. Normally, for medical examinations your pulse is taken for 60 seconds. But to find your pulse while exercising, stopping for this long would lower your pulse and give you a false reading. So taking your pulse for only 10 seconds and multiplying the result by 6 will give you the number of beats in one minute without giving your heart rate a chance to slow down. This will be your exercising pulse rate.

When you first embark on your aerobic exercise sessions, you will need to stop briefly every 10–15 minutes to monitor your pulse. After a while you will become familiar with how the correct pulse rate feels for you. See the chart below to find your exercise heart rate for your age.

Training heart rate zone (while exercising)

Age	65–80% of maximum heart rate	
	(beats in 1 minute)	(beats in 10 seconds)
20	130–160	22–27
22	129–158	22–26
24	127–157	21–26
26	126–155	21–26
28	125–154	21–26
30	124–152	21–25
32	122–150	20–25
34	121–149	20–25
36	120–147	20–25
38	118–146	20–24
40	117–144	20–24
45	114–140	19–23
50	111–136	19–23
55	107–132	18–22
60	104–128	17–21
65	101–124	17–21
70	98–120	16–20

The center column shows how many beats you should have in one minute. Beginners should aim for the lower figure on the left-hand side (that is, 65 percent of their maximum heart rate for their age), then slowly increase to 80 percent of their maximum heart rate. Do not exceed this higher level. The column on the far right gives you how many beats you should have in a 10-second pulse count. Beginners should stay at the lower end of their exercise range.

References: Appendices

1. E. Knight et al., "The Effect of Dietary Protein Intake on Kidney Function in Women with Normal or Mildly Abnormal Kidneys," *Annals of Internal Medicine,* vol. 138(6) (2003), pp. 460–7.

2. D. Feskanich et al., "Protein Consumption and Bone Fractures in Women," *American Journal of Epidemiology,* vol. 143(5) (1996), pp. 472–9.

3. L. Allen et al., "Protein-Induced Hypercalcuria: A Longer-Term Study," *American Journal of Clinical Nutrition,* vol. 32 (1979), pp. 741–9; C. Anand et al., "Effect of Protein Intake on Calcium Balance of Young Men Given 500 mg Calcium Daily," *Journal of Nutrition,* vol. 104 (1974), pp. 695–700.

4. S. Reddy et al., "Effect of Low-Carbohydrate High-Protein-Diets on Acid-Base Balance, Stone-Forming Propensity, and Calcium Metabolism," *American Journal of Kidney Diseases,* vol. 40 (2002), pp. 265–74.

5. "Food, Nutrition and the Prevention of Cancer," World Cancer Research Fund, American Institute for Cancer Research (1997).

6. A. Malin et al., "Evaluation of the Synergistic Effect of Insulin Resistance and Insulin-Like Growth Factors on the Risk of Breast Carcinoma," *Cancer,* vol. 100(4) (2004), pp. 694–700.

7. S. E. Oliver et al., "Screen-Detected Prostate Cancer and IGF," *International Journal of Cancer,* vol. 108(6) (2004), pp. 887–92.

8. H. Seeger, D. Wallwiener, and A. O. Mueck, "Influence of Stroma-Derived Growth Factors on the Estradiol-Stimulated Proliferation of Human Breast Cancer Cells," *European Journal of Gynaecological Oncology,* vol. 25(2) (2004), pp. 175–7.

9. D. W. Voskuil et al., "Insulin-Like Growth Factor (IGF)-System mRNA Quantities in Normal and Tumor Breast Tissue of Women with Sporadic and Familial Breast Cancer Risk," *Breast Cancer Research and Treatment,* vol. 84(3) (2004), pp. 225–33.

10. A. Malin et al., "Evaluation of the Synergistic Effect of Insulin Resistance and Insulin-Like Growth Factors on the Risk of Breast Carcinoma," *Cancer,* vol. 100(4) (2004), pp. 694–700.

11. S. B. Sondike et al., "Effects of a Low-Carbohydrate Diet on Weight Loss and Cardiovascular Risk Factor in Overweight Adolescents," *Journal of Pediatrics,* vol. 142(3), pp. 253–8.

RECOMMENDED READING

CHAPTER 2

Cannon, Geoffrey, *Dieting Makes You Fat*, Sphere (1984).
Plant, Jane, *The Plant Diet*, Virgin (2003).

CHAPTER 4

Haynes, Antony, *The Insulin Factor*, Thorsons (2004).
Steward, Leighton, et al., *Sugar Busters*, Ballantine Books (1995).

CHAPTER 6

Holford, Patrick, *Beat Stress and Fatigue*, Piatkus (1999).

CHAPTER 7

Holford, Patrick, *Say No to Arthritis*, Piatkus (1999).
Holford, Patrick, and Braly, James, *The H Factor*, Piatkus (1999).

CHAPTER 8

Holford, Patrick, *The Optimum Nutrition Bible*, Piatkus (1997, rev. 2004).
Holford, Patrick, *Optimum Nutrition for the Mind*, Piatkus (2003).

CHAPTER 9

Leeds, Anthony, et al., *The GI Factor,* Hodder & Stoughton (1996).

CHAPTER 10

Erasmus, Udo, *Fats That Heal, Fats That Kill,* Alive Books (1987, rev. 1994).

CHAPTER 11

Braly, James, *The Food Allergy and Nutrition Revolution,* Keats Publishing, Inc. (1992).

Braly, James, and Hoggan, Ron, *Dangerous Grains,* Avery Publishing Group (2002).

CHAPTER 12

Holford, Patrick, *The Optimum Nutrition Bible,* Piatkus (1997, rev. 2004).

CHAPTER 13

Ichazo, Oscar, *Master Level Exercise: Psychocalisthenics,* Sequoia Press (1993).

Sharkey, Brian, *Fitness and Health,* Human Kinetics Europe Ltd. (2003).

CHAPTER 19

Durrant-Peatfield, Barry, *The Great Thyroid Scandal and How to Survive It,* Barons Down Publishing (2003).

Neil, Kate, and Holford, Patrick, *Balancing Hormones Naturally,* Piatkus (1998).

Thomas, Gloria, *Apples and Pears,* Orion (1998).

CHAPTER 22

Holford, Patrick, *The Optimum Nutrition Cookbook,* Piatkus (2001).

CHAPTER 25

Holford, Patrick, *The Optimum Nutrition Cookbook*, Piatkus (2001).
Neil, Kate, and Holford, Patrick, *Balancing Hormones Naturally*, Piatkus (1998).

RESOURCES

Organizations and Publications

EATING DISORDERS

If you have a concern about an eating disorder, I recommend you contact the National Eating Disorders Association at 603 Stewart Street, Suite 803, Seattle, WA 98101. Go to www.nationaleatingdisorders.org or contact their Information and Referral Helpline at 800-931-2237.

HOLFORD *WELLNESS ADVISOR* NEWSLETTER

Subscribe to my *Wellness Advisor* newsletter for monthly guidance on achieving super health, including review and analysis of the latest research. A one-year subscription (12 issues) is $39.95. Call 800-809-9610 or order online at www.holfordhealth.com, where you can also sign up for my free health e-letter.

INSTITUTE FOR OPTIMUM NUTRITION

ION is a UK charitable trust, founded by Patrick Holford, whose mission is to help people reach their maximum potential through optimum nutrition. It offers personal consultations with ION-qualified nutritional therapists in the UK. Training courses include Optimum Nutrition Workshops, a Home-study Course, and the three-year Foundation Degree in Nutritional Therapy. ION membership entitles you to the *Optimum Nutrition Magazine,* Nutrition Updates, a Nutrition Resource Center and Information Service which you can access by fax or mail, plus discounts on books and courses. The annual membership fee is $45. To become a member or for further information, write to ION, Blades Court, Deodar Road, London SW15 2NU, England. Tel: 011 44 181 877 9993 Fax: 011 44 181 877 9980, or visit the Web site at www.ion.ac.uk.

NATURAL PROGESTERONE

The best source of information on natural progesterone is Dr. John Lee's Web site, which contains articles, books, details on home testing of hormone levels, natural progesterone products, and much more. For details see www .johnleemd.com.

NUTRITION CONSULTATIONS

One-on-one nutrition consultations are available in the United States with naturopathic physicians, nutritionists, and physicians trained in the optimum nutrition approach. The following organizations can help you find a practitioner in your area.

American Association of Naturopathic Physicians
4435 Wisconsin Ave. NW, Suite 403
Washington, DC 20016
Tel: 866-538-2267
Fax: 202-237-8152
Web: www.naturopathic.org

American College for Advancement in Medicine
23121 Verdugo Drive, Suite 204
Laguna Hills, CA 92653
Tel: 888-439-6891
Fax: 949-455-9679
Web: www.acam.org

American Holistic Medical Association
12101 Menaul Blvd. NE, Suite C
Albuquerque, NM 87112
Tel: 505-292-7788
Fax: 505-293-7582
Web: www.holisticmedicine.org

NUTRITION ASSESSMENT ONLINE

You can have your own personal health and nutrition assessment online using the My Nutrition questionnaire. This gives you a personalized assessment of your current health, and what you most need to change in order to lose weight and feel great. Visit www.patrickholford.com and select "Consultation."

PSYCHOCALISTHENICS®

Psychocalisthenics is an excellent exercise system that takes less than 20 minutes a day. It develops strength, suppleness, and stamina and generates vital energy. The best way to learn it is to do Psychocalisthenics training. The Arica Institute offers one-day training courses. For more information, call 860-927-1006. Also available is an instructional book, *Master Level Exercise: Psychocalisthenics,* and a Psychocalisthenics CD and DVD. Visit www.pcals.com for more information.

Low-GL Foods and Alternatives

COFFEE AND TEA ALTERNATIVES

Two of the best alternatives are Teeccino and Rooibos tea. Teeccino herbal coffee is available in most health food stores; or from Teeccino Caffé, 800-498-3434, www.teeccino.com; or from Daily Vitality Health Products, 800-618-1810, www.holfordhealth.com. Red Rooibos herbal tea is available in most health food stores; or from Daily Vitality Health Products, 800-618-1810, www.holfordhealth.com.

GLUCOMANNAN FIBER

Glucomannan fiber is available as a dissolvable, pleasant-tasting powder from Daily Vitality Health Products, 800-618-1810, or www.holfordhealth.com.

OATCAKE CRACKERS

The brand with the lowest GL is Nairn's Rough Oatcake Crackers. They are available at Whole Foods Market and other good health food stores, as well as from Daily Vitality Health Products, 800-618-1810, or www.holfordhealth.com.

OMEGA NUTRITION

Pumpkin seed butter and Essential Balance Oil are made by Omega Nutrition, 800-661-3529, www.omeganutrition.com.

SUGAR ALTERNATIVES

Although it is best to avoid sugar and sugar alternatives as much as possible, there are two natural sugars that have a very low ⓖⓛ score. One is blue agave syrup, which is used to sweeten healthier drinks. The other is xylitol, which is sold under the brand name Xylosweet. Its GL score is one-seventh that of regular sugar, and it tastes the same. Therefore, if you need to sweeten a food or drink, use xylitol. It's available in health food stores; or from Xlear, Inc., 877-599-5327, www.xlear.com; or from Daily Vitality Health Products, 800-618-1810, www.holfordhealth.com.

HEALTHIER SNACK BARS

Unlike the high-sugar "fad" bars that have recently invaded stores, Organic Food Bars actually give you healthy carboyhdrates and fats to help keep your blood sugar levels balanced. They are available at health food stores or from Daily Vitality Health Products, 800-618-1810, www.holfordhealth.com. CocoChia Snack Bars are another good option. Made from organic coconut and chia seeds, they provide energy, protein, and essential omega-3 fats. They are available from Living Fuel, www.livingfuel.com, 866-580-3835; or from Daily Vitality Health Products, 800-618-1810, www.holfordhealth.com.

Supplements

Creating your own perfect supplement program can be confusing. My Web site, www.holfordhealth.com, offers my top recommendations and product formulations.

Remember, a good supplement program should always include:

- a high-strength multivitamin
- additional vitamin C
- an all-around antioxidant complex
- an essential fat (EFA) supplement containing omega-3 and omega-6 oils.

The following companies produce good-quality supplements that are widely available in the United States:

Daily Vitality

Suppliers of my exclusive formulations, including my Daily Vitality Multi-Nutrient, Vital Brain, Vital EFA, Vital Digestion, Vital Comfort, Vital Mood, Chew-Q® CoQ10, Vital H-Factor, and Vital Liver Support. Call or purchase online: 800-211-7306; www.holfordhealth.com.

Solgar Vitamin and Herb

877-765-4274
www.solgar.com

Enzymatic Therapy, Inc.

800-783-2286
www.enzy.com

Source Naturals

800-815-2333
www.sourcenaturals.com

Products

ENVIRON SKINCARE

Environ products were developed by the cosmetic surgeon Dr. Des Fernandes to help prevent skin cancer and address the damaging effects of the environment on skin. They are formulated with scientifically proven active ingredients—including vitamin A and antioxidant vitamins C, E, and beta carotene—that are used in progressively higher concentrations. Environ products will help you maintain normal, healthy skin and effectively treat and prevent the signs of aging, pigmentation, problem skin, and scarring. To purchase Environ skincare products, contact DermaCare USA at 877-337-6227; or Daily Vitality Health Products at 800-618-1810.

WATER FILTERS

There are many water purification systems on the market. One of the best is the Waterwise 9000 Distiller. It's extremely effective at removing harmful contaminants, including bacteria, viruses, parasites, pesticides, herbicides, chlorine, nitrates, and heavy metals. It's available from Waterwise, 800-874-9028, www.waterwise.com; or Daily Vitality Health Products, 800-618-1810.

The best portable system I've found is the Aquaspace Carafe. It removes 99 percent of lead, 45 volatile organic compounds, and harmful parasites. It's available from Aquaspace Water Systems, 800-319-6776, www.aquaspace.com; or Daily Vitality Health Products, 800-618-1810, www.holfordhealth.com.

Tests

FOOD AND CHEMICAL ALLERGY AND INTOLERANCE TESTS

York Nutritional Laboratories sells home test kits for food and chemical allergies that require a pinprick blood sample—you don't have to go to your doctor. York will test you for a sensitivity to up to 113 foods, including gluten, gliadin, wheat, and yeast. Call them for a Food Intolerance Test kit at 888-751-3388, or visit www.yorkallergyusa.com.

INDEX

Instant Health Information, 24 hours a day!

Visit www.holfordhealth.com to sign up for my free *Health Advisory* e-letter and you'll be the first to learn about my new nutritional and natural health discoveries. Subscribers have instant access to these privileges absolutely FREE!

- ✓ **Dozens of Recipes** From breakfast through dessert, these delicious recipes will nourish your body and delight your senses. Easy to print and share with friends.

- ✓ **Advance Notice of Special Offers** on the best nutritional supplements I recommend.

- ✓ **Customized Information Centers** for your pressing health concerns.

- ✓ **Health FAQs** My answers to your most frequently asked health questions.

- ✓ **Books** Details on the availability of my other titles on nutrition, health and lifestyle.

PLUS, save up to $60 on a print subscription to the *Wellness Advisor*, my monthly journal of optimum health and natural healing information. Don't miss another issue! Visit **www.holfordhealth.com** to subscribe or call 1-800-809-9610.

www.HolfordHealth.com

965

76 protein carb, fat ratio
55
78 1/3 to carbs

GL ⑪

39   104 Saltine Bacon   Avoid rice milk high glycemic Load

Caffeine

@ PS LL
1 mile = 300 cal.

12 K rebapll   GL
                   ⟨328⟩

25/36/19 ⟨18-44⟩ Glycogen

Body mass Index
45,

Half time
Weight Loss   Cortisol
Blood Sugar

Get in bed
154 powder
231

(25) age 150/65 20.

(2) 4,000 Calories = 1 lb fat

5r type O better animal protein

5 type A better as carbohydrate

PS 37 Whey insulin beats plant protein

(75) 74 Glucomannan

6 Quinoa (8) Sugar drug 79 (9)
Caffeine 82 amt 9 how liquid fat 98
80 quit smoking Exercise 9 x 4 Ku
50 better sea salt 104 relaxation 15 his

11g RPA differences

lactic acid 123
[25 weight loss HCA

Boston Children's Hospital

Chromium
[25 polynicotinate

TWO SIMPLE RULES

1. Eat no more than 40 GLs a day
2. Eat protein with carbohydrate

ONE SIMPLE DIET

The Holford Low GL Diet
At its heart, one controlling principle:
If you lose blood sugar control, you gain weight
and feel hungry and tired.
If you gain blood sugar control, you lose weight and
feel happy and full of energy.

THE BOTTOM LINE

When you balance your blood sugar, you'll lose weight fast.

With *The Holford Low GL Diet* you will beat your cravings! You'll enjoy delicious meals, choosing from a wide variety of energy-boosting foods and simple menu plans. The diet is safe and easy to follow, and includes a nutritional supplementation plan to increase your energy and decrease your appetite.

Tried and tested by the Institute for Optimum Nutrition, *The Holford Low GL Diet* is based on the latest medical and nutritional research, made totally accessible. Discover how easy it is to reprogram your body to burn your fat away.

PATRICK **HOLFORD** is founder of the Institute for Optimum Nutrition in London. He is Britain's top nutritionist and author of more than twenty health books, including *The New Optimum Nutrition Bible*, which has sold more than 1 million copies in thirty countries.

ATRIA BOOKS
Cover design by Min Choi

Register online at www.simonsays.com for more information on this and other great books.

$14.95 U.S./$21.00 Can.
ISBN-13: 978-0-7432-8722-7
ISBN-10: 0-7432-8722-3

PRINTED IN THE U.S.A.